ONLINE
DATABASES

IN THE
MEDICAL
AND
LIFE SCIENCES

ONLINE DATABASES

IN THE
MEDICAL
AND
LIFE SCIENCES

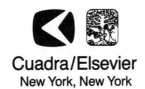

Cuadra/Elsevier
New York, New York

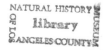

Cuadra/Elsevier
52 Vanderbilt Avenue, New York, New York 10017

Distributors outside the United States and Canada:
Elsevier Science Publishers B.V.
P.O. Box 211, 1000 AE Amsterdam, the Netherlands

Library of Congress Cataloging in Publication Data

Online databases in the medical and life sciences.

Subset of entries contained in the Jan. 1987 plus additions and changes
identified through March 1987 issues of Cuadra/Elsevier's Directory of online
databases.
    Includes indexes.
    1. Medicine — Data bases — Directories.   2. Life sciences — Data bases —
Directories. I. Directory of online databases. [DNLM: 1. Information
Services — directories.   2. Information Systems — directories.   3. Medical
Informatics — directories.   4. Online Systems — directories.
    Z 699.5.M39 058]
R858.055 1987   025'.0661   87-13413
ISBN 0-444-01272-9

Current printing (last digit):
10 9 8 7 6 5 4 3 2 1

Manufactured in the United States of America

CONTENTS

Available from Cuadra/Elsevier

ONLINE DATABASES IN THE MEDICAL AND LIFE SCIENCES

ONLINE DATABASES IN SECURITIES AND FINANCIAL MARKETS

DIRECTORY OF ONLINE DATABASES
Issued quarterly; includes 2 main issues and 2 updates

PREFACE

This **Directory** is designed to provide librarians and other professionals in the life science, health, and allied fields with a comprehensive resource for locating online databases of direct relevance to their particular scientific or service endeavors.

The 686 entries included in this publication represent a carefully selected subset of the 2823 entries contained in the January 1987 issue of the Cuadra/Elsevier **Directory of Online Databases,** plus additions and major changes identified through March 1987. These 686 entries describe 795 databases and distinctly named files within database families, representing about 23 percent of the total number of online databases. The number of online services providing access to one or more of these databases is 148, which represents 28 percent of the total number of online services in the industry.

Because of the frequently overlapping and interdisciplinary nature of information needs, the criteria for inclusion in the development of any subset must necessarily err on the side of "too many" rather than "too few." The primary focus of the selected entries is on the life sciences, biomedical and health-care areas, and related scientific areas of study. Multidisciplinary databases covering biographies, dissertations, conferences and meetings, and legislation, as well as potentially relevant business, social science, news, and health and fitness databases, are also included. In addition, a number of general-interest databases (e.g., for flight schedule data and information on computers and software) of both professional and personal interest have been selected for inclusion in this **Directory.**

In the section that follows, we present a three-part introduction. The first part provides an overview of online database services. It includes definitions of terminology used in the online database industry and provides an explanation of the classification of databases developed by Cuadra Associates and used in this **Directory.** The second part, prepared by Bonnie Snow (DIALOG Information Services, Inc.), focuses on the selection and use of bioscience databases. The third and final section covers the organization and use of this **Directory.**

INTRODUCTION
TO ONLINE DATABASES

Background

The users of online database services include librarians and information specialists; physicians and bioscience researchers; economists, financial analysts, and business planners; engineers and chemists; social science researchers; executives; educators; lawyers; other professionals in a number of areas; and individuals and consumers. A user sits at a computer terminal in the library, office, laboratory, or home, and dials a local telephone number that links the terminal or microcomputer (through the telephone and a coupler or modem) with a computer in some other location. Using a special password, the user gains access to this "host" computer and requests access to the particular system and database of interest. The interaction language of that system, which is designed for use by persons without any computer programming background, permits them to retrieve and display specified information and, in some cases, to do statistical manipulations and other types of processing.

Since the mid-1960s, several streams of technologies and capabilities have come together to support the development and use of online database services. These technologies include the following:

1. Collections of numeric data and/or textual information (**databases**) that are processed by publishers and other organizations in computer-readable form for electronic publishing of printed materials and/or for electronic distribution.
2. Powerful **timesharing computers** that permit a very large number of users to carry on simultaneous interactions with systems through terminals that may be located far from the central computer and its store of data.
3. **Interactive computer programs** (software) that are increasingly efficient, powerful, and user-oriented.
4. Rapid-access **storage devices** that have continued to increase in capacity and reliability and, at the same time, decline in per-character data storage costs.
5. **Computer terminals and microcomputers** that can transmit and receive at various speeds—including 30 characters per second (300 baud), 120 characters per second (1200 baud), and 240 characters per second (2400 baud)—and are more compact, portable, and less expensive than ever before.
6. **Telecommunications networks** that provide local access numbers in cities throughout the world for dialing into a remote computer at far less than the cost of dialing long distance.

During the period in which online database services have been developing, there has been an increased recognition of the role that information can play in meeting the needs of professionals in corporations, educational institutions, public agencies, and other types of research and service organizations. More recently, the role of information in meeting the needs of individuals at home has received considerable attention in the industry. Although online databases have only rarely been subjected to cost-benefit analyses that demonstrate specific savings of time and dollars, user reports leave no doubt that they represent a valuable resource. The use of such databases can help to eliminate duplicative or unnecessary research and development; introduce and promote the transfer of new ideas, services, and technologies; identify baseline data to help support the development of long-range plans; simulate and forecast laboratory and economic situations; bring buyers and sellers together; help individuals to learn about and evaluate choices in educational and leisure-time activities; and identify or provide background and support data in a broad range of problem-solving situations.

The Databases

A number of different types of databases are available online, and they differ in a number of ways: by subject, scope, geographic and chronological coverage, periodicity of release of new information by the producer, and frequency of updating (the addition to the database of newly released information). In addition, they differ in the type of information or data that they contain. A useful way to think about the latter differences is represented in the classification scheme used in this *Directory.*

REFERENCE Databases. Refer or "point" users to another source (e.g., a document, an organization, or an individual) for additional information or for the complete text.

Bibliographic. Contain citations, sometimes with abstracts, of the printed literature, e.g., journal articles, reports, patents, dissertations, conference proceedings, books, or newspaper items.

Referral. Contain references, sometimes with abstracts or summaries, of non-published information. Generally refer users to organizations, individuals, audiovisual materials and other non-print media, for further information.

SOURCE Databases. Those that contain original source data, the full text of original source information, or materials prepared specifically for electronic distribution.

Numeric. Contain original survey data and/or statistically manipulated representations of data. Are generally in the form of time series, which represent measurements (e.g., tons or dollars) over time for a given variable (e.g., production or shipment statistics for a given product or industry).

Textual-Numeric. Are generally databases of records that contain a number of data elements or fields, some of which contain numeric data. Includes those databases with dictionary or handbook-type data typically of chemical and physical properties.

Full Text. Contain records of the complete text of an item, e.g., a newspaper item, a specification, a court decision, or a newsletter.

Software. Contain computer programs that can be downloaded for use with local computers.

The Database Producers

Databases are developed by a group of suppliers referred to as "producers." In some cases, particularly for reference databases, producers are primarily publishers of printed index and abstract journals. These organizations—in both the public and private sectors—acquire, screen, select, index, and sometimes abstract or summarize the primary literature. To produce their printed publications, these organizations have adopted automated systems for phototypesetting and thereby generate a magnetic tape that can be used further for computerized processing, particularly in storage and retrieval systems.

Source databases, on the other hand, are produced by a number of different types of organizations. Some producers of these databases are also publishers of reports and other publications. Others have, as their main line of business, research, consulting, and advisory services in the area covered by the database they produce. Still others are government agencies that, like their counterparts in agencies that produce bibliographic databases,

have a responsibility for the dissemination of information collected or generated in their particular areas. Some producers process and package data into databases that were originally collected by some other source, often the federal government. In their packaging, these producers frequently bring together data from a number of different sources and sometimes increase the value of a collection by including additional data, such as forecasts, that they generate.

Most producers license their databases to other organizations, called "online services" or "host computer services," which provide the computer, software (computer programs), and telecommunications support that enable remote users to access the databases. In such cases, it is easy to differentiate between the organizations that produce and own the data and the organizations that provide online database services. Other producers contract to one or more online services to have their databases distributed online. In some of these cases, the producer also wants to be known as the "online service" and to maintain all contacts with its users, so that the online service is an "invisible" host. And a growing number of producers are, in fact, the online distributors of their own, as well as others', databases. Some producers also provide the software through which their databases are used online.

The Online Services

There are several kinds of organizations that provide online access to databases. The largest group of these organizations are timesharing firms, which provide access primarily to numeric databases. These timesharing firms are also known as "network information services" and as "remote computing services." They provide a number of services, including the use of their computers for the general data processing needs of an organization, consulting and development work in systems, and program development. The provision of database services has been an outgrowth of this tradition. The other online services are generally embedded in organizations that have a commitment to various other information or data processing activities, although a few are organizations completely devoted to the provision of online database services.

In addition to their computers and peripheral equipment, these organizations have one or more special application programs (e.g., database management system, modeling system, report generator, or storage and retrieval system) that are used in conjunction with the databases on which they provide service.

Some companies offer a "main" online service and one or more "special services," each of which is known by a different name. The special services offered by a single organization can differ in terms of the hours of availability, the set of databases that are available, the software that is used to access the databases, and the prices and conditions of access. For example, special services for users at home may have lower evening (non-prime time) charges, simpler software, and fewer databases.

The Gateways

A "gateway" is any computer service that acts as an intermediary between a user and the databases resident on the computers of one or more other organizations. There are several classes of gateways. Some gateways are also online services, i.e., they also have databases resident on their own computers. Others, which do not have resident databases, may simply pass users through to the online service of the user's choice or they may provide a "front-end" (software) interface to help users to select and use the appropriate databases and services. In addition, some gateways are essentially "transparent" to users, who may not know when they have been switched to another computer. In some cases, some of the databases offered through a particular online service may *not* be available to users who access the computer through a gateway service.

From an online user's point of view, gateways represent a potentially important trend, one that offers the promise of helping individuals and institutions manage their access to the growing number of databases available through many more and varied online services. Gateways may give new meaning to the promise of "one-stop" shopping even as the proliferation of intermediary services gives rise to such new complexities as the interconnection of gateways.

CRITERIA FOR INCLUSION IN DIRECTORY

In addition to subject considerations, the criteria applied in selecting a database for inclusion in the **Directory** are as follows:

1. It must be available *online* (i.e., not just available in computer-readable form) for use in an interactive mode.
2. It must be available to the public, or to organizations that can establish their eligibility through subscriptions, membership, or other stated qualifications.

3. It must be accessible through an online service organization that is connected to one or more international telecommunications networks and/or to networks (including direct long-distance communication systems) that serve one country or a limited set of countries.

The **Directory** also includes services that are available only through leased lines or direct long-distance dialing.

PRICING AND PRICES

Pricing policies for access to and use of the online database services are extremely varied. There are a number of components to the prices and they are combined in many different ways. In addition, prices are subject to change with fairly short notice. All of these factors make it extremely difficult to treat the topic in a standard manner in this **Directory.** However, there are some general points that can be made about pricing and prices that can be useful to the potential user.

In at least 39 percent of the entries in this **Directory,** there is an indication that some type of subscription is required for gaining access to the database or that differential charges for subscribers and non-subscribers are available. Subscriptions can range from a few dollars per year to several thousand dollars. In some cases, the user subscribes to a package, which may include access to one or more databases and additional services (e.g., consulting). In other cases, the user has several options, each a combination of a subscription price and associated usage charges.

In general, the major components of the usage prices for online database services differ according to the type of supplier and the type of database (e.g., whether a bibliographic database or a numeric database).

There are two major groups of policies: one for the timesharing firms and their (largely) numeric databases, and one for the others, covering most of the other types of databases. There are, however, exceptions in each group, e.g., where a timesharing firm offers service on a referral database and prices it more like a bibliographic database.

Pricing by Timesharing Firms
(Primarily for Numeric Databases)

Most timesharing firms require a monthly minimum (e.g., $200 per month) that is applied if the total usage charges for a given month do not reach the minimum level. The usage charges include the following components:

Connect Time. An hourly rate, typically ranging from about $4.00 to $45.00, that is charged for the period during which the user is connected to the system. (This figure may or may not include telecommunications charges.)

Compute Resource Units. A rate for actual use of the system that combines charges for use of the central processing unit (CPU), the amount of input/output (I/O) required to read and write to disk and interact with the user's terminal and, sometimes, charges for the user's workspace in the computer memory. The charges for these units (sometimes called CRUs) typically range from $.03 to $.90 per unit. However, they cannot be compared across the online services because the formulas that are used to calculate charges vary from service to service.

Disk Storage. Additional costs are incurred if a user elects to store a selected amount of data from a database, perhaps along with the user's own data, in a "private" file.

These rates can also vary within a specific service, depending upon the speed of the terminal being used (e.g., 300 or 1200 baud) and the time of day in which the processing occurs (e.g., prime time vs. non-prime time). In addition, the CRUs charged for a particular database may be greater than the standard timesharing rates charged for other data processing services. This difference occurs either because the database system that is being used is more demanding of resources, or because a surcharge has been added to the standard rates (by a multiplier or additive factor) as a royalty to the producer of the database.

Pricing by Other Online Services

In most cases, costs for other database services are based on an hourly connect-time rate, plus telecommunications costs for network access, if applicable. The hourly connect-time rates that are cited in the supplier's literature may include the royalty, or the royalty may be cited separately. The typical connect-time rates (including applicable royalties) range from about $15 to $300 per hour. The average is approximately $64 per hour.

For bibliographic and some referral databases, there is an additional charge for offline printing, which is generally based on the number of citations or pages. Typical charges for offline printing range from $.01 to $11.00 per citation, although for a few databases they are considerably higher. The average is about $.38. Additional per-item charges for online printing (i.e., displaying retrieved information directly at the terminal) are becoming more typical, as a means for producers to charge for the information a user is obtaining. Fees typically range from $.04 to $7.00 per item, although they too can be considerably higher. The average is about $.34. Both online and offline printing charges may vary depending on the amount of information that is printed.

In some cases, the use of a service involves a start-up fee, which often covers account setup, initial training, and materials. Occasionally this startup fee also includes the cost of a special terminal and/or leased lines to the online services computer.

Many of the online services that focus on the provision of database access also provide volume discounts or have subscription plans that provide for various levels of connect-time rates, depending upon the expected level of usage.

Selecting an Online Service

With the bibliographic databases, and some reference and textual-numeric databases, one can easily compare prices if the same database is available on more than one service. However, prices do not tell the whole story of costs. There are differences in system capabilities, in the ways in which individual databases are designed for online use on different systems (e.g., the fields that are searchable), in the years of online coverage, and in the response time of the particular system under high user loads.

With the bibliographic databases, particularly, users can estimate total costs of using the online database services by using the concept of a "search." A search of a single database generally takes less than 15 minutes. A search involves the input (typing in) of a formulation to retrieve an initial set of citations, time to review some of the citations after requesting them to be displayed, time to modify the formulation somewhat to increase or limit the number of citations retrieved, and the issuance of a final command to display the results of the search either online or offline. A search of a single database will cost, on the average, about $32. (Averages are, of course, just that. Searches can be done much more quickly—in two or three minutes—or may require much more time.) Most searches that are done to fulfill a particular information need require the use of two or three different databases.

With the numeric databases, it is much more difficult to compare prices when a particular database is available through more than one service. One reason for this difficulty has already been mentioned: the difference in formulas underlying the resource-unit charges. Another reason is that there is great variability across online services in terms of the systems (their capabilities and efficiencies) that are used to operate on these databases. And finally, both comparisons and budgeting are difficult because the uses of numeric databases are extremely varied. There is no comparable "search" measurement in the use of numeric databases. A numeric database can be used simply to retrieve a set of data, or it can be used in conjunction with one's own data to perform sophisticated and demanding statistical manipulations.

Therefore, the selection of an online service will generally be made on the basis of both price and other criteria, including the availability of databases of interest to the organization, system capabilities, and the availability or quality of training, materials, and customer support. To help make these types of evaluations, a potential user will want to review user materials, discuss the overall service, and see a demonstration of the database services for gathering "benchmark-like" data on costs. Although one cannot control all of the factors in a demonstration, e.g., load on the system, one can request from the sales representative of each service that the same types of functions be performed and costed, so that general comparisons can be made.

COPYRIGHT

With the exception of a few databases in the public domain, the databases listed in this **Directory** are copyrighted. This means that, unless the database producer states otherwise, the downloading of data is prohibited. Downloading is the process by which users of online databases capture and store the results of online inquiries (e.g., citations, the full text of items, or time series) in local computer storage devices—either temporarily or permanently—for further computer-based manipulation or reuse of the data.

Users of these databases are encouraged to read their agreements carefully and to contact the database producers, prior to capturing data locally, to make sure that what they want to do represents fair use. Some producers and, on their behalf, the online services, have established policies and prices to cover various types of downloading and reuse. However, both policies and prices can and do vary.

SELECTING AND USING BIOSCIENCE DATABASES

Prepared by **Bonnie Snow**

DIALOG Information Services, Inc.

The publication of this **Directory** serves to remind us that the "information explosion" is more than just rhetoric. Only a decade ago, there were just a handful of life science databases, and an online searcher needed to learn only a few online systems to use these databases. The databases were all computer-readable counterparts of familiar printed products, so that deciding where to look for information online was a minor challenge. In the last five or so years, this picture has changed dramatically. There are now over 380 online databases in this area. This growth has transformed the database selection and use processes.

THE BREADTH AND SPECIALIZATION OF DATABASES

The biosciences can be defined broadly as those sciences concerned with the study of living organisms, including plants, animals, bacteria, viruses, and insects. The life sciences—anatomy, biochemistry, botany, cytology, ecology, forestry, genetics, horticulture, nutrition, pathology, pharmacology, psychiatry, taxonomy, veterinary medicine, and zoology—all fit into this broad group, as do agriculture, aquatic sciences, biomedicine, environment, food science and nutrition, health-care services, and toxicology.

A few online databases, such as BIOSIS PREVIEWS and SCISEARCH, cover literature for virtually every subdivision. Other databases, including such recent additions as AIDS and ANEUPLOIDY, represent efforts to provide customized collections of information aimed at specific user groups. New online database offerings reflect increasing specialization in bioscience research and, to a certain extent, response to social issues. Pollution, alcohol and drug abuse, carcinogens, occupational hazards, asbestos, radiation, health costs, child abuse, bioethics, and birth defects have all been the focus of public concern and questions. Subject-specialty databases have been created to answer information needs in each of these areas, as well as to reduce the growing volume of scientific literature into manageable segments. Ironically, the resulting proliferation of specialty files has itself complicated the research process.

Even when a database is characterized as focusing on a particular life science area, one must take this characterization as being indicative rather than comprehensive. Any given database may cover a wider range of subject matter, and the subject classifications for databases are not mutually exclusive. Cross-references are provided in the subject index of this **Directory** to help users identify relevant databases listed under related terms. For example, aquatic science information is available in many databases listed under "environment," in addition to those compiled under the "aquatic sciences" heading. "Biotechnology" sources offer material on applications in agriculture, forestry, food science, genetic engineering, pharmaceutical products, etc. Many databases on pharmaceutical products provide biomedical and toxicological information, such as physiochemical properties, dosage, indications, and contraindications.

The distinction that is made between "biomedicine" and "health care" deserves special note. The databases listed under "biomedicine" are generally clinically oriented, with an emphasis on professional literature and information in support of patient care. "Health care" databases, on the other hand, tend to deal with political, economic, administrative, and social issues or services, and their source materials and subject matter are primarily nonclinical.

ASSEMBLING THE ARMAMENTARIUM

"One-stop shopping" is rare in information work and, for most searches, more than one database is likely to be needed. To do effective research, one must do a certain amount of advance planning that includes compilation and analysis of data on typical research problems already posed or on the nature of anticipated queries. Database selection for specific inquiries will be dictated not only by subject coverage but also by the format in which information is provided. Careful matching of individual requests with online database resources is important.

For example, a typical biomedical search may begin with a physician asking if a given compound is dialyzable. A textual-numeric database containing factual data would offer the shortest route to providing the answer to that specific question. However, such a request may well lead to further research, to find backup references and background reading. Not all "factual" databases provide supportive documentation or bibliographies and, therefore, such resources may need to be supplemented by searches in bibliographic databases.

On the other hand, the real question in this case may involve how to treat a patient just admitted to the hospital who is suffering from an overdose of the compound, for which yet another type of database—one containing the full text of source materials—may be needed. Although response to such emergency requests is essentially reactive, information management today requires proactive planning. As part of that planning, life science searchers must assemble an armamentarium of online resources that is likely to include the information relevant to their own or their clients' needs.

Time constraints, the origin of an inquiry (who is asking the question), and the ultimate application of the information all affect database selection decisions. Constructing lists or "families" of databases that can answer questions of various types is analogous to setting up a hardcopy reference library. Concentration on one type of resource is usually a mistake. For example, full-text databases offer attractive solutions when time is short, but their scope is necessarily limited, representing only a small fraction of literature published in a given subject area or professional discipline. Bibliographic databases offer breadth to complement the depth of source databases. Thus, they are essential resources in answering most life science research questions.

Content Descriptions

Close examination of content descriptions in the **Directory** entries is particularly important when comparing bibliographic databases. A checklist of items to look for includes:

- number and types of source documents indexed
- geographic origin and language of sources indexed
- availability of abstracts online
- years of coverage available
- frequency with which the database is updated

Familiarity with the *types* of documents covered in a database is crucial, particularly in terms of as-

sessing the timeliness of the database. Scientific communication appears in many forms: patents; meeting, symposia, or conference papers; notes, letters, case reports, and brief research communications; institutional and government technical reports; published theses or dissertations; bibliographies; and monographs.

The most common form of scientific publication, and one of the most timely forms, is journal articles. The number of periodical titles scanned each year for potential references to be included in a given bibliographic database can serve as a rough indicator of its breadth in coverage, although it is important to understand that not all of the scanned journals will be referenced "cover-to-cover." In full-text databases, charts, figures, and selected other materials in a journal may be excluded.

However, other forms of publication can be equally valuable resources, given certain types of problems. For example, conference papers and patents are particularly valuable when information on *new* topics is sought. Monographs, annual reviews, and symposia are helpful in gaining a state-of-the-art overview of past research. Case reports, sometimes conveyed in the form of letters to editors of scientific journals, are a significant means of communication in medicine, pointing to new areas for investigation or new approaches to therapy. Technical reports, by providing information on specific techniques and procedures, assist researchers in the development of new experiments.

Geographic Origin and Language

While this **Directory** is international in scope, the majority of databases contain English-language information. This does *not* mean, however, that non-English material is not indexed. Major bioscience bibliographic databases typically contain references to literature published in at least fifty countries and forty languages. While the online records (i.e., citations and abstracts) are in English, the original source cited may be in another language, a fact that will be noted in the **Directory** entry. In most databases, the language of source documents may be specified as a search parameter. For example, a MEDLINE searcher can specify that references to journal articles on AIDS be restricted to only those in Japanese. The resulting output will be in English, but all sources cited would be in Japanese.

Time Span and Updating

Updating frequencies can be taken as an indication of the emphasis placed on currency in a given database, although the relationship of updating frequency to currency is admittedly tenuous. A database producer may be adding new material to the database every two weeks but that material may actually have been published five months previously. This hidden factor is known as *lag time*—the interval that typically elapses between source document publication and online access or indexing. The average lag time in life science databases is three to four months for bibliographic databases and one month or less for full-text journal or newsletter databases. It is somewhat unpredictable for referral (directory) materials and numeric or textual-numeric databases. Where evaluated, factual data are involved, the compilations can take a considerable amount of time but, on the other hand, the data may not become obsolete.

Online Service

After scanning **Directory** entries and compiling a list of complementary resources, the next order of business in the process is to gain access to those databases. The *Online Service/Gateway Index* will be of particular help to users to gain a perspective on which vendors offer the selected set of databases and, of these, which offer the most.

Generally, one or two online services will be found that can supply most databases on your "shopping list." An illustration here may help to describe possible ways of "coping" when the potentially relevant databases involve use of many more online services. Let's say that a professional organization of registered pharmacists in the United States would like to set up a literature search service for its members. Inquiries will be accepted over the telephone, and results mailed to requesters. Databases are needed that will supply information about drug therapy (indications, contraindications, dosage, interactions, etc.), pharmacy practice issues (e.g., generic substitution, bioequivalency, medication counseling, prescription audits), and new product news. Content descriptions in the **Directory** and advice from experienced pharmacy searchers lead to a list of candidate resources from nearly twenty databases, including: CONSUMER DRUG INFORMATION, DIOGENES, DRUG INFORMATION FULLTEXT, EMBASE, HEALTH PLANNING AND ADMINISTRATION, INTERNATIONAL PHARMACEUTICAL ABSTRACTS, MARTINDALE ONLINE, MEDLINE, THE MERCK INDEX ONLINE, PHARMLINE, PNI, RINDOC, SCISEARCH, SOCIAL SCISEARCH, and TOXLINE.

In an analysis of availability information on this particular set of candidate databases, the staff learns that DIALOG Information Services, Inc. and BRS of-

fer the most databases of interest to this organization. However, another five or so online services, including DATA-STAR, ORBIT Information Technologies, Inc., DIMDI, ESA-IRS, and the National Library of Medicine, also provide access to one or more of the databases, as well as to other potentially relevant ones. Setting up contracts with all nine online services will pose quite a challenge to a startup venture. Subscription, initiation, and/or minimum usage fees required by some of the services must be weighed, along with the "hidden cost" of staff members learning different protocols for using each of the systems and maintaining current documentation (user aids) on each.

Because levels of usage for these potential resources cannot be estimated in advance, our hypothetical organization for pharmacists reexamines its options. In reviewing the content descriptions in the **Directory** in an effort to reduce the candidate list, the staff members note that substantial portions of several databases (e.g., DRUG INFORMATION FULLTEXT, CONSUMER DRUG INFORMATION, MARTINDALE, MEDICAL DRUG AND REFERENCE, and THE MERCK INDEX ONLINE) are found to be available in hardcopy format. It is decided that consultation of these texts "offline" will suffice until demand for the information service can be more accurately estimated. The remaining candidate databases are analyzed to identify the smallest set of services through which those databases can be accessed online.

The bottom line in vendor selection is: does this online service have what I need, or most of what I need? Other points to consider when comparing vendors with similar offerings in a given subject area are listed below.

Cost: What are the rates for individual databases? What, if any, initiation, subscription, or minimum-usage fees apply? Are there telecommunication fees?

Accessibility: What are the hours of availability? Can I access the computer through one of the telecommunications networks or do I have to dial directly?

Capabilities: What can I learn about the service's computer capacity, response time, and "down time"? Critical examination of software is also important. Here are some features to look for:

- keyword searching, combining multiple parameters
- word-proximity searching
- truncation capabilities

- ability to search numbers as well as words and alphanumeric strings of characters
- online sorting (rearrangement of output)
- customized report generation
- online thesauri and online search assistance
- cross-file indexes and other database selection aids
- automatic updating of stored searches
- electronic mail
- document ordering and delivery services

Customer Support: What is the quantity and quality of:

- training
- documentation (hardcopy user aids)
- customer service (toll-free hotlines and hours available; nationwide training sites; regional offices and local representatives)

Reliability and Status: How long has the service been in business, and how successful is it, as measured by number of users, user testimonials, or frequency of citation in the online searching literature?

File Specifications: If a database is available from more than one online service, does your vendor of choice maintain the same time span and frequency of updating? (Tip: contact the database producer and ask how long it takes for each vendor to update the database after the tape is received.)

Other Offerings: How well can the online service meet your unanticipated needs? Although the potential user's initial focus may be on a handful of offerings, later access to a broader spectrum of databases may be needed.

COMMON PROBLEMS AND SOLUTIONS

Problem: Finding Information for the Consumer

Most life science databases are designed for professionals in the bioscience disciplines. Medical databases, for example, cover publications intended for health-care practitioners. The vocabulary employed by biomedical professionals requires "translation" for effective use by consumers/patients.

In selecting databases, note the producers, the type and origin of the source material, and the intended audiences so that you are working with the appro-

priate types of resources. Another clue to the intended audience can be found in the online service: some are focusing on users "at work," whereas others are focusing on users "at home."

Problem: Monitoring Opportunities for Continuing Education

Rapid developments in the sciences necessitate ongoing continuing education. In order to keep up-to-date, subject specialists regularly attend professional meetings to maintain contacts for informal communication among colleagues working in the same field and to take advantage of more formal educational workshops and seminars offered in conjunction with such conferences. Databases that provide schedules or calendars of such events can be found under the "Conferences & Meetings" subject heading.

Problem: Locating Nonprint Information Sources: People, Products, or Projects (Research-in-Progress)

Referral databases (referencing people, products, and ongoing research), as well as selected full-text newsletter databases, offer possible solutions to these types of problems. Sorting through vendor literature for such resources can be quite daunting. With the **Directory** Subject Index, you can readily identify them through such terms as:

- Associations & Foundations-Directories
- Audiovisual Materials-Catalogs
- Biographies
- Forensic Sciences & Services
- Information Systems & Services-Directories
- Publishers & Distributors-Catalogs
- Research-in-Progress

Problem: Identifying Online Counterparts for Hardcopy Sources

Content descriptions in the **Directory** entries for many databases cite hardcopy (non-online) counterparts. One method of preparing for efficient use of an online resource is to review its organization in hardcopy format. Browsing printed counterparts is an inexpensive way to gain familiarity with coverage, editorial, and indexing policies. Although the online version may vary somewhat from cited counterparts, parallels drawn from hands-on hardcopy experience can help in understanding classification and subject indexing schemes.

Costs for maintaining subscriptions to hardcopy sources are escalating. This fact has led many libraries and information and research centers to look for online alternatives. If an expensive printed index is used infrequently, acquiring online access on a pay-as-you-go basis may preclude the necessity for continuing acquisition, processing, and in-house archival storage of that source in hardcopy format. On the other hand, if a reference text is relatively inexpensive and easy to use in non-online format, its retention in a library or personal collection can save online costs and cut down on the number of services needed, as was illustrated above in the example for choosing an online vendor in pharmacy. Potential online users sometimes find that investigating cited counterparts helps them fill in gaps in hardcopy reference collections.

Problem: Knowing Alternatives When In-House Resources Do Not Provide the Answer

In information science, as in the life sciences, to stand still is to go backward. Ongoing continuing education is as important for users of online databases as it is for research biochemists, microbiologists, or physicians. Sometimes just knowing which databases are available can provide partial solutions to information problems. This **Directory** can be used as part of that personal, continuing education self-study program. Through it you can identify new or additional databases that you may not plan to search but need to be aware of, for example, to refer clients to alternative sources when in-house solutions are inadequate.

The next step will be to find organizations or individuals (including, in some cases, the database producer) who have access to the relevant online services and are willing to accept search requests from others. A local online user group in your area may issue directories that identify the online services to which members have access. Establishing contacts ("networking") with other searchers of online databases offers a practical alternative to taking advantage of the wealth of online database resources without having to be direct users of those databases.

ORGANIZATION AND USE OF THE DIRECTORY

The **Directory** is organized into three sections: database descriptions; online service and gateway addresses; and indexes. The content and format of each section are described below.

Descriptions of Online Databases

This main section of the **Directory** is arranged alphabetically by database name. There are a total of 686 entries, which represent approximately 795 databases and distinctly named files in a database family. The uniformly formatted entries are organized according to the fixed set of headings defined below.

Name of Database. The name of the database is given first, without a heading, in bold letters.

Type. This field contains the Cuadra Associates two-level classification described earlier in the *Introduction to Online Databases.*

Reference (Bibliographic or Referral)

Source (Numeric, Textual-Numeric, Full Text, Software)

Subject. This field contains one or more of the terms in an authority list that has been developed to characterize the subject content of the databases.

Producer. This field contains the name of the organization that produces the database. If the database is derived from data supplied by other organizations, all, or an illustrative list, of the original sources are identified in the *Content* section.

Online Service. This field contains the name of each online service through which the database is available. If there is variation in database name from service to service, the name by which the database is known on a particular service is given in parentheses after the service name. In some cases, the online service shown is an organization that operates under contract to a producer that prefers to be listed as the "online service" and to receive all inquiries concerning online access. When the "invisible" online service is known, its name is also included, after the phrase "as a database on. . . ."

Online services may provide "gateway" access to other online services or may themselves be available through one or more gateway services. Check the *Online Service/Gateway Index* to identify specific gateway-only services and online services that provide gateway services to one or more other online services. Please note that some of the databases available on a particular online service may *not* be available through a gateway.

The addresses, telephone and telex numbers for online services are provided in the *Addresses of Online Services and Gateways* section.

Conditions. This field contains information on requirements for gaining access to and using the database. If access is restricted (e.g., to subscribers, to members of certain communities, or to users in certain geographic regions), this information is provided. This field also includes information on subscriptions and subscription costs.

Content. This field provides a description of the subject, coverage, and scope of the database, as well as more detail on the type of information that it contains. If a database comprises more than one file, this fact is noted and the specific content of those files is generally given.

A description may refer to another database that is available separately through one or more other online services. Cross-references are generally provided when a cited database is included in this **Directory.** Descriptions of other cited databases can be found in the **Directory of Online Databases.**

To the extent that the information is known, the names of printed publications that correspond in part or whole to the online database have been included. Sometimes the correspondence is only partial, either because the online database contains more information than the printed product or because the online database does not include certain information, e.g., does not include abstracts or contains only tables of data.

Language. This field contains the language or languages used in bibliographic, referral, and (where applicable) textual-numeric databases.

Coverage. This field describes the geographic coverage of the database, e.g., whether it is international in scope, or limited to a specific country or set of countries.

Time Span. This field contains the starting date for which data have been cumulated, or the closed periods of years represented in the database.

Updating. Updating refers to the frequency with which new or revised information is placed online. This frequency may or may not correspond to the periodicity of the data—the frequency with which new or revised information is released by the producer. For the numeric databases particularly, both periodicity and updating can vary by time series.

For reference databases, this field generally contains the number of records that are added in each update or over the period of a year. Subscribers can estimate the size of the current file on the basis of this information and the period of years given in the **Time Span** field.

Addresses of Online Services and Gateways

The section that follows the *Descriptions of Online Databases* contains the addresses, telephone and telex numbers of the headquarters offices of the online services and gateways. Users may also want to check telephone directories in their area for the numbers of local offices.

Indexes

The final section contains three indexes to the main section of the *Directory.*

Subject Index. In this index, each of the databases is listed alphabetically under the subject heading or headings to which it has been assigned. The subject headings are organized alphabetically, with a number of SEE and SEE ALSO references.

Online Service/Gateway Index. This index is arranged alphabetically by the full name of the online service or gateway. After each online service is the list of databases to which it provides access. As applicable, an online service entry also identifies the gateway(s) through which the online service is available and provides cross references to other, special services provided by the same company. A gateway entry identifies the online service(s) to which it provides access and, as applicable, through which the gateway itself is accessible. Some of the databases listed under a particular online service may not be available through a gateway service.

Master Index. The last section of the *Directory* contains a master alphabetical listing of the databases, online services, and gateways covered in the *Directory*. This listing contains numerous SEE references to help users identify entries for databases or organizations with more than one name and to check alphabetically for them under either acronyms or their fully spelled-out names. Special codes refer users to the *Online Service/ Gateway Index* to identify databases associated with a particular organization.

DESCRIPTIONS OF ONLINE DATABASES

3RD BASE SOFTWARE REGISTRY®

Type: Reference (Referral)
Subject: Computers & Software
Producer: 3rd Base, Division of STEL Enterprises
Online Service: 3rd Base, Division of STEL Enterprises
Conditions: To list a product, vendors pay annual fee of $25 and $20 per product
Content: Contains descriptions of about 15,000 computer software products that are currently available or in development. Includes hardware and operating system requirements, programming language, functions and features, price, and vendor information. Information is provided and maintained by each software vendor.
Language: English
Coverage: Primarily U.S., with some international coverage
Time Span: Current information
Updating: Periodically, as new data become available

AAMSI COMMUNICATION NETWORK

Type: Reference (Bibliographic, Referral); Source (Full Text)
Subject: Biomedicine; Computers & Software; Conferences & Meetings; Health Care; Information Systems & Services
Producer: American Association for Medical Systems and Informatics (AAMSI)
Online Service: CompuServe Information Service
Content: Contains information on the use of computer and information systems in medicine. Includes citations to articles in the current quarter's issues of *Computers in Health Care, Computers in Biology and Medicine, Medical Informatics, Computer Programs in Biomedicine,* and *Journal of Medical Systems,* as well as selected other journals (e.g., *New England Journal of Medicine* and *American Journal of Public Health*). Also includes book reviews; information on vendors of computerized medical systems (including name, address, and product descriptions); a message from the AAMSI President; an editorial; full text of a feature article from the *AAMSI News* newsletter; AAMSI organizational news; a list of such professional activities as workshops and seminars; and a calendar of professional meetings for the coming 2 years. An electronic bulletin board, the AAMSI Medical Forum, is also available.
Language: English
Coverage: International
Time Span: Current information
Updating: Quarterly

ABDA-INTERAKTIONEN

Type: Source (Textual-Numeric)
Subject: Pharmaceuticals & Pharmaceutical Industry
Producer: Bundesvereinigung Deutscher Apothekerverbaende (ABDA), in cooperation with Wissenschaftliche Zentralstelle des Schweizerischen Apothekervereins
Online Service: DIMDI
Content: Contains interaction information for approximately 4200 drugs drawn from the worldwide journal and monographic literature. Covers actions, clinical observations, and recommendations. Corresponds to *Mikropharm I* and *Interaktionskartei.*
Language: German
Coverage: International

Time Span: Current information
Updating: Annually

ABDA-PHARMA

Type: Reference (Referral); Source (Textual-Numeric)
Subject: Pharmaceuticals & Pharmaceutical Industry
Producer: Bundesvereinigung Deutscher Apothekerverbaende (ABDA)
Online Service: DIMDI
Content: Consists of 4 files of information on drug preparations and pharmaceutical substances.
SUBSTANCES. Contains information on approximately 13,000 pharmaceutical substances, including chemical elements and compounds, plant and animal products, and microorganisms. Provides nomenclature from the International Non-Proprietary Names and the International Union of Pure and Applied Chemistry nomenclature, Chemical Abstracts Service Registry Numbers, Arzneimittel-Stoff Katalog numbers, synonyms, molecular formulas, physicochemical properties, substance classifications, drug delivery regulations applicable in the Federal Republic of Germany, maximum dosage that can be prescribed, indications, and dosage. Data are obtained from a variety of journals, books, pharmacopoeias, and chemical handbooks. Corresponds in part to *Pharmazeutische Stoffliste (List of Pharmaceutical Substances).*
DRUGS. Contains data on approximately 18,000 German and 53,000 non-German drugs. For all drugs, includes trade name, active ingredients, dosage forms; for German drugs only, also includes administration and dosage, composition, indications, contraindications, side effects, interactions, producers, shelf life and storage, date of initial marketing, and delivery regulations. Corresponds to *Mikropharm II, Novitaetenkartei* and *Indikationskartei.*
CENTRAL. Contains data on approximately 120,000 drugs available in the Federal Republic of Germany. Includes trade names, dosage forms, indications, drug delivery regulations, shelf life and storage, package sizes, and manufacturers' addresses.
MANUFACTURERS. Contains names and addresses of manufacturers in the Federal Republic of Germany and names of manufacturers outside the country.
Language: German
Coverage: Federal Republic of Germany and international *(see Content)*
Time Span: Current information
Updating: SUBSTANCES and MANUFACTURERS, every 6 weeks; DRUGS, monthly; CENTRAL, twice a month.

ABSTRACTS IN BIOCOMMERCE

Type: Reference (Bibliographic)
Subject: Biotechnology
Producer: BioCommerce Data Ltd.
Online Service: DATA-STAR
Content: Contains over 60,000 citations, with abstracts, to literature on the commercial aspects of biotechnology. Covers industry news, reports of corporate financial developments, research and development projects, personnel changes, and relevant legislation. Sources include more than 100 trade publications, newsletters, and newspapers. Corresponds to *Abstracts in Biocommerce (ABC),* with additional data available online.

Language: English
Coverage: Primarily U.K. and U.S.
Time Span: 1981 to date
Updating: About 300 records every 2 weeks

ABSTRAX 400

Type: Reference (Bibliographic)
Subject: General Interest
Producer: Information Sources, Ltd.
Online Service: BRS; BRS After Dark; BRS/BRKTHRU; BRS/Colleague; TECH DATA
Content: Contains over 152,000 citations, with brief abstracts, to articles in 225 popular (e.g., *Time, Newsweek, Sports Illustrated*) and professional (e.g., *New England Journal of Medicine*) English-language periodicals. Covers current affairs, the arts, sports, personal computing, general science and technology, and popular literature.
Language: English
Coverage: U.S.
Time Span: December 1982 to date
Updating: About 8000 records a month

ACADEMIC AMERICAN ENCYCLOPEDIA®

Type: Source (Full Text)
Subject: Encyclopedias
Producer: Grolier Electronic Publishing, Inc.
Online Service: BRS; BRS After Dark; BRS/BRKTHRU; BRS/Colleague; CompuServe Information Service; DATA-STAR; DIALOG Information Services, Inc.; Dow Jones & Company, Inc.; Knowledge Index; Quantum Computer Services, Inc.; THE SOURCE; STARTEXT, A Division of the Fort Worth Star-Telegram; VU/TEXT Information Services, Inc.
Conditions: Annual subscription to BRS required; annual, semiannual, or monthly subscription to CompuServe required; annual minimum of $12 or monthly minimum of $3 to Dow Jones required; monthly subscription to Quantum Computer Services required; monthly minimum of $10 to THE SOURCE required, with $9 credited toward online usage charges; monthly minimum of $9.95 to STARTEXT required; subscription to VU/TEXT required.
Content: Contains full text of the 20-volume *Academic American Encyclopedia*. Includes about 31,000 articles on a wide variety of subjects. Entries are indexed by subject and include tables, fact boxes, bibliographies, and cross-references.
Language: English
Time Span: 1980 to date
Updating: Quarterly

ACID RAIN

Type: Reference (Bibliographic)
Subject: Environment
Producer: EIC/Intelligence Inc.
Online Service: ESA-IRS
Content: Contains about 1200 citations, with abstracts, to the worldwide literature on the sources of acid rain and its effects on the environment and human life. Covers atmospheric processes, deposition monitoring, impact on aquatic and terrestrial systems, control technologies, economic and health issues, and U.S. policy and planning. Sources include journals, conference proceedings, books, and technical reports from educational institutions, corporations, and governments.

Language: English
Coverage: International
Time Span: 1984 to date
Updating: About 150 records a month

ACIDOC

Type: Reference (Bibliographic)
Subject: Environment
Producer: Acid Rain Information Clearinghouse; Environnement Quebec
Online Service: IST-Informatheque Inc.
Content: Contains approximately 6000 citations, with abstracts, to Canadian, European, and U.S. literature on all aspects, from sources to control, of acid precipitation. Covers air and atmospheric processes, environmental effects, political and socio-economic factors, and technological control. Sources include scientific and general periodicals, monographs, studies, lectures, conference proceedings, and official publications.
Language: English and French
Coverage: International
Time Span: 1975 to date
Updating: Quarterly

ACOG INFORMATION

Type: Reference (Bibliographic, Referral); Source (Textual-Numeric)
Subject: Biomedicine; Conferences & Meetings
Producer: American College of Obstetrics and Gynecology (ACOG)
Online Service: CompuServe Information Service
Content: Contains information on the publications, services, and activities of the American College of Obstetrics and Gynecology (ACOG). Includes a physician referral service; national statistics on the numbers and status (e.g., resident, board-certified) of obstetricians and gynecologists, and on the numbers of nurses and nurse-midwives involved in obstetrical care; guidelines for consumer health practices; and statistics for the latest 4 years on infant natality and mortality, maternal mortality, and procedures (including surgery) performed by obstetricians and gynecologists. Also includes information on continuing education courses and self-study programs for ACOG members, and a schedule of annual and district ACOG meetings. Users may order publications and request searches online.
Language: English
Coverage: U.S.
Time Span: Current information
Updating: Quarterly

ACTIVIDADES FORMATIVAS

Type: Reference (Referral)
Subject: Conferences & Meetings
Producer: Instituto de la Pequena y Mediana Empresa Industrial
Online Service: Ministerio de Industria y Energia
Content: Contains references to about 1000 publicly and privately sponsored courses and training programs of interest to businesses.
Language: Spanish
Coverage: Spain

Time Span: Current information
Updating: Monthly

ADDABASE

Type: Reference (Referral)
Subject: Information Systems & Services-Directories
Producer: Australian Database Development Association (ADDA)
Online Service: ACI Computer Services
Conditions: Monthly minimum to ACI required; fees vary depending on service selected.
Content: Contains descriptions of about 200 publicly available online databases in Australia. Provides database name, producer and online service names and addresses, type of data (bibliographic, factual, full text, numeric, research in progress), file size, frequency of updating, time span, sources of data, corresponding publications, prices and conditions of access, subject terms, and general notes. Also includes descriptions of planned databases. Corresponds to *Directory of Australian Databases*, 2nd edition (1986).
Language: English
Coverage: Australia
Time Span: Current information
Updating: Quarterly

AFEE

Type: Reference (Bibliographic)
Subject: Aquatic Sciences; Environment
Producer: Association Francaise pour l'Etude des Eaux
Online Service: ESA-IRS
Content: Contains about 60,000 citations, with abstracts, to the worldwide literature of books, reports, conference papers, and proceedings on fresh water research and technology. Covers surface and subterranean waters; sea, shore, and coastal areas; water quality, pollution, and treatment; distribution and uses; health, hygiene, and safety; physical, chemical, and microbiological analyses; water policy, planning, and economy; and legislation. Does not include patents. Corresponds to *Information Eaux*.
Language: French
Coverage: International
Time Span: 1970 to date
Updating: About 450 records a month

AGDEX INFORMATION SERVICES

Type: Reference (Bibliographic)
Subject: Agriculture
Producer: Edinburgh School of Agriculture
Online Service: CAB International
Content: Contains about 22,000 citations, with abstracts, to literature relevant in the U.K. to applied agriculture. Covers cereals, root crops, oil crops, sheep, pigs, beef, dairying, farm mechanization, animal health and breeding, weeds, pest, and disease control, horticulture, farm buildings, computers, economics, agricultural policy, forestry, fish farming, horses, and bee keeping. Sources include journals, conference proceedings, technical reports, advisory leaflets, the popular farming press, and grey literature.
Language: English
Coverage: Primarily U.K, with some European coverage
Time Span: 1973 to date
Updating: About 200 records a month

AgeLine

Type: Reference (Bibliographic)
Subject: Gerontology
Producer: American Association of Retired Persons, National Gerontology Resource Center
Online Service: BRS; BRS After Dark; BRS/BRKTHRU; BRS/Colleague
Content: Contains about 18,500 citations, with abstracts, to the literature on social gerontology, with a focus on the social, psychological, and economic aspects of middle age and aging. Covers demographics, economics, employment, health and health care services, housing, intergenerational relationships, social and family relationships, psychological aspects, retirement, transportation, consumer aspects, and leisure. Includes descriptions of programs for older adults, indexed by state. Sources include journal articles, monographs (including chapters of books), reports, dissertations, conference papers, and research projects (including those funded by the U.S. Administration on Aging).
Language: English
Coverage: Primarily U.S., with some coverage of other English-speaking countries
Time Span: Literature, 1978 to date, with selected coverage from 1966; federally funded research projects, 1976 to 1980. Projects funded by U.S. Administration on Aging from 1981 to date will be added in 1986.
Updating: About 500 records every 2 months

AGNET®

Type: Reference (Referral); Source (Numeric, Textual-Numeric, Full Text)
Subject: Agriculture; Aquatic Sciences; Biomedicine; Legislative Tracking; Food Sciences & Nutrition
Producer: AGNET and others
Online Service: AGNET
Conditions: Annual subscription of $50 required
Content: A multi-faceted information service providing access to a variety of databases and computer services of use in operating an agricultural business.
ANIMALREGS. Contains full text of regulations on the importation and movement of animals and livestock. Also lists names and telephone numbers of state and international veterinary officials. Produced by the U.S. Department of Agriculture (USDA), National Center for Animal Health Information System.
FAS. Contains information supplied by the USDA, Foreign Agricultural Service (FAS) on international agricultural production and trade. Includes highlights of U.S. export sales; world production and trade roundups; grain and feed commodity import/export prices for selected ports worldwide; world production estimates; and trade leads for agricultural products from U.S. government attaches worldwide.
FEEDLOT. Contains references to cattle feedlots nationwide. Includes operator's name, address, and telephone number; contract options; types of facilities available (e.g., all concrete, all dirt); types of cattle accommodated; and feedstuffs available. Produced by South Dakota State University.
MARKETS. Contains commodity market data, including daily prices of selected cash markets and of futures markets from the Chicago Board of Trade, Chicago Mercantile Exchange, Kansas City Board of Trade, and Minneapolis Grain Exchange, as well as U.S. production and commodity reports from USDA, Statistical Reporting Service. Includes weekly analyses of markets for livestock and grain commodities. Also contains *World Agricultural Supply & Demand Reports* from the World

Agricultural Outlook Board, providing analyses and forecasts of all major agricultural commodities.

NEBRASKA HEALTHNETWORK. Contains information on medical and laboratory device problems from the Food and Drug Administration. Also provides analyses of the nutritional content of food products. Produced by the Nebraska Department of Health.

NEWSRELEASE. Contains press releases, reports, and analyses on state, regional, national, and international factors affecting the agricultural industry. Includes weather and crop summaries, pest condition reports, and commentaries on major USDA reports.

NMFS. Contains weekly *Fishery Export Opportunities* reports from the Department of Commerce, National Marine Fisheries Service.

PUBSEARCH. Contains citations to publications available to the public from the Nebraska Cooperative Extension.

Users can generate graphs and charts of commodity market data and can use agricultural management models to perform statistical manipulations for crop and livestock production and financial planning. Several electronic services, including mail and classified advertisements, are available.

Language: English

Coverage: Primarily U.S., with some international coverage

Time Span: Varies by database

Updating: Varies by database

AGREP (AGricultural REsearch Projects)

Type: Reference (Referral)

Subject: Agriculture; Research in Progress

Producer: Commission of the European Communities (CEC)

Online Service: Datacentralen; DIMDI; ECHO Service

Content: Contains over 23,000 descriptions of current agricultural research projects in member countries of the European Economic Community (EEC). Covers conservation and natural resources, land use and development, animal production, veterinary medicine, food and nutrition, fisheries, forestry, agricultural economics, and rural sociology. Corresponds to *Permanent Inventory of Agriculture Research Projects*.

Language: English, with titles also in original languages

Coverage: European Economic Community countries (Belgium, Denmark, Federal Republic of Germany, France, Greece, Ireland, Italy, Luxembourg, The Netherlands, and U.K.)

Time Span: Datacentralen, current information; DIMDI, 1975 to date.

Updating: About 200 records a quarter

AGRICOLA

Type: Reference (Bibliographic)

Subject: Agriculture; Food Sciences & Nutrition; Veterinary Sciences

Producer: U.S. Department of Agriculture, National Agricultural Library

Online Service: BRS; BRS After Dark; BRS/BRKTHRU; BRS/Colleague; DIALOG Information Services, Inc.; DIMDI; Knowledge Index; TECH DATA

Content: Contains citations to the journal literature, government reports, serials, monographs, audiovisual resources, and pamphlets in agriculture and related areas that have been acquired by the National Agricultural Library (NAL) for use by the U.S. Department of Agriculture as well as citations contributed by cooperating agencies. Includes agricultural economics and rural sociology, agricultural production, animal sciences,

chemistry and engineering, entomology, food and human nutrition, forestry, natural resources, pesticides, plant science, soils and fertilizers, and water resources. Also covers related areas such as land use, family migration, labor and political movements, and the impact of chemicals on living organisms. Contributing agencies include land grant institutions, the NAL Food and Nutrition Information Center (abstracts available from 1973 on), and the American Agriculture Economics Documentation Center (abstracts available from 1976 on). Corresponds in part to *Bibliography of Agriculture*.

Language: English

Coverage: International

Time Span: BRS, BRS After Dark, BRS/BRKTHRU, BRS/Colleague, and DIALOG, 1970 to date; Knowledge Index, 1979 to date; DIMDI, 1983 to date.

Updating: About 12,000 records a month

AGRIS (International Information System for the Agricultural Sciences and Technology)

Type: Reference (Bibliographic)

Subject: Agriculture

Producer: Food and Agriculture Organization of the United Nations (FAO), Agris Coordinating Centre

Online Service: DIALOG Information Services, Inc. (AGRIS INTERNATIONAL); DIMDI; ESA-IRS; International Atomic Energy Agency (IAEA)

Conditions: Approval of Liaison Office in user's country may be required; contact FAO for complete list of participating countries and addresses of Liaison Offices or consult current issue of *Agrindex*.

Content: Contains approximately 1 million citations, some with abstracts, to the worldwide literature on all aspects of agriculture. Topics covered include geography and history; legislation; education, extension, and advisory work; economics, development, marketing, and rural sociology; plant production; protection of plants and stored products; forestry; animal production; veterinary medicine; aquatic sciences and fisheries; machinery and buildings; natural resources; food science; human nutrition; home economics; and pollution. Corresponds to the monthly *Agrindex*.

Language: English, with titles also in original languages (beginning with 1985, documents have index terms in English, French, and Spanish)

Coverage: International

Time Span: 1975 to date

Updating: About 10,000 records a month

AIDS

Type: Reference (Bibliographic)

Subject: Biomedicine

Producer: Bureau of Hygiene and Tropical Diseases (BHTD)

Online Service: BRS/Colleague; CAB International; DATA-STAR

Content: Contains about 1000 citations, most with abstracts, to the worldwide literature on Acquired Immune Deficiency Syndrome (AIDS), retroviruses, and human T-lymphotropic viruses. Covers etiology of AIDS, transmission, epidemiology, pathology, immunology, serology, treatment and control, and clinical and social aspects of the disease. Sources include journals, books, theses, and reports, with an emphasis on journals in the library of the London School of Hygiene and Tropical Medicine. Corresponds in part to *Abstracts on Hygiene and Communicable Diseases*.

Language: English, with titles also in original languages
Coverage: International
Time Span: Mid-1982 to date
Updating: About 40 records a month

AIDS POLICY AND LAW

Type: Source (Full Text)
Subject: Legislative Tracking
Producer: Buraff Publications, Inc.
Online Service: Executive Telecom System, Inc., Human Resource Information Network
Conditions: Annual subscription to Executive Telecom System required
Content: Contains information on the legal and practical implications of Acquired Immune Deficiency Syndrome (AIDS) on government and private employment policies. Covers rights of stricken employees and their co-workers; fair employment practices; housing; insurance; medical testing and care; schooling; current and pending federal, state, and local legislation and regulations; and litigation and emerging case law.
Language: English
Coverage: U.S.
Time Span: 1986 to date
Updating: Every 2 weeks

AIDS UPDATE

Type: Reference (Bibliographic)
Subject: Biomedicine
Producer: Bureau of Hygiene and Tropical Diseases (BHTD)
Online Service: BRS/Colleague; CAB International; DATA-STAR
Content: Contains about 900 citations, most with abstracts, to the worldwide literature on Acquired Immune Deficiency Syndrome (AIDS), retroviruses, and human T-lymphotropic viruses. Covers etiology, transmission, epidemiology, pathology, immunology, clinical aspects, serology, treatment and control, and social and public aspects. Sources include journals, books, and reports. Corresponds to BHTD AIDS Update Service.
Language: English
Coverage: International
Time Span: Mid-1985 to date
Updating: About 100 records a month

AIM/ARM (Abstracts of Instructional and Research Materials in Vocational and Technical Education)

Type: Reference (Bibliographic)
Subject: Education & Educational Institutions
Producer: The National Center for Research in Vocational Education
Online Service: DIALOG Information Services, Inc.
Content: Contains citations, with abstracts, to instructional materials and research reports in these areas of vocational and technical education: agricultural, business and office, consumer, distributive health occupations, home economics, industrial arts, and trade and industrial education. Also covers manpower economics and development, employment, job training, and vocational guidance. Cited materials include those developed by local school districts, state departments of education, curriculum development laboratories, and industrial

organizations, as well as research reports issued by the U.S. Department of Education, the U.S. Department of Labor, Office of Economic Opportunity, and private foundations. Beginning in 1977, records were submitted for inclusion in the ERIC and RESOURCES IN VOCATIONAL EDUCATION databases *(see)*.
Language: English
Coverage: U.S.
Time Span: September 1967 through 1976 *(see ERIC and RESOURCES IN VOCATIONAL EDUCATION for information from 1977 to date)*
Updating: Not updated

AIR/WATER POLLUTION REPORT

Type: Source (Full Text)
Subject: Environment
Producer: Business Publishers, Inc.
Online Service: NewsNet, Inc.
Conditions: Monthly subscription to NewsNet required; differential charges for subscribers and non-subscribers to *Air/Water Pollution Report*.
Content: Contains full text of *Air/Water Pollution Report*, a newsletter covering air and water pollution. Emphasis is on the Clean Air and Clean Water Acts and other environmental laws and regulations.
Language: English
Coverage: U.S.
Time Span: 1982 to date
Updating: Weekly

AIRLINE ITINERARIES

Type: Source (Textual-Numeric)
Subject: Flight Schedules
Producer: Dittler Airline Data Systems
Online Service: THE SOURCE
Conditions: Monthly minimum of $10 to THE SOURCE required, with $9 credited toward online usage charges
Content: Contains information on direct flights between cities worldwide. The segments of each flight are listed so that users can select airline service between their specific origin and destination cities. Information from this database is also contained in BASELINE.
Language: English
Coverage: International
Time Span: Current month
Updating: Twice a month

AKRON BEACON JOURNAL

Type: Source (Full Text)
Subject: News
Producer: Beacon Journal Publishing Company
Online Service: VU/TEXT Information Services, Inc.
Conditions: Subscription to VU/TEXT required
Content: Contains full text of news items and feature articles from the *Akron Beacon Journal* (Ohio) newspaper. Regional coverage emphasizes the rubber, steel, and automotive industries.
Language: English
Coverage: U.S. (primarily Ohio)
Time Span: 1985 to date
Updating: Daily

ALBANY TIMES-UNION

Type: Source (Full Text)
Subject: News
Producer: Hearst Publishing Group, Capitol Newspapers Division
Online Service: VU/TEXT Information Services, Inc.
Conditions: Subscription to VU/TEXT required
Content: Contains full text of news items and feature articles from the *Times-Union* (New York) newspaper.
Language: English
Coverage: U.S. (primarily Albany, New York area)
Time Span: March 1986 to date
Updating: Daily

ALICE

Type: Reference (Bibliographic)
Subject: Publishers & Distributors-Catalogs
Producer: Editrice Bibliografica s.r.l.
Online Service: CILEA
Conditions: Subscription fee to Editrice Bibliografica required
Content: Contains citations to more than 200,000 currently available and recently out-of-print books published by approximately 1600 publishing companies in Italy. Information for each item includes author, title, subtitle (if any), translator, editor, year of publication, edition, size, pagination, illustrations, price, ISBN number, and publisher. Also includes a maximum of 3 subject terms for each item. Data are provided by Italian publishing societies. Corresponds to the biannual *Catalogo del Libri in Commercio*.
Language: Italian
Coverage: Italy
Time Span: 1978 to date
Updating: Monthly

ALIS (Automated Library Information System)

Type: Reference (Bibliographic)
Subject: Library Holdings-Catalogs
Producer: The National Technological Library of Denmark and others
Online Service: Datacentralen
Content: Consists of 14 files related to the holdings of the National Technological Libraries of Denmark, Finland, Norway, and Sweden, of 2 Danish University Libraries, and of The Danish Veterinary and Agricultural Library. Contains about 225,000 items covering all areas of science and technology, including agriculture, chemistry, physics, mathematics, medicine, engineering, energy, data processing, electronics, and veterinary science.
SMOT (formerly MONO). Contains citations to monographs, dissertations, single issues of series, and conference reports published in 1968 or later. Updated daily.
MONO. Contains holdings information on items listed in SMOT and held by the National Technological Library of Denmark.
REST. Contains holdings information on items listed in SMOT and held by Libraries other than the National Technological Library of Denmark.
SPOT (formerly PERI). Contains holdings information on periodicals and series, including annual reports and yearbooks, held by the National Technological Libraries. Updated daily.
EMNE. Contains the National Technological Library of Denmark's classification scheme (UDC) in Danish. Updated

every 6 to 12 months.
DVJB. Contains approximately 10,500 citations to books, dissertations, conference proceedings, research reports, and other monographic literature covering agriculture, veterinary science, and food science and technology. Corresponds to the holdings of The Danish Veterinary and Agricultural Library. Updated twice a year.
RAPP. Contains citations to reports published by the National Technical Information Service (NTIS) that are held by the National Technological Library of Denmark.
KTHP. Contains holdings information on non-Swedish scientific and technical journals held by about 300 Swedish libraries.
NTHP. Contains holdings information on periodicals and serials held by the Norwegian Technological University Library.
INGE. Contains selected articles from *Ingenioren*.
DTHM. Contains citations to monographs held by institutional libraries of the Technological University of Denmark.
UBMO and UBPE. Contains citations to monographs and periodicals held by the Copenhagen University Library, 2nd Department.
UBIN. Contains citations to books held by the scientific and medical institutional libraries at Copenhagen University.
Coverage: Primarily monographs and serials published in the U.S., U.K., Federal Republic of Germany, France, Denmark, Norway, Sweden, The Netherlands, Belgium, Switzerland, Japan, and the U.S.S.R.
Time Span: Most files, 1968 to date; DVJB, 1979 to date.
Updating: *See Content* (about 20,000 records a year)

ALLENTOWN-THE MORNING CALL

Type: Source (Full Text)
Subject: News
Producer: The Morning Call Newspaper
Online Service: VU/TEXT Information Services, Inc.
Conditions: Subscription to VU/TEXT required
Content: Contains full text of news items, feature stories, and editorials from the Allentown *Morning Call* with emphasis on local and regional news in the Allentown, Bethlehem, and Easton areas of northeastern Pennsylvania. Covers such topics as local business developments, industry news, sports, travel, and the arts. Includes descriptions of maps, charts, graphs, photographs, and other illustrations.
Language: English
Coverage: U.S. (primarily northeastern Pennsylvania area)
Time Span: 1984 to date
Updating: Daily

AMA LIBRARY INFORMATION SERVICE

Type: Reference (Bibliographic, Referral)
Subject: Biomedicine; Conferences & Meetings
Producer: American Medical Association (AMA), Division of Library and Information Management
Online Service: AMA/NET
Conditions: Subscription fee of $50 to AMA/NET required
Content: Contains information about several types of medical information resources.
New Books. Contains citations to recently published books in various subject categories (e.g., pediatrics, psychology, urology).
Search Strategies for SIB and EMPIRES. Contains descriptions of techniques for searching the non-clinical online bibliographic database AMA/NET SOCIO/ECONOMIC BIBLIOGRAPHIC INFORMATION (SIB) *(see)* and the clinical biblio-

graphic database AMA/NET EMPIRES *(see)*.

Meetings and Seminars. Contains a calendar of upcoming AMA-sponsored events, as well as meetings scheduled by other scientific and educational organizations in the medical field.

Language: English
Coverage: Primarily U.S.
Time Span: Current information
Updating: Monthly

AMA/NET^{SM} AP MEDICAL NEWS SERVICE

Type: Source (Full Text)
Subject: Biomedicine; Health Care; News
Producer: American Medical Association (AMA), in conjunction with The Associated Press (AP)
Online Service: AMA/NET
Conditions: Subscription fee of $50 to AMA/NET required
Content: Contains full text of medical-related news stories from AP news wires and U.S. newspapers. Covers people and events; political, legislative, legal, social, and economic issues; medical ethics and education; international medicine; health and fitness, including maternal and child care; drugs and chemicals; toxicology and environmental hazards; disease and diagnosis; medical devices and equipment; surgery and organ transplantation; and hospitals and insurance.
Language: English
Coverage: U.S.
Time Span: Most recent 7 days
Updating: Continuously, throughout the day

AMA/NET^{SM} DISEASE INFORMATION

Type: Source (Full Text)
Subject: Biomedicine
Producer: American Medical Association (AMA)
Online Service: AMA/NET
Conditions: Subscription fee of $50 to AMA/NET required
Content: Contains descriptions of over 3500 diseases, disorders, and conditions. Each description includes nomenclature; etiology; disease course; laboratory, radiological, and pathological findings; and signs and symptoms. Corresponds in part to *Current Medical Information and Terminology*, 5th edition (1981).
Language: English
Time Span: Current information
Updating: Quarterly

AMA/NET^{SM} EMPIRES®

Type: Reference (Bibliographic)
Subject: Biomedicine
Producer: Elsevier Science Publishers b.v.
Online Service: AMA/NET
Conditions: Subscription fee of $50 to AMA/NET required
Content: Contains citations, with some abstracts, to articles in 320 key medical journals. Articles are coded by medical specialty according to a customized version of the American Medical Association (AMA) Specialty Classification Codes. Citations include full bibliographic information, subject indexing, drug terminology, and drug manufacturers. In the Current Awareness Service, access is by Specialty Codes. In the Reference Service, current and retrospective access is available by individual citation elements.

Language: English
Coverage: International
Time Span: 1984 to date
Updating: About 1200 records a week

AMA/NET^{SM} MEDICAL PROCEDURE CODING AND NOMENCLATURE

Type: Source (Textual-Numeric)
Subject: Health Care
Producer: American Medical Association (AMA)
Online Service: AMA/NET
Conditions: Subscription fee of $50 to AMA/NET required
Content: Provides identification codes and descriptions of over 6000 procedures in the areas of medicine, surgery, and diagnostic services. Codes can be used by physicians to report medical services and procedures on patient bills and by insurance companies in processing claims. Corresponds to current edition of *Physicians' Current Procedural Terminology*.
Language: English
Coverage: U.S.
Time Span: Current information
Updating: Annually

AMA/NET^{SM} SOCIO/ECONOMIC BIBLIOGRAPHIC INFORMATION

Type: Reference (Bibliographic)
Subject: Health Care
Producer: American Medical Association (AMA), Division of Library and Information Management
Online Service: AMA/NET
Conditions: Subscription fee of $50 to AMA/NET required
Content: Contains citations to articles on the non-clinical aspects of health care, including economics, education, ethics, international relations, legislation, political science, psychology, public health, medical practices, and sociology. Includes such topics as cost containment, insurance reimbursement, medical staff relations, and practice management. Covers legislative reports, monographs, newspapers, and over 700 journals. Corresponds in part to *Socioeconomic Research Resources (MEDSOC)*, with current information available online.
Language: English
Time Span: 1981 to date
Updating: Monthly

AMERICAN AIRLINES EAASY SABRE®

Type: Reference (Referral)
Subject: Flight Schedules
Producer: American Airlines
Online Service: Dialcom, Inc.; General Electric Information Services Company (GEISCO); Quantum Computer Services, Inc.
Conditions: Monthly subscription of $9.95 to Quantum Computer Services required; flight reservations can be made online only by members of American Airlines AAdvantage (frequent flyer) program.
Content: Contains domestic and international flight schedules and fares for over 600 airlines. Users can reserve flights on more than 300 carriers, order tickets to be sent through the mail or relayed to a travel agent, arrange and confirm hotel and motel reservations, and reserve rental cars through major agencies worldwide. American Airlines AAdvantage members can also check the status of their bonus miles online, and travel agents can access selected Rand McNally publications.

Language: English
Coverage: International
Time Span: Current information
Updating: Daily

AMERICAN MEN AND WOMEN OF SCIENCE

Type: Reference (Referral)
Subject: Biographies
Producer: Jaques Cattell Press, a division of R.R. Bowker Company
Online Service: BRS; BRS/BRKTHRU; BRS/Colleague; DIALOG Information Services, Inc.; TECH DATA
Content: Contains approximately 130,500 biographies of scientists and engineers in the biological and physical sciences. Includes full names, place and date of birth, disciplines, education and honorary degrees, professional experience, concurrent positions, memberships in scientific societies, research interests, and mailing address. Corresponds to *American Men and Women of Science, Physical and Biological Sciences*, 15th Edition.
Language: English
Coverage: U.S. and Canada
Time Span: Current information
Updating: Every 3 years

AMILIT

Type: Reference (Bibliographic)
Subject: Occupational Safety & Health
Producer: Swedish National Board of Occupational Safety and Health
Online Service: ARAMIS (a cooperative service of the Swedish Center for Working Life, Swedish National Board of Occupational Safety and Health, and The Swedish National Environmental Protection Board)
Content: Contains about 8000 citations to Swedish research reports on occupational safety and health and related topics.
Language: Swedish and English
Coverage: Sweden
Time Span: 1982 to date
Updating: About 1500 records a year

ANCHORAGE DAILY NEWS

Type: Source (Full Text)
Subject: News
Producer: Advanced Search Concepts
Online Service: VU/TEXT Information Services, Inc.
Conditions: Subscription to VU/TEXT required
Content: Contains full text of news items and feature articles from the *Anchorage Daily News* (Alaska) newspaper.
Language: English
Coverage: U.S. (primarily Anchorage, Alaska area)
Time Span: October 1985 to date
Updating: Daily

ANEUPLOIDY

Type: Reference (Bibliographic)
Subject: Biomedicine
Producer: Oak Ridge National Laboratory, Environmental Mutagen Information Center

Online Service: National Library of Medicine (NLM) (as a TOXLINE database *(see)*)
Content: Contains approximately 2800 citations to literature on research in aneuploidy (numerical chromosome abnormalities) in humans and experimental systems. Citations are classified into one of the following groups: (1) population studies covering spontaneous incidence of aneuploidy in human populations; (2) screening studies covering the testing of chemicals or physical agents for the induction of aneuploidy; and (3) general studies that do not fit into the other categories.
Language: English
Coverage: International
Time Span: 1970 to date
Updating: Twice a year

ANIMAL DISEASE OCCURRENCE

Type: Reference (Bibliographic); Source (Textual-Numeric)
Subject: Veterinary Sciences
Producer: CAB International
Online Service: DIMDI
Content: Contains about 4500 records on the incidence of animal diseases worldwide. Data include the country of occurrence, number of animals affected, duration of the disease, number of deaths, and economic effects. Each record includes a citation to the source publication. Corresponds to *Animal Disease Occurrence*.
NOTE: On BRS, CISTI, DIALOG, DIMDI, and ESA-IRS, citations are included in CAB ABSTRACTS *(see)*.
Language: English
Coverage: International
Time Span: 1980 to date
Updating: Twice a year

ANNAPOLIS–THE CAPITAL

Type: Source (Full Text)
Subject: News
Producer: The Capital-Gazette Newspapers, Inc.
Online Service: VU/TEXT Information Services, Inc.
Conditions: Subscription to VU/TEXT required
Content: Contains full text of news items, feature stories, and editorials from *The Capital*, with an emphasis on regional news in the Annapolis, Maryland area. Regional coverage includes news of the U.S. Naval Academy, environmental issues affecting the Chesapeake Bay, and Maryland state government.
Language: English
Coverage: U.S. (primarily Annapolis, Maryland area)
Time Span: June 1986 to date
Updating: Daily

ANTIC ONLINE

Type: Reference (Bibliographic); Source (Full Text)
Subject: Computers & Software
Producer: Antic Publishing Inc.
Online Service: CompuServe Information Service
Content: Contains summaries and selected full-text articles from *Antic*, a magazine providing news and information of interest to users of Atari computers. Includes synopses of reviews of software and hardware products, letters to the editor, a weekly opinion survey of the "product of the week", and information on user group events.

Language: English
Coverage: U.S.
Time Span: Current information
Updating: Weekly

AP NEWS

Type: Source (Full Text)
Subject: News
Producer: The Associated Press (AP)
Online Service: DIALOG Information Services, Inc.; Mead Data Central, Inc. (AP) (as part of NEXIS WIRE SERVICES *(see))*; NewsNet, Inc. (AP DATASTREAM BUSINESS NEWS WIRE); VU/TEXT Information Services, Inc.
Conditions: Subscription to Mead Data Central required; monthly subscription to NewsNet required; subscription to VU/TEXT required.
Content: Contains full text of more than 132,000 items from AP's DataStream newswire service. Covers international news; U.S. general, financial and business, political, and Washington, D.C.-area news; and sports and entertainment news.
NOTE: On NewsNet, news items are accessible only through NewsFlash, a selective dissemination service, and are retained 2 weeks for each user.
Language: English
Coverage: International
Time Span: Mead Data Central, 1977 to date; DIALOG, July 1984 to date; VU/TEXT, 1985 to date; NewsNet, most current 2 weeks.
Updating: Most services, about 500 stories a day, 48 hours after publication; NewsNet, 15 minutes after publication.

AP VIDEOTEX

Type: Source (Full Text)
Subject: News
Producer: The Associated Press (AP)
Online Service: AgriData Network (NEWSFINDER) (as an AgriData Network database); Dialcom, Inc.; General Videotex Corporation/DELPHI (ASSOCIATED PRESS VIDEOTEX NEWSWIRE); THE SOURCE
Conditions: Subscription to AgriData Network required; monthly minimum of $100 to Dialcom, Inc. required; monthly minimum of $10 to THE SOURCE required, with $9 credited toward online usage charges.
Content: Contains full text of news stories covering international, national, sports, business, and weather news. Articles are specially edited by AP to fit 40-character terminal displays.
Language: English
Coverage: International
Time Span: Current information
Updating: About 250 records a day

APPLE II/III SIG

Type: Source (Full Text, Software)
Subject: Computers & Software
Producer: THE SOURCE
Online Service: THE SOURCE
Conditions: Monthly minimum of $10 to THE SOURCE required, with $9 credited toward online usage charges
Content: Contains news and information for users of Apple II and Apple III personal computers. Provides announcements and reviews of new products and services, including notices of discounts from vendors; a directory of bulletin boards; and software available for downloading.

Language: English
Coverage: U.S.
Time Span: Current information
Updating: Daily

APPLIED SCIENCE & TECHNOLOGY INDEX℠

Type: Reference (Bibliographic)
Subject: Science & Technology
Producer: The H.W. Wilson Company
Online Service: WILSONLINE
Content: Contains about 82,000 citations to articles, book reviews, interviews, new product reviews, and selected editorials and letters to the editor in 336 English-language publications in the applied sciences and technology. Covers aeronautics and space science, chemistry, computer science, construction industry, electric and electronics industry, energy resources and research, fire and fire prevention, food industry, geology, machinery, mathematics, mineralogy, metallurgy, oceanography, physics, plastics, textiles, transportation, and the following engineering fields: chemical, civil, electrical, environmental, industrial, mechanical, mining, nuclear, and telecommunications. Corresponds to *Applied Science & Technology Index.*
Language: English
Coverage: Canada, Ireland, The Netherlands, Switzerland, U.K., and U.S.
Time Span: November 1983 to date
Updating: Twice a week; about 5000 articles a month.

APTIC (Air Pollution Technical Information Center)

Type: Reference (Bibliographic)
Subject: Environment
Producer: U.S. Environmental Protection Agency (EPA), Air Pollution Technical Information Center
Online Service: DIALOG Information Services, Inc.
Content: Contains citations, with abstracts, to literature related to the sources, effects, prevention, and control of air pollution. The social, political, economic, legal, and administrative aspects of environmental issues are also covered in these areas: atmospheric interaction; methods of measurement and control; effect on human health, plants, livestock, and materials; emission sources; and air quality and emissions data. Contains all references from *Air Pollution Abstracts*, which is no longer published.
Language: English
Coverage: U.S.
Time Span: 1966 through September 1976, with some materials through 1978
Updating: Not updated

AQUACULTURE

Type: Reference (Bibliographic)
Subject: Aquatic Sciences
Producer: National Oceanic and Atmospheric Administration, National Environmental Data Referral Service
Online Service: DIALOG Information Services, Inc.
Content: Contains citations, with some abstracts, to literature on the growing of marine, brackish, and freshwater organisms. Subjects covered include disease, economics, engineering, feed and nutrition, growing requirements, legal aspects, and life history. Hydroponic techniques are not included.

Language: English
Coverage: International
Time Span: 1970 to March 1984
Updating: Not updated

AQUALINE®

Type: Reference (Bibliographic)
Subject: Aquatic Sciences; Environment
Producer: Water Research Centre (WRC)
Online Service: Pergamon InfoLine
Content: Contains about 96,000 citations, with abstracts, to the worldwide literature on every aspect of water, wastewater, and the aquatic environment. Topics covered include groundwater, surface waters, wastewater treatment, instrumentation, control and computing, resource development and management, water sampling and analysis, water treatment, distribution systems, drinking water quality, river management, sludge utilization, tidal waters, sewerage systems, and other water-related topics. Corresponds to *Aqualine Abstracts*.
Language: English
Coverage: International
Time Span: 1960 to date
Updating: About 800 records a month

AQUAREF (Canadian Water Resource References)

Type: Reference (Bibliographic)
Subject: Aquatic Sciences; Environment
Producer: Environment Canada, WATDOC, Inland Waters Directorate
Online Service: CISTI, Canadian Online Enquiry Service (CAN/OLE)
Conditions: CISTI accessible only in Canada
Content: Contains over 60,000 citations, with abstracts, to scientific, technical, and general-interest literature on Canadian water resources and such other environmental topics as wildlife, lands, fisheries, forestry, air, and baseline studies. Covers more than 200 Canadian and foreign journals; conference proceedings; French and English reports and publications of Environment Canada; publications of other federal, provincial, territorial, and municipal government departments and agencies; universities; and research centers.
Language: English and French
Coverage: Canada
Time Span: 1972 to date
Updating: About 1000 records every 2 months

AQUATIC INFORMATION RETRIEVAL DATA BASE

Type: Reference (Bibliographic); Source (Textual-Numeric)
Subject: Environment
Producer: U.S. Environmental Protection Agency (EPA), Office of Pesticides and Toxic Substances
Online Service: Chemical Information Systems, Inc., a subsidiary of Fein-Marquart Associates (CIS); Information Consultants, Inc. (ICI) (as part of The Integrated Chemical Information System)
Conditions: Annual subscription fee of $300 to CIS required but fee is waived for educational institutions and non-profit public libraries worldwide; differential charges for subscribers and non-subscribers to ICI.

Content: Contains data on acute, chronic, bioaccumulative, and sublethal effects of chemical substances on freshwater and saltwater organisms (excluding bacteria, birds, and aquatic mammals). Each record covers a single experiment and includes chemical substance information, description of test organism, study protocol, test results, and bibliographic reference.
NOTE: On CIS, this file contains 68,338 records on 4179 chemical substances.
Language: English
Coverage: International
Time Span: 1970 to date
Updating: Periodically, as new data become available

AQUATIC SCIENCES AND FISHERIES ABSTRACTS

Type: Reference (Bibliographic)
Subject: Aquatic Sciences
Producer: Cambridge Scientific Abstracts, on behalf of the Food and Agriculture Organization (FAO) of the United Nations, Fishery Information, Data and Statistics Service; Intergovernmental Oceanographic Commission; United Nations, Department of International Economic and Social Affairs, Ocean Economics and Technology Branch
Online Service: BRS; BRS After Dark; BRS/BRKTHRU; BRS/Colleague; CISTI, Canadian Online Enquiry Service (CAN/OLE) (ASFA) (through a contract with the Canadian Department of Fisheries and Oceans); DIALOG Information Services, Inc. (through a contract with Cambridge Scientific Abstracts); DIMDI (ASFA) (through a contract with Bundesforschungsanstalt fuer Fischerei); ESA-IRS
Conditions: CISTI accessible only in Canada
Content: Contains about 200,000 citations, with abstracts, to worldwide literature on the science, technology, and management of marine, brackish, and freshwater environments. Includes the following and related subjects: aquaculture; aquatic biology; biological oceanography; chemical oceanography; coastal zone management; commerce, trade, and economics; diving; ecology and ecosystems; environmental studies; fisheries (harvesting, processing, and marketing); fish products; geological oceanography; law of the sea; limnology; marine biology, policy, pollution and technology; meteorology and climatology; ocean engineering; ocean resources; offshore activities; physical oceanography; underwater acoustics and optics; vessels, underwater vessels, and buoys; and water pollution. Corresponds to *Aquatic Sciences and Fisheries Abstracts, Part 1: Biological Sciences and Living Resources, Part 2: Ocean Technology, Policy and Non-Living Resources,* and *ASFA Aquaculture Abstracts*.
Language: English, with titles also in original languages
Coverage: International
Time Span: Most services, 1975 to date; DIALOG, 1978 to date.
Updating: About 3000 records a month

ARIZONA BUSINESS GAZETTE

Type: Source (Full Text)
Subject: News
Producer: Phoenix Newspapers, Inc.
Online Service: VU/TEXT Information Services, Inc.
Conditions: Subscription to VU/TEXT required
Content: Contains full text of news items and feature articles from the *Arizona Business Gazette*, a newspaper covering commercial, industrial, and agricultural development in

Arizona. Regional coverage emphasizes high-technology industries, resort and real estate financing and development, and water rights in the southwest U.S. Includes legal notices and summaries of decisions from Arizona courts.

Language: English

Coverage: U.S. (primarily Arizona)

Time Span: June 1986 to date

Updating: Weekly

THE ARIZONA REPUBLIC

Type: Source (Full Text)

Subject: News

Producer: Phoenix Newspapers, Inc.

Online Service: VU/TEXT Information Services, Inc.

Conditions: Subscription to VU/TEXT required

Content: Contains full text of news items and feature articles from *The Arizona Republic* newspaper. Regional coverage emphasizes the aerospace, high technology, and tourism industries.

Language: English

Coverage: U.S. (primarily southwestern states)

Time Span: April 1986 to date

Updating: Daily

ARTHUR D. LITTLE/ONLINE

Type: Reference (Bibliographic); Source (Full Text)

Subject: Health Care

Producer: Arthur D. Little Decision Resources

Online Service: DIALOG Information Services, Inc.

Conditions: Surcharge of $100 required on selected Executive Summaries and full text reports

Content: Contains more than 900 citations to, or full text of, non-exclusive publications produced by Arthur D. Little, Inc., its divisions and subsidiaries. Includes industry forecasts, technology assessments, product and market overviews, corporate profiles and assessments, and opinion research. Covers these industries: information processing, including computers and office automation; telecommunications; electronics; health care, including pharmaceuticals, medical equipment and supplies, diagnostic products, and health care services; chemicals, including specialty chemicals, petrochemicals, packaging, plastics, and fibers; transportation; energy, including energy management, and alternative energy sources; construction and building products; biotechnology. Each record contains the table of content and/or the list of tables and figures from each document. Full text of Executive Summaries are available from *Industry Outlook Reports*, *Research Letters*, *Marketing Index Reports*, and the *Public Opinion Index Reports*. Full text of articles from *Futurescope*, the *International Health Care Portfolio*, and the *International InfoTran Portfolio* are also available. Corresponding programs include IMPACT, INFOTRAN, HEALTH CARE INDUSTRY SERVICE, WORLD TELECOMMUNICATIONS INFORMATION PROGRAM, and the PUBLIC OPINION INDEX of Opinion Research Corporation.

Language: English

Coverage: Primarily U.S., with some international coverage

Time Span: 1977 to date

Updating: About 60 records every 2 months

ASBESTOS

Type: Reference (Bibliographic)

Subject: Biomedicine

Producer: University of Sherbrooke, Informatheque-PRAUS (Programme de Recherche et de Developpement sur l'Amiante)

Online Service: QL Systems Limited

Content: Contains citations, with abstracts, to the worldwide literature on all aspects of asbestos, including technology, chemistry, geology, mineralogy, construction, economics, biology, mining, patents, production, products, pollution control, laws and regulations, health and safety, statistics, and medical research concerning asbestos-related diseases. Sources include over 3000 journals, books, government publications, research reports, trade literature, bibliographies, and selected databases.

Language: English

Coverage: International

Time Span: Technological documents, 1970 to date; medical documents, 1890 to date.

Updating: Quarterly

ASI® (American Statistics Index)

Type: Reference (Bibliographic)

Subject: Government-U.S. Federal

Producer: Congressional Information Service, Inc. (CIS)

Online Service: DIALOG Information Services, Inc.

Content: Contains citations, with abstracts, to publications containing social, economic, demographic, and other statistical data collected and analyzed by the U.S. government. Covers statistical publications (or publications containing substantial statistical data) generated by executive, legislative, and judicial departments; research, administrative, and regulatory agencies; and special bodies created by the Congress or the President. Corresponds to *American Statistics Index*.

Language: English

Coverage: U.S.

Time Span: 1973 to date, with selected coverage of publications issued during the 1960s

Updating: About 1000 records a month

AUSTRALASIAN MEDICAL INDEX

Type: Reference (Bibliographic)

Subject: Biomedicine

Producer: National Library of Australia; Department of Health

Online Service: Australian Medline Network

Conditions: Permission of the National Library of Australia required

Content: Contains over 9000 citations, with abstracts, to the biomedical literature of Australia and New Zealand. Covers clinical practice, research, policy, health services, drug abuse, the biology of aging, and Aboriginal health. Sources include periodicals (excluding those covered in MEDLINE *(see)*), monographs, conference proceedings, and abstracts.

Language: English

Coverage: Australia, New Zealand, and Fiji

Time Span: 1980 to date

Updating: About 500 records a month

AUSTRALIAN BIBLIOGRAPHY OF AGRICULTURE

Type: Reference (Bibliographic)

Subject: Agriculture

Producer: CSIRO

Online Service: ACI Computer Services

Conditions: Monthly minimum to ACI required; fees vary depending on service selected.

Content: Contains citations, with some abstracts, to journals, reports, monographs, and pamphlets in the field of agriculture that have been published in Australia or produced by Australian organizations. Topics covered include fisheries; forestry; food technology; human nutrition; soil, plant, and animal sciences; agricultural economics; and rural sociology.

Language: English

Coverage: Australia

Time Span: 1975 to date

Updating: About 500 records a month

AUSTRALIAN GOVERNMENT PUBLICATIONS

Type: Reference (Bibliographic)

Subject: Publishers & Distributors-Catalogs

Producer: National Library of Australia

Online Service: ACI Computer Services (to be available in 1987)

Conditions: Monthly minimum to ACI required; fees vary depending on service selected.

Content: Contains over 25,000 citations to publications produced by the government of the Commonwealth of Australia and its states and territories. Covers all subjects within the scope of government activity, including agriculture, economics and financial institutions, small business, trade and export, law and legislation, health services, public service administration, transportation engineering, technology, and the environment. Sources include books, pamphlets, leaflets, and serials. Also covers compilations of parliamentary debates, transcripts of proceedings of parliamentary committees, and proceedings of courts and tribunals. Corresponds to *Australian Government Publications*.

Language: English

Coverage: Australia

Time Span: 1983 to date

Updating: About 2500 records a quarter

AUSTRALIAN LEISURE INDEX

Type: Reference (Bibliographic)

Subject: General Interest

Producer: Australian Clearinghouse for Publications in Recreation, Sport, and Tourism (ACHPIRST)

Online Service: ACI Computer Services

Conditions: Monthly minimum to ACI required; fees vary depending on service selected.

Content: Contains about 16,000 citations, with abstracts, to Australian literature in the fields of recreation, leisure, sports, physical education, fitness, health, tourism, and other related fields. Covers journal articles, monographs, conference papers, theses, research reports, audiovisual items, and unpublished reports. Corresponds to *Australian Leisure Index* (1982 to date) and *Australian Leisure Bibliography* (pre-1982 monographs only) .

Language: English

Coverage: Australia

Time Span: 1982 to date, with earlier monographs

Updating: About 1000 records twice a year (June and December)

AUSTRALIAN NATIONAL BIBLIOGRAPHY

Type: Reference (Bibliographic)

Subject: Publishers & Distributors-Catalogs

Producer: National Library of Australia

Online Service: ACI Computer Services

Conditions: Monthly minimum to ACI required; fees vary depending on service selected.

Content: Contains bibliographic information on books and pamphlets published in Australia. Also includes selected government publications, new serial titles, and foreign publications that are authored by Australians or that have Australian subject content. Each record includes author, title, language, publisher and place of publication, form of reproduction (e.g., Braille) , and the issue of *Australian National Bibliography* in which the item appeared.

Language: English

Coverage: Australia

Time Span: 1972 to date

Updating: About 1000 records a month

AUSTRALIAN SCIENCE INDEX

Type: Reference (Bibliographic)

Subject: Science & Technology

Producer: CSIRO

Online Service: ACI Computer Services

Conditions: Monthly minimum to ACI required; fees vary depending on service selected.

Content: Contains citations to Australian scientific and technical literature, including the physical, biological, and applied sciences. Covers journals, research and technical reports, monographs, geological surveys, and conference proceedings that have been published in Australia. Topics covered include agriculture, astronomy and astrophysics, botany, chemistry, computer science, earth sciences, engineering, environment, general science, mathematics, microbiology, physics, and zoology. Corresponds to *Australian Science Index*.

Language: English

Coverage: Australia

Time Span: 1976 to 1983

Updating: Not updated

AVLINE (AudioVisuals onLINE)

Type: Reference (Referral)

Subject: Audiovisual Materials-Catalogs; Biomedicine; Education & Educational Institutions; Library Holdings-Catalogs

Producer: National Library of Medicine

Online Service: National Library of Medicine (NLM)

Content: Contains references to over 13,000 audiovisual and other non-print teaching materials cataloged by NLM. Primarily clinical in scope, covers items used for health sciences education and for continuing education of practitioners. Selected records added prior to July 31, 1981 may contain critical appraisals resulting from peer review that was conducted (until March 1982) by the Association of American Medical Colleges. Information for obtaining each item is also included.

Language: English
Coverage: Primarily U.S.
Time Span: All audiovisual materials cataloged by NLM since 1975
Updating: About 100 records a month

AZURTEL℠

Type: Source (Full Text)
Subject: News
Producer: SEMI
Online Service: SEMI
Content: Contains full text of general, regional, and local news items, sports articles, and Paris stock market reports from *Le Provencal* newspaper.
Language: French
Coverage: France (primarily Marseilles area)
Time Span: Current information
Updating: Daily

BEILSTEIN ONLINE℠

Type: Reference (Bibliographic); Source (Textual-Numeric)
Subject: Chemistry-Properties; Chemistry-Structure & Nomenclature
Producer: Beilstein Institute; Springer-Verlag
Online Service: DIALOG Information Services, Inc. (to be available in 1987)
Content: Contains data from the *Beilstein Handbook of Organic Chemistry, Series H to EIV* (1830-1959), the *Fifth Supplementary Series of the Beilstein Handbook of Organic Chemistry* (1960-1980), and material abstracted from primary literature since 1980. At present, structural and factual data for approximately 700,000 heterocyclic compounds are available in 2 files: a structural file conforming to the Beilstein Registry Connection Table in which users can search by stereochemical specifications, and a factual file containing as many as 400 data items for each compound, including physical properties, molecular formula, keywords (e.g., spectra), literature citations, comments about preparation, Chemical Abstracts Service Registry Number, and Beilstein Registry Number (Beilstein Prime Key).
NOTE: The entire Beilstein database, which covers approximately 3.5 million heterocyclic, acyclic, and isocyclic compounds, is expected to be online by 1991.
Language: English
Coverage: International
Time Span: 1830 to date

BHTD

Type: Reference (Bibliographic)
Subject: Biomedicine
Producer: Bureau of Hygiene and Tropical Diseases (BHTD)
Online Service: CAB International
Content: Contains about 27,000 citations, with abstracts, to the worldwide literature on tropical and communicable diseases. Covers bacterial, viral, fungal, and protozoal infections and helminthiases (e.g., Acquired Immune Deficiency Syndrome, Legionnaires' disease). Also covers occupational hygiene and medicine, toxicology, cancer epidemiology, medical entomology, and primary health care. Corresponds to *Tropical Diseases Bulletin* and *Abstracts on Hygiene and Communicable Diseases*.
Language: English, with titles in original languages

Coverage: International
Time Span: Mid-1982 to date
Updating: About 750 records a month

BIBLAT

Type: Reference (Bibliographic)
Subject: Science & Technology
Producer: Universidad Nacional Autonoma de Mexico, Centro de Informacion Cientifica y Humanistica
Online Service: Telesystemes-Questel
Content: Contains about 35,000 citations to articles on Latin America and articles with Latin American first authors, from over 6000 journals published outside Latin America. Covers a wide variety of subjects, including agriculture, astronomy, biomedicine, chemistry, earth sciences, economics, engineering, life sciences, mathematics, physics, psychology, and the social sciences and humanities. Corresponds to *Bibliografia Latinoamericana I* and *Bibliografia Latinoamericana II*.
Language: English
Coverage: Latin America
Time Span: 1977 to date
Updating: About 3000 records twice a year

BIBLIO-DATA

Type: Reference (Bibliographic)
Subject: Publishers & Distributors-Catalogs
Producer: Deutsche Bibliothek
Online Service: FIZ Karlsruhe; GID-SfT
Content: Contains more than 1.4 million references to books, periodicals, theses, maps, and audiovisual materials published in the Federal Republic of Germany. Also contains references to German-language materials published in other countries. Corresponds in part to *Deutsche Bibliographie*, the national bibliography of the Federal Republic of Germany.
Language: German
Coverage: Austria, Federal Republic of Germany, German Democratic Republic, and the German-speaking part of Switzerland
Time Span: 1966 to date
Updating: About 4000 records every 2 weeks

BIBLIOGRAFIA ESPECIALIZADA SOBRE MATERIAS ESPECIFICAS

Type: Reference (Bibliographic)
Subject: Science & Technology
Producer: Instituto Nacional de la Administracion Publica, Centro de Estudios y Documentacion; Universidad Complutense de Madrid, Facultad de Ciencias de la Informacion
Online Service: Ministerio de Cultura, Secretaria General Tecnica
Content: Contains over 59,000 citations to books and journal articles published in Spain on advertising, information science, and science and technology. Also covers worldwide literature on public administration.
Language: Spanish
Coverage: Public administration, international; other topics, Spain.
Time Span: Varies by topic, with earliest data from 1900
Updating: Annually

BIBLIOGRAPHIC INDEX℠

Type: Reference (Bibliographic)

Subject: Bibliographies

Producer: The H.W. Wilson Company

Online Service: WILSONLINE

Content: Contains citations to bibliographies with 50 or more citations that are published separately as books and pamphlets or that appear in other publications. Covers scholarly and general-interest topics. Sources include approximately 2600 periodicals. Corresponds to *Bibliographic Index*.

Language: English

Coverage: International

Time Span: November 1984 to date

Updating: Twice a week

BILLCAST℠ LEGISLATIVE FORECASTS

Type: Reference (Referral)

Subject: Legislative Tracking

Producer: George Mason University, Center for Study of Public Choice

Online Service: Mead Data Central, Inc. (BLCST) (as a Reference Service database) ; West Publishing Company

Conditions: Subscription to Mead Data Central required; subscription to West Publishing Company required.

Content: Contains information on public bills introduced in the U.S. Congress. Includes bill number, title, sponsor, date of introduction, and legislative stages (i.e., Senate or House of Representatives, committee or floor) . Provides statistical forecast of the chance of success for a bill to pass each of its legislative stages.

Language: English

Coverage: U.S.

Time Span: Current legislative session

Updating: Weekly

BILLTRAK℠

Type: Reference (Referral)

Subject: Legislative Tracking

Producer: Capitol Information Management, A division of Electronic Data Systems

Online Service: Capitol Information Management, A division of Electronic Data Systems

Conditions: Initiation fee and subscription required

Content: Contains legislative information on bills, resolutions, and constitutional amendments introduced in the California State Legislature. For each measure, includes full text and synopsis as well as such information as name of sponsor, title, date of introduction, code sections affected, amendments, fiscal impact, and appropriations. Also covers committee hearing schedules, legislator voting records, and campaign contributions. Users can search by author, subject, code section, and date (e.g., introduced, set for hearing, amended, enrolled, chaptered, vetoed) . Source of information is the California State Legislature.

Language: English

Coverage: U.S. (California)

Time Span: Current session

Updating: Daily

BioBusiness℠

Type: Reference (Bibliographic)

Subject: Biotechnology; Life Sciences

Producer: BioSciences Information Service (BIOSIS)

Online Service: DATA-STAR; DIALOG Information Services, Inc.; Mead Data Central, Inc. (BIOBUS) (as a Reference Service database)

Conditions: Subscription to Mead Data Central required

Content: Contains about 30,000 citations, with abstracts, to the worldwide periodical literature on business applications of biological and biomedical research. Covers agriculture and forestry, food technology, genetic engineering, pharmaceutical products, and other industries affected by biotechnological developments. Also covers patents in such areas as immunological testing, food processes, and fishing. For each patent record, includes inventor's name and address, patent title and number, patent classes, date granted, and assignee. Sources are BIOSIS PREVIEWS *(see)* and MANAGEMENT CONTENTS.

Language: English

Coverage: International

Time Span: 1985 to date

Updating: About 2500 records a month

BIODOC℠

Type: Reference (Referral)

Subject: Biographies

Producer: SERVI-TECH s.p.r.l.

Online Service: G.CAM Serveur

Content: Contains biographies of more than 40,000 contemporary European personalities. Includes name, occupation, place and date of birth, family, education, academic honors, languages spoken, career history, publications, memberships, hobbies and interests, private and business addresses, and business telephone number. Corresponds to *Who's Who in Europe* and *Nouveau Dictionnaire Biographique Europeen*.

Language: French

Coverage: Europe

Updating: Quarterly

BIOETHICSLINE

Type: Reference (Bibliographic)

Subject: Health Care; Sociology

Producer: Kennedy Institute of Ethics, Georgetown University

Online Service: National Library of Medicine (NLM)

Content: Contains citations to the literature on abortion, euthanasia, human experimentation, recombinant DNA research, and numerous other ethical, legal, and public policy issues of concern to the medical community. Relevant articles are drawn from 66 indexes, 74 journals, 4 online databases, and selected other reference tools. Corresponds to the annual *Bibliography of Bioethics*.

Language: English

Coverage: International

Time Span: 1973 to date

Updating: About 300 to 500 records every 2 months

BIOGRAFIAS

Type: Reference (Referral)

Subject: Biographies; Science & Technology

Producer: Ministerio de Cultura, Secretaria General Tecnica

Online Service: Ministerio de Cultura, Secretaria General Tecnica

Content: Contains over 13,000 biographies of Spanish painters, writers, musicians, and scientists. Also covers musicians and scientists from other countries. Biographies include lists of major works and bibliographies.

Language: Spanish

Coverage: Primarily Spain

Time Span: Painters born prior to 1900; writers born in the 20th century; musicians born prior to 1940; and scientists born prior to 1930.

Updating: Periodically, as new data become available

BIOGRAPHY INDEX℠

Type: Reference (Bibliographic)

Subject: Biographies

Producer: The H.W. Wilson Company

Online Service: WILSONLINE

Content: Contains references to biographies available in current books of biography, autobiography, critical studies, and biographical fiction; about 2600 periodicals; newspaper obituaries; bibliographies; and other printed material. Both current and historical persons are included. Information includes the name of the person, dates of birth (and death), profession, and the names and dates of biographical source publications that list the individual. Corresponds to *Biography Index*.

Language: English

Coverage: International

Time Span: July 1984 to date

Updating: Twice a week

BIOGRAPHY MASTER INDEX

Type: Reference (Bibliographic)

Subject: Biographies

Producer: Gale Research Company

Online Service: DIALOG Information Services, Inc.

Content: Provides master index to biographical information in over 500 source publications and 1150 publication editions, including English-language general and geographical Who's Who-type publications, major biographical dictionaries, handbooks, and directories. Both current and historical persons are included. Corresponds to *Biography and Genealogy Master Index*, 2nd edition and its annual updates. Information includes the name of the person, date of birth (and death), and the names and dates of biographical source publications that list the individual.

Language: English

Coverage: International

Time Span: Current information

Updating: Irregularly

BIOLOGICAL & AGRICULTURAL INDEX℠

Type: Reference (Bibliographic)

Subject: Agriculture; Aquatic Sciences; Environment; Food Sciences & Nutrition; Life Sciences; Veterinary Sciences

Producer: The H.W. Wilson Company

Online Service: WILSONLINE

Content: Contains about 72,000 citations to articles, book reviews, symposia and conference papers, and selected letters to the editor in over 200 English-language periodicals on biology and agriculture. Covers zoology, veterinary medicine, soil science, plant pathology, physiology, nutrition, microbiology, marine biology and limnology, genetics and cytology, horticulture, forestry, food science, entomology, environmental sciences, ecology, biology, biochemistry, botany, animal husbandry, agricultural research, agricultural engineering, agricultural economics, and agricultural chemicals. Corresponds to *Biological & Agricultural Index*.

Language: English

Coverage: International

Time Span: July 1983 to date

Updating: Twice a week; about 4500 articles a month.

BIOMEDICAL SAFETY AND STANDARDS

Type: Reference (Referral); Source (Full Text)

Subject: Conferences & Meetings; Health Care; Safety

Producer: Quest Publishing Company

Online Service: NewsNet, Inc.

Conditions: Monthly subscription to NewsNet required; differential charges for subscribers and non-subscribers to *Biomedical Safety and Standards*.

Content: Contains full text of *Biomedical Safety and Standards*, a newsletter on safety and accident-prevention issues related to medical equipment and devices. Covers equipment for medical diagnosis and treatment; Food and Drug Administration-defined "critical devices" (e.g., surgical implants and life-support systems); patient-care equipment (e.g., electric beds, gurneys, radiant infant warmers); and hospital safety problems. Includes new product announcements and reports of malfunctions, safety hazard notices, and product recalls, with information on model, serial, and lot numbers of recalled products or devices. Also covers legal and regulatory actions, including the development and promulgation of standards, and outcomes of lawsuits related to medical device safety. Provides notices of meetings and a calendar of events.

Language: English

Coverage: U.S. and Canada

Time Span: December 1985 to date

Updating: Every 2 weeks

BIOMEDICAL TECHNOLOGY INFO SERVICE

Type: Reference (Referral); Source (Full Text)

Subject: Biotechnology; Conferences & Meetings; Health Care

Producer: Quest Publishing Company

Online Service: NewsNet, Inc.

Conditions: Monthly subscription to NewsNet required; differential charges for subscribers and non-subscribers to *Biomedical Technology Information Service*.

Content: Contains full text of *Biomedical Technology Information Service*, a newsletter on technological, regulatory, and professional developments in the medical instrumentation industry. Covers advances in biomedical technology, including patient monitoring and diagnostics, computer applications, medical electronics, prosthetics, and surgical procedures. Also covers regulatory activity, legal developments, and relevant information sources, including government reports and manuals. A calendar of professional and business events is also provided.

Language: English

Coverage: U.S. and Canada

Time Span: December 1985 to date

Updating: Every 2 weeks

BIOSIS PREVIEWS®

Type: Reference (Bibliographic)

Subject: Agriculture; Aquatic Sciences; Bioengineering; Environment; Food Sciences & Nutrition; Life Sciences; Toxicology; Veterinary Sciences

Producer: BioSciences Information Service (BIOSIS)

Online Service: BRS; BRS After Dark; BRS/BRKTHRU; BRS/Colleague; Central Institute for Scientific and Technical Information; CISTI, Canadian Online Enquiry Service (CAN/OLE); Council of Scientific Research, Scientific Documentation Center; DATA-STAR; DIALOG Information Services, Inc.; DIMDI; ESA-IRS; The Japan Information Center of Science and Technology (JICST); Knowledge Index; Mead Data Central, Inc. (as a Reference Service database); STN International; University of Tsukuba

Conditions: CISTI accessible only in Canada; subscription to Mead Data Central required; access through University of Tsukuba limited to affiliates of the University of Japan.

Content: Contains about 4.7 million citations, with abstracts, to the worldwide literature on research in the life sciences: microbiology; plant and animal science; experimental medicine; agriculture; pharmacology; ecology; biochemistry; bioengineering; and biophysics. Covers original research reports, reviews of original research, history and philosophy of biology and biomedicine, and documentation and retrieval of biological information. Also covers patents in such areas as immunological testing, food processes, and fishing. For each patent record, includes inventor's name and address, patent title and number, patent classes, date granted, and assignee. Approximately 9000 periodicals, as well as books, patents, monographs, conference proceedings, research communications, and symposia are screened. Corresponds in coverage to *Biological Abstracts* (BA) and *Biological Abstracts/RRM* (BA/RRM) (formerly *BioResearch Index*).

NOTE: Abstracts from July 1976 to date (from BA on Tape) are available online through BRS, DATA-STAR, DIALOG, DIMDI, ESA-IRS, and STN International. Abstracts from 1978 to date are available through Central Institute for Scientific and Technical Information. Abstracts from 1982 to date are available through CISTI.

Language: English

Coverage: International

Time Span: CISTI, DIALOG, ESA-IRS, Knowledge Index, STN International, and Tsukuba, 1969 to date; BRS, BRS After Dark, BRS/BRKTHRU, BRS/Colleague, DATA-STAR, and DIMDI, 1970 to date; Central Institute for Scientific and Technical Information, 1978 to date; JICST, 1979 to date; Mead Data Central, 1980 to date; Council of Scientific Research, 1984 to date.

Updating: About 19,500 records from BA a month; about 19,500 records from BA/RRM a month.

BIOTECHNOLOGY

Type: Reference (Bibliographic)

Subject: Biotechnology

Producer: Derwent Publications Ltd.

Online Service: ORBIT Information Technologies Corporation

Conditions: Subscription to *Biotechnology Abstracts* required

Content: Contains citations, with abstracts and indexing, to the worldwide journal and patent literature on biotechnology, including microbiology, genetic manipulation, biochemical engineering, fermentation, down-stream processing, pharmaceuticals, industrial uses of micro-organisms, plant breeding, cell hybridization, and industrial waste management. Corresponds to *Biotechnology Abstracts*.

Language: English

Coverage: International

Time Span: June 1982 to date

Updating: About 1000 records a month

BIRD (Banque d'Information Robert Debre)

Type: Reference (Bibliographic)

Subject: Families & Family Life; Health Care

Producer: Centre International de l'Enfance

Online Service: G.CAM Serveur

Content: Contains approximately 70,000 citations, with abstracts, to the worldwide literature on the health of children and families. Covers nutrition, sanitation, health education, emotional health, and social factors relating to child and family health, particularly in developing countries. Sources include reports, theses, books, periodicals, government publications, and publications of international organizations (e.g., United Nations Educational, Scientific, and Cultural Organization, United Nations Childrens Fund, and Food and Agriculture Organization of the United Nations).

Language: English, French, and Spanish

Coverage: International

Time Span: 1980 to date

Updating: About 1000 records a month

BIRTH DEFECTS INFORMATION SYSTEM

Type: Source (Textual-Numeric, Full Text)

Subject: Biomedicine

Producer: Center for Birth Defects Information Services, Inc.

Online Service: BRS/Colleague (to be available in 1987)

Conditions: Authorization required for use of BDIS Diagnostic Assist and BDIS Unknowns Registry. Subscribers are not billed for use of the Unknowns Registry.

Content: Consists of 3 separate databases relating to birth defects.

BDIS Information Retrieval. Contains full text of articles on over 1000 birth defects and malformation syndromes, written for this database by 400 specialists from 22 countries. Each article summarizes clinical features of a condition, its natural history, complications, major diagnostic criteria, treatment, prognosis and, if known, mode of inheritance. Selected references are included.

BDIS Diagnostic Assist. A database system designed to assist in differential diagnosis of complex birth defect syndromes, for use by qualified professionals in human genetics. Contains data on over 600 of the more complex birth defects and malformation syndromes. On the basis of clinical case descriptions input by the user, along with user's answers to pertinent questions, the system provides a list of the best possible matches from the syndromes contained in the database.

BDIS Unknowns Registry. A database containing clinical, demographic, and epidemiological information on cases that have been processed through the Diagnostic Assist facility for which there is no clear diagnosis. The database is analyzed regularly for cases that have strong similarities, and users who registered cases are notified of any matches.

A directory of about 150 voluntary organizations in medical genetics and maternal and child health will be added.

Language: English

Coverage: International

Time Span: Current information
Updating: Periodically, as new data become available

BNA EXECUTIVE DAY
Type: Source (Full Text)
Subject: Health Care
Producer: The Bureau of National Affairs, Inc. (BNA)
Online Service: Dialcom, Inc.; Executive Telecom System, Inc., Human Resource Information Network; NewsNet, Inc.
Conditions: Annual subscription to Executive Telecom System required; monthly subscription to NewsNet required.
Content: Consists of 9 files of business news and information.
BNA AGRIBUSINESS REPORT. Contains summaries of U.S. Department of Agriculture activities. Updated daily.
DAILY TAX ALERT. Contains news of developments in individual and corporate taxation.
EXECUTIVE DIGEST. Contains news of financial and regulatory developments affecting corporate business. Updated daily.
HEALTHLINE. Contains information on general health care issues, including drug abuse, epidemics, illness prevention, and health-related legislative and regulatory activity. Updated weekly.
LABORLINE. Covers labor and employee relations, including pension benefits, contract negotiations, arbitration awards, and relevant decisions of federal and state courts and of the National Labor Relations Review Board. Updated daily.
LAWLINE. Contains judicial decisions and developments of general interest. Covers criminal law, civil proceedings (e.g., child custody, divorce), and client-attorney privilege. Updated weekly.
MANAGEMENT TRENDS. Contains information on trends and developments in employer-employee relations. Covers compensation, fringe benefits, workplace safety, and employee assistance. Updated weekly.
MONEYLINE. Covers general financial topics (e.g., credit regulations, consumer protection, child support, alimony). Updated weekly.
WOMEN'S PORTFOLIO. Contains information on labor, financial, legal, and health issues of interest to women. Covers employment practices (e.g., job training and sharing, flex time), Equal Employment Opportunity Commission (EEOC) and court decisions, divorce law, saving and spending patterns, pay equity, and financial planning. Updated weekly.
Language: English
Coverage: U.S.
Time Span: Current week
Updating: Varies by file *(see Content)*

BOOK REVIEW DIGEST℠
Type: Reference (Bibliographic)
Subject: General Interest
Producer: The H.W. Wilson Company
Online Service: WILSONLINE
Content: Contains citations, each with excerpts of reviews, to more than 32,500 current reviews of English-language books. Each citation also contains references to the reviews. Covers popular and scholarly works of fiction and non-fiction works, as well as juvenile literature. Sources include over 80 periodicals published in Canada, the U.K., and the U.S. in the humanities, social sciences, and general science. Corresponds to *Book Review Digest*.
Language: English

Coverage: Canada, U.K., and U.S.
Time Span: April 1983 to date
Updating: Twice a week; about 1500 books a month.

BOOKNET
Type: Reference (Referral)
Subject: Publishers & Distributors-Catalogs
Producer: ACI Computer Services
Online Service: ACI Computer Services
Conditions: Monthly minimum to ACI required; fees vary depending on service selected.
Content: Contains bibliographic and price information for all English-language books in print in Australia, New Zealand, U.K., and U.S. including paperback books and books on cassette. Sources of data include *Books in Print, British Books in Print, Australian Books in Print,* and *New Zealand Books in Print.* Users can place book orders online.
Language: English
Coverage: International
Time Span: Current information

BOOKS IN PRINT
Type: Reference (Bibliographic)
Subject: Publishers & Distributors-Catalogs
Producer: R.R. Bowker Company
Online Service: BRS; BRS After Dark; BRS/BRKTHRU; BRS/Colleague; DIALOG Information Services, Inc.; Knowledge Index; TECH DATA
Content: Contains citations to over one million books currently in print or declared out of print (from July 1979 to date), and soon-to-be-published titles from more than 18,000 publishers. Includes scholarly, popular, adult, juvenile, reprint, and other books on all subjects published by U.S. publishers or exclusively distributed in the U.S. and available to the trade or general public for single- or multiple-copy purchases. Such items as government publications, Bibles, free books, and subscription-only titles are excluded. Corresponds to *Books in Print, Forthcoming Books in Print, Books in Print Supplement,* and data that appear in other Bowker bibliographies (e.g., *Scientific and Technical Books in Print, Medical Books in Print, Business and Economics Books in Print, Paperbound Books in Print*). Subject classification scheme utilizes over 80,000 Library of Congress subject headings as well as Sears headings and *Paperbound Books in Print* headings.
Language: English
Coverage: U.S.
Time Span: 1900 to date
Updating: About 5500 records a month

BOOKSINFO
Type: Reference (Bibliographic)
Subject: Publishers & Distributors-Catalogs
Producer: Brodart Co.
Online Service: BRS; BRS/BRKTHRU; BRS/Colleague; TECH DATA
Content: Contains citations, prices, status, International Standard Book Number (ISBN), Library of Congress (LC) number, and LC subject headings on about 950,000 English-language books currently in print. Covers monographs from 10,000 U.S. publishers, including academic and small publishers, and 200 foreign presses. Juvenile books, textbooks, monographs, and series are included.

Language: English
Coverage: Primarily U.S.
Time Span: 1950 to date
Updating: About 2000 records a month

BOSTON CitiNet℠

Type: Reference (Referral); Source (Full Text)
Subject: General Interest; Government-U.S. State; News
Producer: Applied Videotex Systems
Online Service: Applied Videotex Systems
Conditions: There is no charge for this service.
Content: Contains information of interest in New England, particularly in the Boston area. Includes weather, classified advertisements, employment and investment opportunities, museum calendar, hotel guide, television program schedules, World Trade Center (Boston) information and upcoming events, lottery information, movie schedules and reviews, and federal, state, and local news.
RealNet. Contains commercial and residential listings of properties for sale or rent, current mortgage rates, references to service providers (e.g., plumbers, contractors, inspectors), community information (e.g., on parks, taxes, schools), and classified advertisements. Includes the bulletin board of the Boston Computer Society, Real Estate Special Interest Group.
SkiData. Contains information on snow conditions, weather, lodgings, and facilities at New England ski resorts. Also includes advice on selecting ski equipment. Source of data is the New England Ski Areas Council. Updated twice a day during the ski season.
The State House News Service. Provides information on topics under discussion in Massachusetts courts. Produced by the State House News Service. Covers December 1984 to date. Updated daily.
Also contains a variety of bulletin boards, an electronic mail service, and an online shopping service.
Language: English
Coverage: U.S. (New England, with emphasis on the Boston area)
Time Span: Current information
Updating: Periodically, as new data become available

THE BOSTON GLOBE

Type: Source (Full Text)
Subject: News
Producer: Globe Newspaper Company
Online Service: VU/TEXT Information Services, Inc.
Conditions: Subscription to VU/TEXT required
Content: Contains full text of news items and feature stories from *The Boston Globe* (Massachusetts) newspaper. Also includes the special sections on science, food, entertainment, and sports.
Language: English
Coverage: U.S. (primarily New England area)
Time Span: 1980 to date
Updating: Daily

BREV

Type: Reference (Bibliographic)
Subject: Patents
Producer: Belgian Ministry of Economic Affairs, DHNE-SPIC
Online Service: BELINDIS

Content: Contains citations, with abstracts (since 1984), to Belgian patents and other European patents valid in Belgium. Each record includes International Patent Classification code. Corresponds to *Recueil/Verzameling*. Sources include the European Patent Office and the Belgian Ministry of Economic Affairs.
Language: Dutch, English, and French
Coverage: Belgium
Time Span: 1973 to date
Updating: Periodically, as new data become available

BRITISH EXPERTISE IN SCIENCE AND TECHNOLOGY (BEST)

Type: Reference (Referral)
Subject: Biographies; Science & Technology
Producer: Longman Cartermill Limited
Online Service: Longman Cartermill Limited
Conditions: Annual subscription required
Content: Contains information on about 14,000 sources of expertise, research, and services available in over 250 scientific and technical areas in the U.K. 'Expertise' records on individual researchers include name and address, qualifications, professional memberships, positions held, descriptions of completed research and current grants, and relevant publications and patents. 'Service' records on academic and government institutions (e.g., universities, polytechnics, research councils) include available services and facilities, equipment, number of personnel, and contact information.
Language: English
Coverage: U.K.
Time Span: Current information
Updating: Monthly

BRITISH MEDICAL ASSOCIATION'S PRESS CUTTINGS

Type: Reference (Bibliographic)
Subject: Biomedicine; News
Producer: British Medical Association
Online Service: DATA-STAR
Content: Contains summaries of news items of interest to the medical profession. Sources of information include national and regional newspapers, as well as television and radio stations.
Language: English
Coverage: Primarily U.K.
Time Span: 1984 to date
Updating: About 20 records a day

BRS/FILE

Type: Reference (Referral)
Subject: Information Systems & Services-Directories
Producer: BRS
Online Service: BRS; BRS/BRKTHRU
Content: Contains descriptions and cost information for all databases publicly available through BRS.
Language: English
Time Span: Current information
Updating: Monthly

BSI STANDARDLINE

Type: Reference (Bibliographic)
Subject: Standards & Specifications
Producer: British Standards Institution (BSI)
Online Service: Pergamon InfoLine
Content: Contains citations, with abstracts, to approximately 10,000 standards promulgated by the British Standards Institution (BSI). Includes the BSI general, automobile, marine, and aerospace standards, codes of practice, drafts under development, and drafts for public comment (DPC). Covers such areas as building and construction materials, electronics testing, and equipment safety and reliability. BSIH, a historical file, contains references to standards that have lapsed or have been withdrawn. Corresponds in part to *BSI Catalogue*.
Language: English
Coverage: U.K.
Time Span: Current information; BSIH, standards withdrawn or lapsed since November 1985, with some older withdrawn items; DPC, 1986 to date.
Updating: Monthly

BULLETIN BOARD SYSTEMS

Type: Reference (Referral); Source (Full Text)
Subject: Information Systems & Services; Information Systems & Services-Directories
Producer: Meckler Publishing Co.
Online Service: NewsNet, Inc.
Conditions: Monthly subscription to NewsNet required; differential charges for subscribers and non-subscribers to *Bulletin Board Systems*.
Content: Contains full text of *Bulletin Board Systems*, a newsletter covering news on uses, users, and legal issues of interest to electronic bulletin board operators and users. Also provides a listing of approximately 1000 available services and profiles of selected bulletin boards, including hours of operation, telephone number, and notes on special features.
Language: English
Coverage: International
Time Span: October 1983 to date
Updating: Monthly

CA SEARCH®

Type: Reference (Bibliographic)
Subject: Chemistry
Producer: Chemical Abstracts Service (CAS)
Online Service: BRS; BRS After Dark; BRS/BRKTHRU; BRS/Colleague; CISTI, Canadian Online Enquiry Service (CAN/OLE) (CAS); DATA-STAR (CHEM); DIALOG Information Services, Inc. (CA SEARCH); ESA-IRS (CHEMABS); The Japan Information Center of Science and Technology (JICST) (CA SEARCH); ORBIT Information Technologies Corporation (CAS); STN International (CA FILE); TECH DATA; Telesystemes-Questel (CAS)
Conditions: CISTI accessible only in Canada
Content: Contains citations to the worldwide literature in chemistry: organic, analytical, physical, applied, macromolecular, biochemical, and chemical engineering. Covers journal articles, monographs, conference proceedings, technical reports, dissertations, and patents. Contains bibliographic information and keyword index entries from the printed *Chemical Abstracts* and CAS-assigned subject terms and Registry Numbers.
NOTE: Through DIALOG, Telesystemes-Questel, ORBIT, and

STN, users can retrieve systematic names by transferring retrieved Registry Numbers to the REGISTRY NOMENCLATURE AND STRUCTURE SERVICE *(see)*. Backfiles of citations only are available through BRS (for 1970-1976) and CISTI (for July 1973-1976) under the name CA CONDENSATES.
NOTE: On STN International, contains some abstracts from 1967 to mid-1975 and all abstracts from mid-1975 to date.
Language: English
Coverage: International
Time Span: DATA-STAR, DIALOG, ESA-IRS, ORBIT, STN International, and Telesystemes-Questel, 1967 to date; BRS, BRS After Dark, BRS/BRKTHRU, BRS/Colleague, CISTI, and JICST, 1977 to date.
Updating: BRS, BRS After Dark, BRS/BRKTHRU, BRS/Colleague, and CISTI, about 40,000 records a month; DATA-STAR, DIALOG, ESA-IRS, JICST, ORBIT, STN International, and Telesystemes-Questel, about 19,000 records every 2 weeks.

CAB ABSTRACTS

Type: Reference (Bibliographic)
Subject: Agriculture; Food Sciences & Nutrition; Veterinary Sciences
Producer: CAB International
Online Service: BRS (CABA); BRS After Dark (CABA); BRS/BRKTHRU (CABA); BRS/Colleague (CABA); CAB International; CISTI, Canadian Online Enquiry Service (CAN/OLE); DIALOG Information Services, Inc.; DIMDI; ESA-IRS; The Japan Information Center of Science and Technology (JICST); University of Tsukuba
Conditions: CISTI accessible only in Canada; access through University of Tsukuba limited to affiliates of the University of Japan.
Content: Contains about 2 million citations, with abstracts, to the worldwide literature in the agricultural sciences and related areas of applied biology. Corresponds to the 27 main journals and 20 specialized journals published by CAB International. Subjects covered include animal breeding, engineering, bees, dairy science, crops, forestry, helminthology, horticulture, veterinary medicine, plant breeding, protozoology, applied entomology, mycology, plant pathology, rural development and sociology, soils and fertilizers, weeds, agricultural economics, leisure and recreation, tourism, human and animal nutrition, and arid lands (1980 to 1982). Coverage of veterinary medicine begins in 1972.
NOTE: On CISTI, DIALOG, DIMDI, and ESA-IRS, also contains citations from ANIMAL DISEASE OCCURRENCE *(see)*.
NOTE: On all BRS services, 2 subsets are available separately: on agricultural economics and rural development and sociology (ECON) and on leisure, recreation, and tourism (TOUR).
Language: English
Coverage: International
Time Span: CISTI, DIALOG, and DIMDI, 1972 to date; ESA-IRS and Tsukuba, 1973 to date; BRS, BRS After Dark, BRS/BRKTHRU, and BRS/Colleague, 1980 to date; JICST, 1981 to date; CAB, 1984 to date.
Updating: About 12,000 records a month

CALL-APPLE

Type: Reference (Referral); Source (Software)
Subject: Computers & Software
Producer: Apple Pugetsound Program Library Exchange (A.P.P.L.E.)

Online Service: THE SOURCE

Conditions: Available to members of A.P.P.L.E. only; monthly minimum of $10 to THE SOURCE required, with $9 credited toward online usage charges.

Content: A shopping service for publications and products for Apple and Apple-compatible computers. Includes software and hardware, e.g., disk drives, modems, fans, disk-controller cards, and printers. Users can order products online and can download computer programs that were listed in the 6 most recent issues of *Call-A.P.P.L.E.* magazine.

Language: English

Time Span: Current information

Updating: At least twice a month

CANADIAN BUSINESS AND CURRENT AFFAIRS

Type: Reference (Bibliographic)

Subject: News

Producer: Micromedia Limited

Online Service: CISTI, Canadian Online Enquiry Service (CAN/OLE); DIALOG Information Services, Inc.; IST-Informatheque Inc.

Conditions: CISTI accessible only in Canada; accessible through IST-Informatheque only in Canada.

Content: Contains over 475,000 citations to articles in 175 English-language business periodicals, 200 popular periodicals, and 10 daily newspapers published in Canada. Articles cover product, company, and industry information; national, provincial, and local news; editorials and selected letters to the editor; government activities; labor news; crime; sports; obituaries; biographies; reviews; art; children's literature; cooking; education; health; history; hobbies; music; nature; recreation; science; social issues; and travel. Corresponds to *Canadian News Index (see CNI)*, *Canadian Business Index*, and *Canadian Magazine Index (see CMI)*.

Language: English

Coverage: Canada

Time Span: DIALOG, July 1980 to date; CISTI and IST-Informatheque, 1982 to date.

Updating: About 13,000 records a month

CANADIAN PRESS NEWSTEX™

Type: Source (Full Text)

Subject: News

Producer: The Canadian Press (CP)

Online Service: QL Systems Limited

Content: Contains the full text of over 2 million English-language news stories from the CP news wire service. Includes stories from CP bureaus in Canada, CP reporters abroad, and local stories from CP's 100 member newspapers. Broadcast News Limited, which serves 450 private radio and television broadcasters, contributes to coverage of Canada. International stories are also obtained from The Associated Press, Reuters, and Agence France Presse.

Language: English

Coverage: International

Time Span: 1981 to date

Updating: About 500 items a day

CANCERLIT™

Type: Reference (Bibliographic)

Subject: Biomedicine

Producer: U.S. National Institutes of Health (NIH), National Cancer Institute, International Cancer Research Data Bank

Online Service: DATA-STAR; DIALOG Information Services, Inc.; DIMDI; The Japan Information Center of Science and Technology (JICST); MIC-KIBIC; National Library of Medicine (NLM); University of Tsukuba

Conditions: Access through University of Tsukuba limited to affiliates of the University of Japan

Content: Contains more than 500,000 citations, with abstracts, to the worldwide literature on oncological epidemiology, pathology, treatment, and research. Prior to 1976, the database corresponded to *Cancer Therapy Abstracts* from 1967, and *Carcinogenesis Abstracts*, from 1963. Since then, the database has covered the primary literature directly, including articles selected from over 3500 journals pertaining to cancer and carcinogens, monographs, technical reports, conference proceedings, and theses.

Language: English

Coverage: International

Time Span: Most services, 1963 to date; Tsukuba, 1974 to date.

Updating: About 5000 records a month

CANCERNET (International Database on Oncology)

Type: Reference (Bibliographic)

Subject: Biomedicine

Producer: CANCERNET/Centre National de la Recherche Scientifique (CNRS)

Online Service: University of Tsukuba

Content: Contains citations, with abstracts, to literature on oncology. Covers clinical and experimental carcinology, epidemiology, public health, and fundamental sciences (e.g., immunology, virology). Corresponds to *Cancer/Oncology, Bulletin Signaletique 251*.

Language: English and French

Coverage: International

Time Span: 1968 to 1984; abstracts from some articles, from 1981 to 1984.

Updating: Not updated; *see PASCAL: ONCOLOGY for current information (1985 to date).*

CANCERPROJ (Cancer Research Projects)

Type: Reference (Referral)

Subject: Biomedicine; Research in Progress

Producer: Current Cancer Research Project Analysis Center (CCRESPAC) for the U.S. National Institutes of Health (NIH), National Cancer Institute, International Cancer Research Data Bank

Online Service: DIMDI; National Library of Medicine (NLM); University of Tsukuba

Conditions: Access through University of Tsukuba limited to affiliates of the University of Japan

Content: Contains about 10,000 summaries of ongoing and recently completed cancer research projects. Includes U.S. federal and non-federal, and non-U.S. supported projects that are solicited through various international collaborating organizations by CCRESPAC for the ICRDB.

Language: English
Coverage: International
Time Span: National Library of Medicine and University of Tsukuba, 1984 to date; DIMDI, 1985 to date.
Updating: Quarterly

CANPLAINS DATA BASE

Type: Reference (Referral)
Subject: Research in Progress
Producer: Canadian Plains Research Center, University of Regina
Online Service: CISTI, Canadian Online Enquiry Service (CAN/OLE)
Conditions: CISTI accessible only in Canada
Content: Contains over 24,000 references to current, recently completed, published and unpublished research, including master and doctoral theses, relevant to the 3 Canadian prairie provinces (Manitoba, Saskatchewan, and Alberta). Covers natural sciences, social sciences, and the humanities, with emphasis on the environment, the land, the people, and resources of the region.
Language: English
Coverage: Canada
Time Span: 1976 to date
Updating: About 1000 new records a quarter; records of current research are updated approximately every 2 years on a revolving basis throughout the year.

CAOLD FILE

Type: Reference (Referral)
Subject: Chemistry
Producer: Chemical Abstracts Service (CAS)
Online Service: STN International
Content: Contains CAS Registry Numbers for documents abstracted in *Chemical Abstracts* prior to 1967 *(see CA SEARCH)* that cite substances registered in the REGISTRY FILE *(see REGISTRY NOMENCLATURE AND STRUCTURE SERVICE)*. Corresponds in part to the *6th* and *7th Collective Formula Index*.
Coverage: International
Time Span: 1962 to 1966
Updating: Weekly, with substances from previous editions of the *Index*

CASSI® (Chemical Abstracts Service Source Index)

Type: Reference (Bibliographic, Referral)
Subject: Publishers & Distributors-Catalogs; Chemistry
Producer: Chemical Abstracts Service (CAS)
Online Service: ORBIT Information Technologies Corporation
Content: Contains bibliographic information on about 60,000 serial and non-serial publications held by over 350 libraries worldwide, and includes, for each title, National Union Catalog (NUC) codes to indicate libraries that have copies of the publication and codes for document suppliers from whom individual papers are available. Covers scientific and technical literature relevant to chemistry, chemical engineering, and the chemical sciences. Includes bibliographic information for titles cited in *Chemical Abstracts* since 1907, titles published in Beilstein's *Handbuch der Organischen Chemie* from its inception to 1965, and titles covering the pure and theoretical chemical literature

from 1830 to 1940 from *Chemisches Zentralblatt*. Corresponds to *Chemical Abstracts Service Source Index* and its quarterly supplements.
NOTE: A companion file, NUC/CODES, provides name and address information for each holding library or supplier source listed by NUC code in CASSI.
Language: English
Coverage: International
Time Span: Primarily 1900 to date, with earliest data from the 1700s
Updating: Quarterly

CATLINE™ (CATalog onLINE)

Type: Reference (Bibliographic)
Subject: Biomedicine; Library Holdings-Catalogs
Producer: National Library of Medicine
Online Service: Australian Medline Network; National Library of Medicine (NLM)
Content: Contains citations to over 590,000 monographs and serials in the NLM collection.
Language: English
Coverage: International
Time Span: 1801 to date
Updating: About 300 records a week

CENSO DE BIBLIOTECAS

Type: Reference (Referral)
Subject: Information Systems & Services-Directories
Producer: Ministerio de Cultura, Biblioteca Nacional
Online Service: Ministerio de Cultura, Secretaria General Tecnica
Content: Contains references to over 4000 public libraries in Spain. Descriptions include address and telephone number, type of library, date established, number of works by type (e.g., books, periodicals, encyclopedias, dictionaries), hours of service, conditions of access, other services available (e.g., photocopying), and interlibrary connections.
Language: Spanish
Coverage: Spain
Time Span: Current information
Updating: Annually

CENTERS FOR DISEASE CONTROL INFORMATION SERVICE

Type: Reference (Referral); Source (Full Text)
Subject: Biomedicine; Conferences & Meetings
Producer: American Medical Association (AMA); U.S. Department of Health and Human Services, Public Health Service, Centers for Disease Control (CDC)
Online Service: AMA/NET
Conditions: Subscription fee of $50 to AMA/NET required
Content: Contains news and information on disease and health care in the U.S.
AIDS INFORMATION SERVICE. Contains definitions, statistics, and facts on Acquired Immune Deficiency Syndrome (AIDS). Includes references to sources of additional information and notices of upcoming conferences and meetings.
CDC INFO UPDATE. Provides titles of publications available from CDC, announcements of upcoming symposia, and descriptions of current research.
CONTINUING EDUCATION PROGRAMS. Contains announcements of training and seminars for physicians and other health professionals offered or sponsored by CDC.
MORBIDITY & MORTALITY WEEKLY REPORT. *(see)*

Language: English
Coverage: U.S.
Time Span: Current information
Updating: Weekly

CESARS (Chemical Evaluation Search and Retrieval System)

Type: Source (Textual-Numeric)
Subject: Chemistry-Properties; Toxicology
Producer: State of Michigan, Department of Natural Resources, Office of Materials Control
Online Service: Chemical Information Systems, Inc., a subsidiary of Fein-Marquart Associates (CIS)
Conditions: Annual subscription fee of $300 to CIS required but fee is waived for educational institutions and non-profit public libraries worldwide
Content: Contains toxicological data on approximately 195 chemicals. Each record, representing one chemical, may provide up to 120 data items, covering physical and chemical properties, toxicity, carcinogenicity, mutagenicity, teratogenicity, and, when available, environmental fate. Data are obtained from literature and references to source documents are provided.
Language: English
Coverage: International, with most data extracted from English-language research papers
Time Span: 1962 to date
Updating: Periodically, as new data become available

THE CHARLOTTE OBSERVER

Type: Source (Full Text)
Subject: News
Producer: Knight Publishing Co.
Online Service: VU/TEXT Information Services, Inc.
Conditions: Subscription to VU/TEXT required
Content: Contains full text of news items and feature articles from *The Charlotte Observer* (North Carolina) newspaper. Regional coverage emphasizes the banking, textile, and transportation industries.
Language: English
Coverage: U.S. (primarily Charlotte, North Carolina area)
Time Span: July 1985 to date
Updating: Daily

CHEMICAL BUSINESS NEWSBASE

Type: Reference (Bibliographic)
Subject: News
Producer: The Royal Society of Chemistry
Online Service: DATA-STAR; DIALOG Information Services, Inc.; Finsbury Data Services Ltd.; Pergamon InfoLine
Content: Contains approximately 30,000 citations, with abstracts, to news and literature on trends and developments in the European chemical industry and in the related agricultural, food processing, electronics, pharmaceutical, and textile industries. Also covers major developments in the U.S., Japan, and other world areas. Includes such topics as company takeovers and mergers; plant commissioning, upgrading, and capacity reports; and chemical costs, production, supplies, and demand. Sources include periodicals, annual reports and other company literature, press releases, government reports, and brokerage firm and market research reports. Corresponds to 14 *Chemical Business Bulletins*, each providing news of specific areas (e.g., pharmaceuticals, agrochemicals).

Language: English, with titles also in original languages
Coverage: International, with emphasis on Western Europe
Time Span: DIALOG, October 1984 to date; DATA-STAR, EDS, and Pergamon InfoLine, 1985 to date.
Updating: About 1000 records a week

CHEMICAL CARCINOGENESIS RESEARCH INFORMATION SYSTEM

Type: Reference (Bibliographic); Source (Textual-Numeric)
Subject: Toxicology
Producer: U.S. National Institutes of Health (NIH)
Online Service: Chemical Information Systems, Inc., a subsidiary of Fein-Marquart Associates (CIS); Information Consultants, Inc. (ICI) (as part of The Integrated Chemical Information System)
Conditions: Annual subscription fee of $300 to CIS required but fee is waived for educational institutions and non-profit public libraries worldwide; differential charges for subscribers and non-subscribers to ICI.
Content: Contains bibliographic references and data extracted from the worldwide literature on test conditions and results of the carcinogenicity, co-carcinogenicity, mutagenicity, and tumor promotion of chemical substances. Both positive and negative results are reported. Sources of data include environmental surveys, NIH-sponsored studies, monographs of the International Agency for Research in Cancer, and international journals on cancer research.
NOTE: On CIS, the database contains 1269 records on 1088 chemical substances.
Language: English
Coverage: International
Time Span: 1971 to date
Updating: Twice a year, with data added on about 100 chemicals each update

CHEMICAL EXPOSURE

Type: Reference (Bibliographic); Source (Textual-Numeric)
Subject: Toxicology
Producer: Science Applications International Corporation, Health and Environmental Information
Online Service: DIALOG Information Services, Inc. (CHEMICAL EXPOSURE)
Content: Contains over 11,000 citations to the worldwide literature on over 1000 chemicals that have been identified in human and animal biological media (e.g., tissues, body fluids) and reported effects of drugs (through 1984 only), metals, pesticides, and other substances on the body. Each record covers information about one chemical on a particular tissue; there may be more than one record for articles on multiple chemicals and/or multiple tissues. Each record includes bibliographic information, Chemical Abstracts Service systematic name and Registry Number, chemical properties, formulas, synonyms, tissue levels measured, analytical method used, number and sex of cases, demographic information on sources of samples, health effects, geographic location, and animal studied. Corresponds to *Chemicals Identified in Human Biological Media* and *Chemicals Identified in Feral and Food Animals*.
Language: English
Coverage: International
Time Span: 1974 to date
Updating: About 2000 records a year

CHEMICAL HAZARDS IN INDUSTRY

Type: Reference (Bibliographic)

Subject: Occupational Safety & Health

Producer: The Royal Society of Chemistry

Online Service: DATA-STAR; Pergamon InfoLine

Content: Contains over 5000 citations, with abstracts, to the worldwide literature on hazards and safe working practices in the chemical and related industries. Covers accident prevention, chemical engineering, epidemiology, environmental health, hazardous waste management, legislation (primarily U.K.), safety, and toxicology. Sources include more than 200 journals, as well as reports, monographs, booklets, and films.

Language: English

Coverage: International

Time Span: 1984 to date

Updating: Monthly; about 2500 records a year.

CHEMICAL HAZARDS RESPONSE INFORMATION SYSTEM (CHRIS)

Type: Source (Textual-Numeric)

Subject: Chemistry-Properties; Environment

Producer: U.S. Coast Guard

Online Service: Chemical Information Systems, Inc., a subsidiary of Fein-Marquart Associates (CIS)

Conditions: Annual subscription fee of $300 to CIS required but fee is waived for educational institutions and non-profit public libraries worldwide

Content: Contains information on about 1000 chemical substances for use in spill situations. Includes chemical names and synonyms, molecular formula, biological and fire hazard potential, and chemical and physical properties.

Language: English

Coverage: U.S.

Time Span: Current information

Updating: Periodically, as new data become available

CHEMICAL INDUSTRY NOTES®

Type: Reference (Bibliographic)

Subject: News

Producer: Chemical Abstracts Service (CAS)

Online Service: DATA-STAR (CHEMICAL INDUSTRY NOTES); DIALOG Information Services, Inc. (CHEMICAL INDUSTRY NOTES); ORBIT Information Technologies Corporation (CIN)

Content: Contains citations, with abstracts, to the worldwide business literature on chemical processing in the chemical, pharmaceutical, petroleum, paper and pulp, and agriculture industries. Topics covered include production, pricing, sales, facilities, products, processes, corporate and government activities, and people. Corresponds to *Chemical Industry Notes*.

Language: English

Coverage: International

Time Span: December 1974 to date

Updating: DIALOG, about 2000 records every 2 weeks; DATA-STAR and ORBIT, about 1000 records a week.

CHEMICAL JOURNALS ONLINE (CJO)

Type: Source (Full Text)

Subject: Chemistry

Producer: American Chemical Society (ACS) (ACS Journals Online); John Wiley & Sons, Inc. (Wiley Polymer Journals Online)

Online Service: STN International

Content: Consists of 2 files of information on chemistry and polymer science.

ACS Journals Online. Contains full text of over 45,000 articles (including captions, references, and footnotes, but excluding illustrations) from 19 primary journals published by the American Chemical Society. Covers *Accounts of Chemical Research, Analytical Chemistry* (research papers only), *Biochemistry, Chemical Reviews, Environmental Science & Technology* (research papers only), *I&EC Fundamentals, I&EC Process Design and Development, I&EC Product Research and Development, Inorganic Chemistry, Journal of Agricultural and Food Chemistry, Journal of the American Chemical Society, Journal of Chemical and Engineering Data, Journal of Chemical Information and Computer Sciences, Journal of Medicinal Chemistry, Journal of Organic Chemistry, Journal of Physical Chemistry, Langmuir, Macromolecules,* and *Organometallics.* Registry Numbers, assigned by Chemical Abstracts Service, are included for the *Journal of the American Chemical Society, Journal of Organic Chemistry, Inorganic Chemistry,* and *Organometallics.*

Wiley Polymer Journals Online. Contains full text of over 3000 articles (including captions, references, and footnotes, but excluding illustrations) from 3 journals published by John Wiley & Sons, Inc. Covers the *Journal of Applied Polymer Science,* the *Journal of Polymer Science* (consisting of *Polymer Chemistry, Polymer Letters,* and *Polymer Physics*), and *Biopolymers.* To be available in 1987.

Language: English

Coverage: International

Time Span: ACS journals, 1982 to date (*Lanqmuir,* 1985 to date); Wiley journals, 1984 to date.

Updating: ACS journals, about 350 articles every 2 weeks; Wiley journals, about 150 articles a month.

CHEMICAL REGULATION REPORTER

Type: Source (Full Text)

Subject: Environment

Producer: The Bureau of National Affairs, Inc. (BNA)

Online Service: Mead Data Central, Inc. (as part of LEXIS ENERGY LIBRARY and LEXIS ENVIRONMENTAL LIBRARY); West Publishing Company (to be available in 1987)

Conditions: Subscription to Mead Data Central required; subscription to West Publishing Company required.

Content: Contains full text of the current developments section of *Chemical Regulation Reporter,* covering legislative, regulatory, and industry activities related to control of chemicals in the air, water, land, and workplace. Includes control of pesticides, chemical testing, transportation of hazardous materials, waste disposal, and recordkeeping. Primary source is the U.S. Environmental Protection Agency.

Language: English

Coverage: U.S.

Time Span: 1982 to date

Updating: Weekly

CHEMICAL REGULATIONS AND GUIDELINES SYSTEM

Type: Reference (Bibliographic)

Subject: Environment; Legislative Tracking

Producer: CRC Systems, Inc. (under contract to the U.S. Environmental Protection Agency)

Online Service: DIALOG Information Services, Inc.

Content: Contains citations, with abstracts, to U.S. government statutes, promulgated regulations, and federal guidelines, standards, and support documents on chemical substances. Covers the *U.S. Code* and its supplements, *Statutes at Large, Code of Federal Regulations, Federal Register*, and other materials obtained directly from federal agencies. Covers federal, state, and international information, including tariffs, health and safety regulations, registration requirements, and any other restrictions placed on chemical substances. Each record includes document type and status; promulgation and effective dates; geographic area covered; promulgating agency and office; source citation; and Chemical Abstracts Service Registry Number for the cited substances. Also includes chemical role tags that indicate the context in which the substances appear in the document. Links are made between statutes and regulations promulgated under the statutes, and with support documents generated prior to the promulgation of a regulation.

Language: English

Coverage: Primarily U.S.

Time Span: All regulatory information in effect through June 1982

Updating: Not updated

CHEMICAL RIGHT-TO-KNOW REQUIREMENTS

Type: Source (Full Text)

Subject: Legislative Tracking; Occupational Safety & Health

Producer: The Bureau of National Affairs, Inc. (BNA)

Online Service: Executive Telecom System, Inc., Human Resource Information Network

Conditions: Annual subscription to Executive Telecom System required

Content: Contains information on the legal and practical aspects of disclosure information on hazardous chemicals required of businesses and government agencies. Covers state and federal right-to-know laws and the federal Hazard Communication Standard from the Occupational Safety and Health Administration as they relate to worker training, labeling, recordkeeping and posting, and trade secrets and confidentiality. Also includes a discussion of legal challenges, funding and compliance problems, inspection requirements, and potential regulatory changes. For 25 states with comprehensive right-to-know laws, provides effective date and description of law; employers, employees, and chemicals covered; community provisions; penalties for violations; and guidelines for specific requirement compliance. Corresponds to *Right-To-Know: A Regulatory Update on Providing Chemical Hazard Information*.

Language: English

Coverage: U.S.

Time Span: 1985 only

Updating: Not updated

CHEMICAL SAFETY DATA GUIDE

Type: Source (Full Text)

Subject: Occupational Safety & Health

Producer: The Bureau of National Affairs, Inc. (BNA)

Online Service: Executive Telecom System, Inc., Human Resource Information Network

Conditions: Annual subscription to Executive Telecom System required

Content: Contains full text of *Chemical Safety Data Guide*, covering the identification, handling, and regulation of substances covered by the Occupational Safety and Health Administration (OSHA) Hazard Communication Standard and state right-to-know laws. Includes physical hazard (e.g., flammability, explosibility) and health hazard (e.g., long- and short-term exposure limits, known or suspected carcinogenicity) data; use and safe handling precautions; spillage, leakage, and disposal procedures; and protective equipment requirements or recommendations. Also provides and defines respirator codes.

Language: English

Coverage: U.S.

Time Span: Current information

Updating: Periodically, as new data become available

CHEMICAL SUBSTANCES CONTROL

Type: Source (Full Text)

Subject: Occupational Safety & Health

Producer: The Bureau of National Affairs, Inc. (BNA)

Online Service: Executive Telecom System, Inc., Human Resource Information Network

Conditions: Annual subscription to Executive Telecom System required

Content: Contains full text of *Chemical Substances Control*, a newsletter providing news and analyses of government and private activities relating to regulatory compliance and management of chemicals, including toxic and hazardous chemicals, pesticides, and other substances. Also covers reporting and recordkeeping, labeling and packaging, testing, transportation, and disposal.

Language: English

Coverage: U.S.

Time Span: November 1985 to date

Updating: Every 2 weeks

CHEMLINE

Type: Source (Textual-Numeric)

Subject: Chemistry-Structure & Nomenclature

Producer: National Library of Medicine, Toxicology Information Program

Online Service: DIMDI; National Library of Medicine (NLM)

Content: Contains nomenclature and structure information for over 659,000 chemical substances found in other NLM databases and the Toxic Substances Control Act (TSCA) Inventory of the U.S. Environmental Protection Agency. Includes Chemical Abstracts Service (CAS) Registry Numbers, molecular formulas, and systematic nomenclature taken from CA SEARCH *(see)* and Chemical-Biological Activities (CBAC) *(see TOXLINE)*. Also includes synonyms (generic and trivial names) from the CA Index Guide, and, when applicable, number of rings, ring size, ring elemental analysis, and component line formula. Users can search by chemical name or name fragments, molecular formula or formula fragments, and ring analysis terms. Users can also retrieve generic compound classes by searching at the chemical substructure level.

Language: English
Time Span: Current information
Updating: Every 2 months

CHEMREG

Type: Reference (Bibliographic)
Subject: Legislative Tracking; Occupational Safety & Health
Producer: The Bureau of National Affairs, Inc. (BNA)
Online Service: Information Consultants, Inc. (ICI) (as part of The Integrated Chemical Information System)
Conditions: Differential charges for subscribers and non-subscribers to ICI
Content: Contains citations to federal regulations covering the manufacture, processing, use, storage and handling, transportation, workplace exposure, and disposal of chemical substances. Covers regulations published in the *Code of Federal Regulations* and the *Federal Register* of various government departments, including Department of Transportation, Food and Drug Administration, Occupational Safety and Health Administration, Department of Energy, National Institute for Occupational Safety and Health, Nuclear Regulatory Commission, and the Department of Commerce. Corresponds in part to *Index to Government Regulation*.
Language: English
Coverage: U.S.
Time Span: Current regulations in force
Updating: Every 2 months

CHEMSEARCH℠

Type: Source (Textual-Numeric)
Subject: Chemistry-Structure & Nomenclature
Producer: DIALOG Information Services, Inc. (from data provided by Chemical Abstracts Service (CAS))
Online Service: DIALOG Information Services, Inc.
Content: Contains nomenclature information for substances not yet entered in CHEMNAME *(see REGISTRY NOMENCLATURE AND STRUCTURE SERVICE)* or CHEMSIS *(see)* that have appeared in the most recent 3 updates of CA SEARCH *(see)*. Elements of data include CAS Registry Number, molecular formula, and systematic names from the Chemical Abstracts Substance Index. Ring data and synonyms are not included. Any identified substance, whether named one or more times in CA SEARCH, is present unless it is already included in CHEMNAME or CHEMSIS.
Time Span: Most recent 3 updates of CA SEARCH
Updating: Every 2 weeks

CHEMSIS℠ (CHEM Singly Indexed Substances)

Type: Source (Textual-Numeric)
Subject: Chemistry-Structure & Nomenclature
Producer: DIALOG Information Services, Inc. (from data provided by Chemical Abstracts Service (CAS))
Online Service: DIALOG Information Services, Inc.
Content: Contains nomenclature information for chemical substances cited only one time in a given collective index period (e.g., the 10th Collective Index, 1977-1981) of *Chemical Abstracts (see CA SEARCH)*. Includes the same elements of data as CHEMNAME *(see REGISTRY NOMENCLATURE AND STRUCTURE SERVICE)*: CAS Registry Number, molecular formula, systematic names from the Chemical Abstracts Substance Index, synonyms, and ring data. Additional search terms generated by DIALOG for this database are also included. *See also CHEMNAME (under REGISTRY NOMENCLATURE AND STRUCTURE SERVICE), CHEMSEARCH, AND CHEMZERO.*

CHEMZERO℠

Type: Source (Textual-Numeric)
Subject: Chemistry-Structure & Nomenclature
Producer: DIALOG Information Services, Inc. (from data provided by Chemical Abstracts Service (CAS))
Online Service: DIALOG Information Services, Inc.
Content: Contains nomenclature information for over 1.6 million chemical substances that are not cited in *Chemical Abstracts (see CA SEARCH)*. The following data items from the REGISTRY NOMENCLATURE AND STRUCTURE SERVICE *(see)* are included: CAS Registry Number, molecular formula, systematic names from the Chemical Abstracts Substance Index, and synonyms. Additional search terms generated by DIALOG for this database are also included. *See also CHEMNAME (listed under REGISTRY NOMENCLATURE AND STRUCTURE SERVICE), CHEMSEARCH, and CHEMSIS.*
Time Span: 1965 to date
Updating: Irregularly

CHICAGO TRIBUNE

Type: Source (Full Text)
Subject: News
Producer: Chicago Tribune Company
Online Service: VU/TEXT Information Services, Inc.
Conditions: Subscription to VU/TEXT required
Content: Contains full text of news items and feature articles from the *Chicago Tribune* (Illinois) newspaper. Regional coverage emphasizes local government and agriculture, energy, financial services, manufacturing, and transportation industries.
Language: English
Coverage: U.S. (primarily Chicago, Illinois area)
Time Span: 1985 to date
Updating: Daily; items appear within 24 hours of publication.

CHILD ABUSE AND NEGLECT

Type: Reference (Bibliographic, Referral)
Subject: Research in Progress; Social Services
Producer: U.S. Department of Health and Human Services, National Center on Child Abuse and Neglect
Online Service: DIALOG Information Services, Inc.
Content: Contains citations, with abstracts, to materials concerned with the definition, identification, prevention, and treatment of child abuse and neglect. Includes references to the general literature and audiovisual materials; excerpts of current state laws; current research in progress; listings of U.S. service programs; and court case decisions.
Language: English
Coverage: U.S.
Time Span: 1965 to date (research projects and service programs cover the most current 2 years)
Updating: Research projects, audiovisual materials, service programs, and legal citations, annually; literature, including court case decisions, twice a year.

CHRONOLOG® NEWSLETTER

Type: Source (Full Text)
Subject: Information Systems & Services
Producer: DIALOG Information Services, Inc.
Online Service: DIALOG Information Services, Inc.
Content: Contains full text of the international edition of the monthly newsletter of DIALOG Information Services, Inc. Provides information on new and reloaded databases, DIALOG special services, database search aids, telecommunications, DIALOG user meetings and workshops, regional service activities, and new system features. Also includes tips on searching techniques. Does not include search examples.
Language: English
Coverage: International
Time Span: 1981 to date
Updating: Monthly, with each newsletter available about the 20th day of the month and precedes availability of the *Chronolog*

CHUNICHI

Type: Reference (Bibliographic)
Subject: News
Producer: Chunichi Shimbun Company
Online Service: Chunichi Shimbun Company (as an ACE database on Nippon Telegraph and Telephone Corporation)
Content: Contains over 70,000 citations, with some abstracts, to news articles from 2 daily newspapers: the *Chunichi Shimbun* (morning and evening editions) and the *Mid-Japan Economist*. Covers international, national, and regional news, with an emphasis on business and industry in the Nagoya area of central Japan.
Language: Japanese
Coverage: Japan
Time Span: 1984 to date
Updating: Daily, 4 days after publication of original article

CIBERPAT

Type: Reference (Bibliographic)
Subject: Patents
Producer: Registro de la Propiedad Industrial
Online Service: Registro de la Propiedad Industrial
Content: Contains approximately 325,000 references to patents granted in Spain. Includes international classification, applicant, significant dates, and priority information. References to patents granted after 1983 also include an abstract of the patented work.
Language: Spanish
Coverage: Spain
Time Span: 1964 to date
Updating: Every 2 weeks

CIS® (CIS/INDEX)

Type: Reference (Bibliographic)
Subject: Government-U.S. Federal
Producer: Congressional Information Service, Inc. (CIS)
Online Service: DIALOG Information Services, Inc. (CIS/INDEX)
Content: Contains citations, with abstracts, to publications produced by the committees and subcommittees of the U.S. Congress. The types of publications covered are Hearings, Reports, Committee Prints, House and Senate Documents, and Executive and Treaty Documents. Legislative histories of Public Laws are available through 1983. Records of Hearings comprise several sub-records (analytics), each of which contains abstracts of testimony given by individual witnesses or groups of witnesses. Covers a broad range of subjects of interest to the Congress in its oversight, investigatory, and legislative activities, including the areas of commerce, labor, economics, technology, health, education, welfare, defense, energy, conservation, and transportation. Corresponds to the *CIS/Index to Publications of the U.S. Congress*.
Language: English
Coverage: U.S.
Time Span: 1970 to date
Updating: About 1050 records a month

CISDOC; CISILO

Type: Reference (Bibliographic)
Subject: Occupational Safety & Health
Producer: International Occupational Safety and Health Information Centre (CIS), International Labour Office
Online Service: ARAMIS (a cooperative service of the Swedish Center for Working Life, Swedish National Board of Occupational Safety and Health, and The Swedish National Environmental Protection Board) (CISILO); ESA-IRS (CISDOC); National Library of Medicine (NLM) (as a TOXLINE database*(see)*) (INTERNATIONAL LABOUR OFFICE); Telesystemes-Questel (CISILO)
Content: Contains citations, with abstracts, to the worldwide literature on occupational safety and health. Topics covered include pathology and medicine of work in many industries and professions, education, ergonomy, statistics, and the organization, inspection, and risks of safety systems.
Language: English and French
Coverage: International
Time Span: ESA-IRS, 1972 to date; other services, 1974 to date.
Updating: About 300 records 7 or 8 times a year

CLAIMS®/CITATION

Type: Reference (Bibliographic)
Subject: Patents
Producer: IFI/Plenum Data Company
Online Service: DIALOG Information Services, Inc.
Content: Contains references to every U.S. and non-U.S. patent (over 12 million patent numbers) cited in U.S. patents. Each of the more than 3 million references identifies, by patent number, all later U.S. patents in which an earlier patent is cited. Each patent record contains the patent number of each later patent (both U.S. and non-U.S.) that cites it.
Language: English
Coverage: Primarily U.S.
Time Span: Cited patents, 1836 to date; citing patents, 1947 to date.
Updating: About 16,000 records a quarter

CLAIMS®/CLASS

Type: Reference (Referral)
Subject: Patents
Producer: IFI/Plenum Data Company
Online Service: DIALOG Information Services, Inc.; ORBIT Information Technologies Corporation; STN International (IFIREF)
Content: Contains classification codes and titles for classes and subclasses provided in the U.S. Patent Office *Manual of Classification*. Covers approximately 400 main classes and 105,000 subclasses that pertain to patents issued for mechanical, electrical, and chemical inventions.

Language: English
Coverage: U.S.
Time Span: Current information
Updating: STN, replaced twice a year; DIALOG, replaced annually.

CLAIMS®/COMPOUND REGISTRY

Type: Source (Textual-Numeric)
Subject: Chemistry-Structure & Nomenclature; Patents
Producer: IFI/Plenum Data Company
Online Service: DIALOG Information Services, Inc.; ORBIT Information Technologies Corporation
Content: Contains a listing of approximately 14,000 chemical compounds referenced 5 or more times since 1950 in patents covered by the CLAIMS/UNITERM database *(see)*. Each record includes the IFI compound term number, main compound name, available synonyms, molecular formula, element count, fragment codes, and fragment terms. Corresponds to the *Compound Term List Name/Number Order for the IFI Chemical Patent Databases* and *Compound Term List Molecular Formula Order for the IFI Chemical Patent Databases.*
Time Span: 1950 to date
Updating: Annually, with complete reload

CLAIMS®/COMPREHENSIVE DATABASE

Type: Reference (Bibliographic)
Subject: Patents
Producer: IFI/Plenum Data Company
Online Service: DIALOG Information Services, Inc.; STN International
Content: A set of 3 databases (2 historical and 1 current) that contain enhanced indexing of the U.S. chemical and chemically related patents included in the CLAIMS/UNITERM databases *(see)*. Each patent record has the same set of general and compound terms selected from the controlled vocabulary (uniterms) used in CLAIMS/UNITERM. In addition, all fragment terms include roles to indicate the function (e.g., reactants, products, non-reactants) of each chemical substance. Also includes systematic indexing of polymers and the substructure fragmentation system used in indexing Markush structures.
Language: English
Coverage: Primarily U.S.
Time Span: Historical, 1950 to 1962 and 1963 to 1970; current, 1971 to date.
Updating: Monthly

CLAIMS®/REASSIGNMENT & REEXAMINATION

Type: Reference (Bibliographic)
Subject: Patents
Producer: IFI/Plenum Data Company
Online Service: DIALOG Information Services, Inc.; ORBIT Information Technologies Corporation (to be available in 1987)
Content: Contains approximately 36,000 citations to patents for which ownership has been transferred from one party to another (reassigned patents) or for which the patentability has been reviewed and rejected or reaffirmed by the U.S. Patent and Trademark Office (reexamined patents). Includes bibliographic data for all patents. For reassigned patents, also includes names of former and new assignees, date of reassignment, and type of reassignment (e.g., quarter interest). For reexamined patents, also includes name and location of reexamination requestor, request number and date, reexamination certificate date, and text from the certificate describing the results of the reexamination.

Language: English
Coverage: U.S.
Time Span: Reassigned patents, 1980 to date; reexamined patents, 1981 to date.
Updating: Annually

CLAIMS®/U.S. PATENTS

Type: Reference (Bibliographic)
Subject: Patents
Producer: IFI/Plenum Data Company
Online Service: DIALOG Information Services, Inc.; ORBIT Information Technologies Corporation; STN International (IFIPAT)
Content: Contains about 1.6 million citations to granted U.S. utility patents, reissued patents, and defense publications announced in the U.S. Patent Office *Official Gazette*. Equivalent patents issued by Belgium, Federal Republic of Germany, France, Great Britain, and The Netherlands are also included for chemical patents. Covers patents in these areas of science and technology: aerospace and aeronautical engineering, agricultural engineering, biomedical technology, chemistry, chemical engineering, civil engineering, electronics and electrical engineering, electromagnetic technology, mechanical engineering, medicine, nuclear science, and telecommunications. Contains records previously contained in CLAIMS/CHEM. Abstracts are included for chemical patents since 1950 and for all others since 1965.
Language: English
Coverage: Primarily U.S.
Time Span: Chemical patents, 1950 to date; all others, 1963 to date.
Updating: CLAIMS/U.S. PATENTS 63-70 is not updated. CLAIMS/U.S. PATENT ABSTRACTS 71- is updated monthly with about 5500 records. Weekly updates are available in CLAIMS/U.S. PATENT ABSTRACTS WEEKLY before they are merged into the main database.

CLAIMS®/UNITERM

Type: Reference (Bibliographic)
Subject: Patents
Producer: IFI/Plenum Data Company
Online Service: DIALOG Information Services, Inc.; ORBIT Information Technologies Corporation (CLAIMSU); STN International (IFIUDB)
Conditions: Subscribers to *Uniterm Index* have unlimited use; non-subscribers are limited to 12 hours of use per calendar year.
Content: A set of 3 databases (2 historical and 1 current), that contain about 1.6 million citations to all U.S. chemical and chemically-related patents. In addition to the information in CLAIMS/U.S. PATENTS *(see)*, each patent in these databases has been assigned a set of at least 20 descriptors (uniterms) selected from a controlled vocabulary consisting of general terms, fragment terms, and compound terms. *Chemical Abstracts* references and foreign patent equivalents from Belgium, Federal Republic of Germany, France, Great Britain, and The Netherlands are included. Covers all patents listed in the Chemical Section of the *Official Gazette* of the U.S. Patent Office. Abstracts are included for records since 1950.
Language: English
Coverage: Primarily U.S.
Time Span: Historical, 1950 to 1962 and 1963 to 1970; current, 1971 to date.
Updating: STN, about 1400 records a week; DIALOG and ORBIT, about 4500 records a quarter.

CLINICAL ABSTRACTS

Type: Reference (Bibliographic)
Subject: Biomedicine
Producer: Medical Information Systems, Reference & Index Services, Inc.
Online Service: DIALOG Information Services, Inc.
Content: Contains approximately 9000 citations, with abstracts, to English-language clinical medicine literature. Covers pediatrics, family practice, internal medicine, general surgery, and cardiovascular surgery. Sources include 300 medical journals. Corresponds to *Abstracts in Internal Medicine*.
Language: English
Coverage: International
Time Span: 1981 to date
Updating: Monthly

CLINICAL LAB LETTER

Type: Reference (Referral); Source (Full Text)
Subject: Biomedicine; Conferences & Meetings
Producer: Quest Publishing Company
Online Service: NewsNet, Inc.
Conditions: Monthly subscription to NewsNet required; differential charges for subscribers and non-subscribers to *Clinical Lab Letter*.
Content: Contains full text of *Clinical Lab Letter*, a newsletter on medical technology developments. Covers new products and procedures (e.g., a test for Acquired Immune Deficiency Syndrome antibodies in donated blood); safety hazard notices and product recalls; regulatory actions, including the promulgation of new standards; legal actions, including outcomes of lawsuits related to clinical laboratory tests; and business news on the manufacturers of products for clinical laboratories. Also provides news of professional activities (e.g., deadlines for certification examinations); announcements of continuing education courses, meetings, and events; and lists of new literature, brochures, and bulletins.
Language: English
Coverage: Primarily U.S., with some international coverage of meetings and conferences
Time Span: November 1985 to date
Updating: Every 2 weeks

CLINICAL NOTES ON-LINE

Type: Source (Full Text)
Subject: Biomedicine
Producer: Elsevier-IRCS Ltd.
Online Service: DATA-STAR
Content: Contains full text of physicians' observations (clinical notes, classified according to the Systematized Nomenclature of Medicine) on patients in hospitals and general practices. Covers all fields of medicine, including surgery, dentistry, and ophthalmology. Case records submitted by physicians include name and institutional address of attending physician, patient's history and symptoms, diagnosis, descriptive case notes, treatment, and outcome. Records are updated with editorially reviewed comments submitted by the originators, users of the database, and invited authorities.
Language: English
Coverage: International
Time Span: 1984 to date
Updating: Monthly

CLINPROT (Clinical Cancer Protocols)

Type: Reference (Referral)
Subject: Biomedicine
Producer: U.S. National Institutes of Health (NIH), National Cancer Institute, International Cancer Research Data Bank
Online Service: DIMDI; National Library of Medicine (NLM); University of Tsukuba
Conditions: Access through University of Tsukuba limited to affiliates of the University of Japan
Content: Contains summaries of clinical investigations on the use of new anticancer agents and treatment modalities. Provides descriptions of clinical trials, including patient entry criteria, the therapy regimen, and special study parameters. Covers over 5300 open (active) and closed protocols.
Language: English
Coverage: International
Time Span: April 1977 to date
Updating: Quarterly; more than 500 records a year.

CMI (Canadian Magazine Index)

Type: Reference (Bibliographic)
Subject: General Interest
Producer: Micromedia Limited
Online Service: CISTI, Canadian Online Enquiry Service (CAN/OLE); DIALOG Information Services, Inc.; QL Systems Limited; Telesystemes-Questel
Conditions: CISTI accessible only in Canada
Content: Contains citations to articles in over 200 Canadian English-language popular and special interest periodicals (e.g., *Autosport Canada, Beautiful British Columbia, Toronto Life*). Covers art, business, children's literature, computers, cooking, education, geography, health, history, hobbies, music, nature, recreation, regions of Canada, science, social and women's issues, and travel. Also includes citations to 15 U.S. popular magazines and 9 Canadian business publications. Corresponds to *Canadian Magazine Index. (See also CANADIAN BUSINESS AND CURRENT AFFAIRS)*
Language: English
Coverage: Primarily Canada, with some coverage of U.S.
Time Span: 1985 to date
Updating: About 3000 records a month

CNI (Canadian News Index)

Type: Reference (Bibliographic)
Subject: News
Producer: Micromedia Limited
Online Service: QL Systems Limited
Content: Contains citations to items in 7 major Canadian newspapers: *Montreal Gazette, Toronto Globe & Mail, Toronto Star, Vancouver Sun, Winnipeg Free Press, Calgary Herald*, and *Halifax Chronicle-Herald* and 27 national or regional news and public affair magazines. Subjects included are national (Canadian) and international news, provincial affairs, editorials, government and labor activities, reviews, and biographical information. Corresponds to *Canadian News Index. (see also CANADIAN BUSINESS AND CURRENT AFFAIRS)*
Language: English
Coverage: Canada
Time Span: 1977 to date
Updating: About 8000 records a month

CNRS-SHS

Type: Reference (Referral)

Subject: Research in Progress; Social Sciences & Humanities

Producer: Centre National de la Recherche Scientifique, Centre de Documentation Sciences Humaines

Online Service: Centre National de la Recherche Scientifique, Centre de Documentation Sciences Humaines (CNRS/CDSH)

Content: Contains descriptions of current research in the social sciences and humanities by the more than 600 research centers sponsored by CNRS/CDSH. Descriptions include name and address of research center, research topics, publications, names of researchers, geographical code, and keywords. Covers research in anthropology, archaeology, demography, development, ecology, economics, education, employment, aesthetics, ethnology, geography, health, history, history of science and technology, law, linguistics, literature, musicology, philosophy, political science, prehistory, psychology, religion, and sociology. Corresponds to *Annuaire CNRS Sciences de l'homme et de la societe*.

Language: French

Coverage: France

Time Span: Current information

Updating: Quarterly

COFFEELINE℠

Type: Reference (Bibliographic)

Subject: Agriculture

Producer: International Coffee Organization

Online Service: DIALOG Information Services, Inc.

Content: Contains about 16,000 citations, with abstracts, to the worldwide literature on all aspects of the production, trade, and consumption of coffee from the farming of coffee plants to production, packaging, marketing, and health aspects of coffee. Corresponds to *International Coffee Organization Library Monthly Entries*.

Language: English, French, Portuguese, and Spanish

Coverage: International

Time Span: 1973 to date

Updating: About 200 records a month

COLLEAGUE MAIL SERVICES

Type: Reference (Referral); Source (Full Text)

Subject: Biomedicine; Conferences & Meetings; Health Care

Producer: BRS/Colleague and others

Online Service: BRS/Colleague

Content: Contains a variety of electronic services for medical professionals, including electronic mail, a calendar of medical events, and tips for online searching of bibliographic and full-text databases available through BRS/Colleague. Also provides the following bulletin boards: Anesthesia Safety and Technology, Cellforum (for comments and questions from pathologists, cell biologists, and molecular biologists), Clinical Drug Information, Computer Software for Medical Office Management, Dermatology, Geriatrics and Gerontology, Hackers' Q & A (for information on microcomputer products and applications), Human Genetics, Immunology, Interventional Cardiology, Medical Education Forum (for discussion of information technology in medical schools), Medical Ethics, Neurology, Pediatric Psychiatry, and Sickle-Cell Disease. These forums may include notices of available positions, positions wanted, and equipment sources.

Language: English

Coverage: U.S.

Time Span: July 1986 to date

Updating: Twice a week

THE COLLEGE BOARD

Type: Reference (Referral); Source (Full Text)

Subject: Education & Educational Institutions

Producer: The College Board

Online Service: CompuServe Information Service

Content: Contains information on U.S. colleges, admission requirements, and financial aid, to assist users in selecting an appropriate college based upon individual interests, needs, and academic standing. Includes an interactive program for estimating eligibility for financial aid.

Language: English

Coverage: U.S.

Time Span: Current academic year

Updating: Twice a year (fall and spring), with some items updated as needed

THE COLUMBUS DISPATCH

Type: Source (Full Text)

Subject: News

Producer: The Dispatch Printing Company

Online Service: VU/TEXT Information Services, Inc.

Conditions: Subscription to VU/TEXT required

Content: Contains full text of news items and feature articles from *The Columbus Dispatch* (Ohio) newspaper. Regional coverage emphasizes the banking and insurance industries, information technologies research, and state government and legislative activity.

Language: English

Coverage: U.S. (primarily Columbus, Ohio area)

Time Span: July 1985 to date

Updating: Daily

COMBINED HEALTH INFORMATION DATABASE

Type: Reference (Bibliographic); Source (Full Text)

Subject: Biomedicine; Health Care

Producer: Combined Health Information Database and others

Online Service: BRS; BRS After Dark; BRS/BRKTHRU; BRS/Colleague; TECH DATA

Content: Contains 5 files of information on health education and health promotion topics for health professionals and the general public.

ARTHRITIS. Contains citations, with abstracts, to journal articles, books, pamphlets, and audiovisual materials on arthritis and related musculoskeletal diseases. Covers 1978 to date. Produced by Arthritis Information Clearinghouse.

DIABETES. Contains citations, with abstracts, to journal articles, brochures, books, and audiovisual materials on diabetes. Covers 1973 to date. Produced by National Diabetes Information Clearinghouse.

DIGESTIVE DISEASES. Contains full text of information on digestive diseases prepared by the Digestive Diseases Clearinghouse and citations, with abstracts, to professional and patient education literature. Covers 1980 to date. Produced by National Digestive Diseases Information Clearinghouse.

HIGH BLOOD PRESSURE. Contains citations, with abstracts,

to books, journal articles, pamphlets, reports, and educational materials on blood pressure. Covers 1981 to date. Produced by High Blood Pressure Information Center.

HEALTH EDUCATION. Contains citations, with abstracts, to curricular materials, reports, monographs, journal articles, conference proceedings, unpublished documents, and program descriptions on health education and health promotion methods and activities. Covers such topics as patient education, school and community health education, occupational health education, risk reduction education, professional training, and research and evaluation. Covers 1977 to date. Produced by Centers for Disease Control, Center for Health Promotion and Education. Corresponds to *Current Awareness in Health Education.*

Language: Primarily English, with some coverage of materials in other languages

Coverage: Primarily U.S., with some international coverage

Time Span: Varies by file *(see Content)*

Updating: Quarterly

COMITE DES TRAVAUX HISTORIQUES ET SCIENTIFIQUES (CTHS)

Type: Reference (Referral)

Subject: Associations & Foundations-Directories

Producer: Ministere de l'Education Nationale, Comite des Travaux Historiques et Scientifiques

Online Service: Serveur Universitaire National de l'Information Scientifique et Technique (SUNIST)

Content: Contains information on about 2000 French learned societies in the fields of archaeology, history, and science. Provides address and telephone number, publications and subscription prices, and a description of activities.

Language: French

Coverage: France

Time Span: Current information

Updating: Periodically, as new data become available

COMPENDEX® (Computerized Engineering Index)

Type: Reference (Bibliographic)

Subject: Bioengineering

Producer: Engineering Information, Inc.

Online Service: BRS; BRS/BRKTHRU; BRS/Colleague; Centre de Documentation de l'Armement (CEDOCAR); CISTI, Canadian Online Enquiry Service (CAN/OLE); DATA-STAR; DIALOG Information Services, Inc.; ESA-IRS; Knowledge Index (ENGINEERING LITERATURE INDEX); ORBIT Information Technologies Corporation; Pergamon InfoLine; STN International; TECH DATA

Conditions: CISTI accessible only in Canada

Content: Contains about 1.5 million citations, with abstracts, to the worldwide literature (excluding patents) in engineering and technology. Fields of engineering include: civil, water and waterworks, sanitary and waste, fuel, bioengineering, geology and mining, petroleum, metallurgical, mechanical, industrial, aerospace, automotive, marine, railroad, electrical, electronics and communications control, chemical, and agricultural. Related subject areas covered include construction materials, properties and testing of materials, transportation, pollution, ocean and underwater technology, nuclear technology, fluid flow, heat and thermodynamics, computers and data processing, light and optical technology, sound and acoustical technology, food technology, applied physics, instruments, measurements, and information science. Conference review records

contain conference code numbers which are links to complete coverage of all individual papers in Ei ENGINEERING MEETINGS *(see)*. Corresponds to *The Engineering Index Monthly.*

Language: Primarily English, with about 30% of the documents in other languages; all abstracts in English.

Coverage: International

Time Span: ESA-IRS and STN, 1969 to date; DIALOG and ORBIT, 1970 to date; CISTI, 1970 to date, with abstracts from 1982 to date; CEDOCAR and Pergamon InfoLine, 1973 to date; Knowledge Index, 1975 to date; BRS, BRS/BRKTHRU, BRS/Colleague, DATA-STAR, and TECH DATA, 1976 to date.

Updating: About 12,000 records a month

COMPREHENSIVE CORE MEDICAL LIBRARY

Type: Source (Full Text)

Subject: Biomedicine

Producer: BRS

Online Service: BRS; BRS/Colleague

Content: Contains full text of major medical textbooks and medical journals. Includes the American College of Obstetricians and Gynecologists' *Standards for Obstetric-Gynecologic Services* (6th edition); Boucek's *Coronary Artery Disease, Pathological and Clinical Assessment;* Brenner and Stein's *Acid Base and Potassium Homeostasis, Acute Renal Failure, Chronic Renal Failure,* and *Hypertension;* Chapman's *Acute Renal Failure;* Charnley's *The Closed Treatment of Common Fractures;* Cohen's *Emergencies in Obstetrics and Gynecology;* Conn's *Current Therapy;* Copass' *The Paramedic Manual;* Eisenberg's *Emergency Medical Therapy;* Grenvik and Safar's *Brain Failure and Resuscitation;* Griffith's *Instructions for Patients;* Hollingworth's *Pregnancy, Diabetes, and Birth;* Karliner's *Coronary Care;* Larson and Eisenberg's *Manual of Admitting Orders and Therapeutics;* Mandell, Douglas, and Bennett's *Principles and Practice of Infectious Diseases;* Margulies and Thaler's *The Physician's Book of Lists;* Michaelson's *Textbook of the Fundus of the Eye;* Ogilvie's *Birch's Emergencies in Medical Practice;* Parillo's *Major Issues in Critical Care Medicine;* Percival's *Holland and Brews Manual of Obstetrics;* Sabiston's *Textbook of Surgery* (12th edition); Schiff's *Diseases of the Liver;* Schwartz's *Principles and Practice of Emergency Medicine;* Smillie's *Injuries of the Knee Joint;* and Williams' *Gray's Anatomy.* Publishers include Churchill Livingstone, J.B. Lippincott, and W.B. Saunders. Also includes the serials *Cardiology Clinics, Emergency Medicine Clinics of North America,* and *Medical Clinics of North America,* published by W.B. Saunders, and the full text of *Annals of Internal Medicine* (September 1984 to date), *Annals of Surgery* (February 1985 to date), *American Journal of Psychiatry* (August 1985 to date), *American Journal of Public Health* (July 1985 to date), *Archives of Diseases in Childhood* (July 1985 to date), *British Medical Journal* (1984 to date), *Cancer Treatment Reports* (June 1985 to date), *Clinical Orthopaedics* (May 1985 to date), *Clinical Pediatrics* (June 1985 to date), *Clinical Pharmacology and Therapeutics* (July 1985 to date), *Emergency Medicine Reports* (November 11, 1985 to date), *Journal of Bone & Joint Surgery* (July 1985 to date), *Journal of the National Cancer Institute* (1985 to date), *Lancet* (May 1983 to date), *Medical Letter on Drugs and Therapeutics* (1982 to date), *Medicine* (November 1985 to date), *Nature* (October 31, 1985 to date), *New England Journal of Medicine* (1983 to date), *Pediatrics* (July 1985 to date), *Seminars in Respiratory Medicine* (July 1985 to date), and *Sexually Transmitted Diseases* (April 1985 to date).

Language: English

Coverage: Primarily English-speaking countries
Time Span: Textbooks, current editions; journals *(see Content)*.
Updating: Periodically, as new textbook editions and journal issues become available

COMPUTER EXPRESS

Type: Reference (Referral)
Subject: Computers & Software
Producer: Computer Express
Online Service: CompuServe Information Service (as part of THE ELECTRONIC MALL); General Videotex Corporation/DELPHI; THE SOURCE
Content: Contains about 500 descriptions of computer hardware, software, and peripherals available for IBM, Amiga, Apple, Commodore, and McIntosh computers. Includes software in such areas as home management, business, education, and recreation. Users can place orders online.
Language: English
Coverage: U.S.
Time Span: Current information
Updating: About 50 records every 2 weeks

COMPUTERIZED AIDS INFORMATION NETWORK (CAIN)

Type: Reference (Bibliographic, Referral); Source (Full Text)
Subject: Health Care
Producer: Los Angeles Gay and Lesbian Community Services Center
Online Service: General Videotex Corporation/DELPHI
Content: Contains information related to Acquired Immune Deficiency Syndrome (AIDS): general information, including definitions of terms, health agency recommendations for reducing risks of infection, requirements for reporting diagnosed cases, and advice on dealing with the social ramifications of the disease; relevant news from the Associated Press wire service; references to organizations and funding sources supporting AIDS-related projects; research and clinical data, including epidemiological statistics, reports on behavioral and research studies, information on test protocols and diagnostics, and infection control guidelines; and citations to relevant scientific and medical literature, including journal articles, audiovisual materials, brochures, newsletters, and reports. Also includes references to organizations providing medical, psychological, dental, financial, insurance, legal, or religious/spiritual services. Electronic mail, bulletin board, and conferencing services are also available.
Language: English
Coverage: Primarily U.S., with some international coverage
Time Span: Late 1984 to date
Updating: Periodically, as new data become available

COMPUTERPAT

Type: Reference (Bibliographic)
Subject: Patents
Producer: Pergamon InfoLine Inc.
Online Service: Pergamon InfoLine
Content: Contains citations, with abstracts, to approximately 8000 U.S. patents issued in the fields of digital computers and data processing. Covers all patents issued since 1942 for U.S. Patent and Trademark Office subclasses 364/200 and 364/900.

Language: English
Coverage: U.S.
Time Span: 1942 to date
Updating: Weekly

COMPUTING TODAY!

Type: Source (Full Text)
Subject: Computers & Software
Producer: Computing Today!
Online Service: NewsNet, Inc.
Conditions: Monthly subscription to NewsNet required
Content: Contains news of computer industry developments and reviews of new hardware and software products for microcomputers, minicomputers, and mainframe computers. Covers vendor news (e.g., licensing and distribution agreements, changes in pricing or trade-in policies, major sales) and announcements of new or upgraded products for the Apple II family, Macintosh, IBM microcomputers and compatibles, and other types and classes of computers. Includes reviews of software products for accounting, word processing, education, and entertainment; reviews of graphics programs and printers; information on training programs and computer-oriented publications; and suggestions for improving programming skills.
Language: English
Coverage: Primarily U.S.
Time Span: February 1986 to date
Updating: Weekly

CONF

Type: Reference (Referral)
Subject: Conferences & Meetings; Science & Technology
Producer: Fachinformationszentrum Energie, Physik, Mathematik GmbH
Online Service: STN International
Content: Contains announcements of approximately 40,000 past, present, and future conferences in the areas of science and engineering, including physics, mathematics, computer science, astronomy and astrophysics, aeronautics and astronautics, and energy. Information for each conference includes title, sponsoring organization, conference location and dates, contacts for further information, notes on related publications, and keywords describing the conference topic.
Language: English and German
Coverage: International
Time Span: 1976 to date
Updating: About 100 conferences a week

CONFERENCE PAPERS INDEX

Type: Reference (Bibliographic)
Subject: Science & Technology
Producer: Cambridge Scientific Abstracts
Online Service: DIALOG Information Services, Inc.; ESA-IRS
Content: Contains over 1 million citations to scientific and technical papers presented at regional, national, and international meetings. Separate references to conferences are included from 1982 to date. Is a source of information on current research and development, primarily in the life sciences, medicine, chemistry, physical sciences, and engineering. Records include names and addresses of authors, conference title, location, date, sponsors, and the information required to order available proceedings, preprints, reprints, and abstracts. Corresponds to *Conference Papers Index*.

Language: English
Coverage: International
Time Span: 1973 to date
Updating: About 3000 records a month

CONFERENCE PROCEEDINGS INDEX

Type: Reference (Bibliographic)
Subject: Library Holdings-Catalogs; Conferences & Meetings; Science & Technology
Producer: The British Library
Online Service: BLAISE-LINE
Conditions: Annual subscription of 49 pounds (UK) for U.K. users or 56 pounds (UK) for other users to BLAISE Online Services required
Content: Contains approximately 200,000 citations to proceedings of conferences, congresses, symposia, workshops, and seminars in British Library Document Supply Centre's collection. Includes proceedings published as monographs or parts of reports, and in journals. Covers all subject areas, but emphasis is on the sciences. Information for each item includes subject coverage, sponsors, location, date and, if available, ISSN or ISBN. Corresponds to *Index of Conference Proceedings Received*.
Language: Citations in original language, with notes in English
Coverage: International
Time Span: 1964 to date, with some information from the 19th century
Updating: About 1000 records a month

CONGRESSIONAL ACTIVITIES

Type: Reference (Referral); Source (Full Text)
Subject: Conferences & Meetings; Government-U.S. Federal; Legislative Tracking
Producer: Oliphant Washington News Service
Online Service: NewsNet, Inc.
Conditions: Monthly subscription to NewsNet required; differential charges for subscribers and non-subscribers to *Congressional Activities*.
Content: Contains full text of the *Congressional Activities*, a newsletter providing a calendar of forthcoming U.S. Congressional activities, with an emphasis on energy and environmental matters. Taxes and general subjects are covered as well. Also includes summaries of bills and resolutions, information on their status, and brief citations to selected speeches and debates contained in the *Congressional Record*.
Language: English
Coverage: U.S.
Time Span: March 1984 to date
Updating: 40 to 45 times a year

CONGRESSIONAL RECORD ABSTRACTS©

Type: Reference (Bibliographic)
Subject: Government-U.S. Federal
Producer: National Standards Association
Online Service: BRS (to be available in 1987); BRS After Dark (to be available in 1987); BRS/BRKTHRU (to be available in 1987); BRS/Colleague (to be available in 1987); DIALOG Information Services, Inc. (CONGRESSIONAL RECORD ABSTRACTS); ORBIT Information Technologies Corporation

Content: Provides citations, with abstracts, to the *Congressional Record* (House, Senate, Extension of Remarks, and Digest sections), the official diary of the activities of the U.S. Congress. Records describe bills and resolutions, amendments, committee and subcommittee reports, public laws, floor actions, schedules of committee and floor activities, executive communications, speeches, and materials inserted into the Record by members of Congress. Corresponds to the daily CSI publication *Congressional Record Abstracts--Master Edition*.
Language: English
Coverage: U.S.
Time Span: 1981 to date
Updating: About 1000 records a week

CONSUMER DRUG INFORMATION℠

Type: Source (Full Text)
Subject: Pharmaceuticals & Pharmaceutical Industry
Producer: American Society of Hospital Pharmacists
Online Service: BRS; BRS After Dark; BRS/BRKTHRU; BRS/Colleague; DIALOG Information Services, Inc.; Knowledge Index; Mead Data Central, Inc. (as a MEDIS database *(see)*)
Conditions: Subscription to Mead Data Central required
Content: Contains full text of *Consumer Drug Digest*, covering most drugs prescribed in the U.S. Provides a general description of each drug and information on possible side effects, precautions, instructions on dosage and use, and advice on storage.
Language: English
Coverage: U.S.
Time Span: Current information
Updating: Quarterly

CQ WASHINGTON ALERT SERVICE

Type: Reference (Referral); Source (Full Text)
Subject: Legislative Tracking
Producer: Congressional Quarterly Inc.
Online Service: Congressional Quarterly Inc., Washington Alert Service (as a database on General Electric Information Services Company)
Conditions: Initiation fee of $180 and monthly maintenance fee of $18 to Congressional Quarterly Inc. required
Content: Contains information on legislative activities in the current and previous U.S. Congress. Includes committee and floor schedules from the current day through the next 3 months; summaries of floor actions; legislative histories of all bills introduced; listing of congressional documents; all roll-call votes taken in the current and previous Congress; support/opposition voting analysis profiles of members of Congress; and the full text of *CQ Weekly Report*. Sources include the *Congressional Record* and several publications of Congressional Quarterly, Inc.
Language: English
Coverage: U.S.
Time Span: 1983 to date
Updating: Daily

CREATIVE COMPUTING FORUM

Type: Source (Full Text, Software)
Subject: Computers & Software
Producer: Creative Computing

Online Service: CompuServe Information Service

Content: Contains full text of selected articles from *Creative Computing* magazine. Also includes an index of current high and low prices for retail computer equipment in various regions of the U.S. and a file of popular programs, program modifications, and enhancements that can be downloaded for personal use. Users can submit questions and receive answers online from the magazine's staff.

Language: English

Coverage: U.S.

Time Span: Articles, July 1984 to date, with selected coverage of earlier materials; other data, current information.

Updating: Daily

CRIS/USDA (Current Research Information System)

Type: Reference (Referral)

Subject: Agriculture; Research in Progress

Producer: U.S. Department of Agriculture (USDA), Current Research Information System

Online Service: DIALOG Information Services, Inc.

Content: Contains about 35,000 descriptions of ongoing and recently completed research projects related to agriculture. Covers research sponsored or conducted by USDA research agencies, state agricultural experiment stations, state forestry schools, and other cooperating state institutions in those biological, physical, social, and behavioral sciences related to agriculture, including natural resource conservation and management; crop and livestock protection; production management systems; product development; marketing and economics; food and nutrition; consumer health and safety; family life; housing; rural development; environmental protection; forestry; outdoor recreation; and community, area, and regional development.

Language: English

Coverage: U.S.

Time Span: Most recent 2 years; terminated projects are retained for 2 years and are purged annually.

Updating: About 450 new and revised projects a month

CRYSTMET® (NRC Metals Crystallographic Data File)

Type: Reference (Bibliographic); Source (Textual-Numeric)

Subject: Chemistry-Structure & Nomenclature

Producer: CISTI, Canadian Scientific Numeric Database Service

Online Service: CISTI, Canadian Scientific Numeric Database Service (CAN/SND); FIZ Karlsruhe

Conditions: Accessible in the Federal Republic of Germany only through FIZ Karlsruhe

Content: Contains published crystallographic data for metallic structures determined by diffraction methods. Includes approximately 6000 references to atoms with positional, thermal, and occupational parameters determined since 1913. Also includes 4500 references to metals and intermetallic compounds assigned to known structure types since 1975 where the composition is clearly defined and the space group and unit cell have been determined. Each entry contains empirical formula and structure type; structure data, including specimen (powder or single crystal), reflections, reliability factor, intensity, radiation, and temperature and pressure of data collection; mineral names and location of origin; and bibliographic citations, including cross references to works with contrary findings.

Language: English

Coverage: International

Time Span: 1913 to date

Updating: Annually

CTCP (Clinical Toxicology of Commercial Products)

Type: Source (Textual-Numeric)

Subject: Toxicology

Producer: Dartmouth Medical School; University of Rochester

Online Service: Chemical Information Systems, Inc., a subsidiary of Fein-Marquart Associates (CIS)

Conditions: Annual subscription fee of $300 to CIS required but fee is waived for educational institutions and non-profit public libraries worldwide

Content: A database system that contains chemical and toxicological information on over 20,000 commercial products (excluding food products) derived from 3000 chemicals. Records can be retrieved by manufacturer, trade name, manufacturer's approved usage, date of most recent change in chemical formulation, chemical names of ingredients, and Chemical Abstracts Service Registry Number. Includes data on toxicity, symptoms, and treatments. Corresponds to *Clinical Toxicology of Commercial Products* by Gosselin, Hodge, Smith and Gleason, 5th edition (1984).

Language: English

Time Span: 1984 (5th edition)

Updating: Twice a year

CUADRA DIRECTORY OF DATABASES

Type: Reference (Referral)

Subject: Information Systems & Services-Directories

Producer: Cuadra/Elsevier

Online Service: DATA-STAR; DataArkiv AB; Telesystemes-Questel; West Publishing Company

Conditions: Subscription to West Publishing Company required

Content: Contains descriptions of more than 3400 publicly available online databases worldwide. Each entry provides the names by which a database is known, a type classification of Source (Numeric, Textual-Numeric, Full Text, or Software) or Reference (Bibliographic or Referral), name of database producer, names of online services and gateways through which the database can be accessed, description of content, subject, language, geographic coverage, time span, frequency of updating and, if applicable, conditions of access. Also provides addresses and telephone numbers for database producers, online services and gateways. Corresponds to *Directory of Online Databases*.

Language: English

Coverage: International

Time Span: Current information

Updating: Quarterly

CUMULATIVE BOOK INDEX℠

Type: Reference (Bibliographic)

Subject: Publishers & Distributors-Catalogs

Producer: The H.W. Wilson Company

Online Service: WILSONLINE

Content: Contains citations to English-language books published worldwide. Also covers books that are partially in English, including dictionaries, phrase books, and others aids

to language learning. For books available in more than one country, the publisher, distributor, and price in local currency are given for each country of issue. Also contains names and addresses of publishers and distributors and book status (e.g., in-print, out-of-print). Corresponds to *Cumulative Book Index*.
Language: English
Coverage: International
Time Span: 1982 to date
Updating: Twice a week; about 50,000 records a year.

CURRENT AWARENESS IN BIOLOGICAL SCIENCES
Type: Reference (Bibliographic)
Subject: Life Sciences
Producer: Pergamon Press Ltd.
Online Service: Pergamon InfoLine
Content: Contains approximately 290,000 citations to the worldwide literature on biology. Covers selected articles from approximately 3000 journals. Subjects include biochemistry, cell and developmental biology, genetics and molecular biology, immunology, microbiology, neurosciences, pharmacology and toxicology, and physiology. Includes an indication of whether articles are reviews or editorials and whether published in a language other than English. Corresponds to *Current Awareness in Biological Sciences*.
Language: English
Coverage: International
Time Span: 1983 to date
Updating: Monthly

CURRENT BIOTECHNOLOGY ABSTRACTS
Type: Reference (Bibliographic)
Subject: Biotechnology
Producer: The Royal Society of Chemistry
Online Service: DATA-STAR; ESA-IRS; Pergamon InfoLine
Content: Contains about 12,000 citations, with abstracts, to the worldwide literature on biotechnology. Covers techniques (e.g., genetic manipulation, monoclonal antibodies, enzymology, fermentation technology) and relevant industry activities in such areas as pharmaceuticals, energy production, agriculture, chemicals, and food. Sources include books, monographs, technical and government reports, proceedings, newspapers, patents, and about 200 journals. Users may access citations by subject, substance, or organization name.
Language: English
Coverage: International
Time Span: April 1983 to date
Updating: About 400 records a month

CURRENT CONTENTS SEARCH℠
Type: Reference (Bibliographic)
Subject: Biomedicine; Life Sciences; Science & Technology
Producer: Institute for Scientific Information (ISI)
Online Service: BRS After Dark; BRS/BRKTHRU; BRS; BRS/Colleague
Content: Contains approximately 168,000 citations to articles listed in the tables of contents of leading scientific journals. Covers clinical medicine and life sciences; engineering, technology, and applied sciences; agriculture, biology, and environmental sciences; and physical, chemical, and earth sciences. Includes title, authors, bibliographic data, and, when available, authors' addresses. Corresponds to *Current Contents*.

Language: English
Coverage: International
Time Span: Current 3 months
Updating: About 14,000 records a week

DAILY NEWS, LOS ANGELES
Type: Source (Full Text)
Subject: News
Producer: Tribune Newspapers West, Inc.
Online Service: VU/TEXT Information Services, Inc.
Conditions: Subscription to VU/TEXT required
Content: Contains full text of news items and feature articles from the Los Angeles (California) *Daily News* newspaper. Regional coverage emphasizes the entertainment, high technology, and aerospace industries.
Language: English
Coverage: U.S. (primarily Los Angeles, California area)
Time Span: October 1985 to date
Updating: Daily

DAILY WASHINGTON ADVANCE
Type: Source (Full Text)
Subject: Legislative Tracking
Producer: The Bureau of National Affairs, Inc. (BNA)
Online Service: Dialcom, Inc. (as an AdvanceLine database)
Conditions: Monthly minimum of $10 or $25 to Dialcom, Inc. required
Content: Contains full text of selected articles from *Daily Report for Executives*, covering legal, regulatory, financial, and economic developments in the U.S. courts, Congress, and government agencies. Covers such topics as securities regulation, federal budget information, import and export controls, energy developments, anti-trust and trade regulations, and environmental controls. Sources of information include the *Federal Register*, federal court opinions, and executive department and agency memoranda and proposed and final regulations. Corresponds to Sections A, L, and N of *Daily Report for Executives*.
Language: English
Coverage: U.S.
Time Span: Most recent 6 months
Updating: Daily, by 7:00 A.M. Eastern Time

DARC
Type: Source (Textual-Numeric)
Subject: Chemistry-Structure & Nomenclature
Producer: Telesystemes-Questel
Online Service: Telesystemes-Questel
Content: A database system that provides access to more than 10 million substances contained in the Chemical Abstracts Service (CAS) REGISTRY NOMENCLATURE AND STRUCTURE SERVICE *(see)* and other databases.
EURECAS. Contains all structures, excluding polymers, covered in the Registry Nomenclature and Structure Service (RNSS), from 1965 to date.
POLYCAS. Covers polymers from RNSS, from 1965 to date.
MINICAS. Contains every hundredth compound from EURECAS.
UPCAS. Contains monthly updates to EURECAS and POLYCAS.
INDEX CHEMICUS ONLINE. Contains over 3 million structures

described in the literature since 1962. *(see)*

JANSSEN. *(see)*

Structure searches are entered by typing commands on the keyboard or using a graphics tablet and stylus, to specify substance structures or portions of structures. Users can search for exact structures; substructures, which allow unlimited attachment of atoms or groups of atoms to a partial structure; and generic structures, which allow the user to specify up to 20 atoms or groups of atoms that may be attached to a partial structure. Searches can also specify CAS Registry Numbers, to retrieve the structure diagram and molecular formula. Users can transfer Registry Numbers of retrieved substances to CAS *(see CA SEARCH)* or INDEX CHEMICUS ONLINE *(see)* for subject or bibliographic searching.

Time Span: All substances registered by CAS since 1965

Updating: Over 28,000 new substances a month

DATA BASE DIRECTORY SERVICE® (DBDS)

Type: Reference (Referral)

Subject: Information Systems & Services-Directories

Producer: Knowledge Industry Publications, Inc., in cooperation with the American Society for Information Science

Online Service: BRS; BRS After Dark; BRS/BRKTHRU; BRS/Colleague

Conditions: Annual subscription of $215 to Knowledge Industry Publications includes semiannual printed directory and monthly newsletter updates

Content: Contains descriptions of about 2700 online databases, with an emphasis on databases available in Canada and the U.S. Includes database name, subject, summary of content, producer, vendor, prices, corresponding printed sources, language, original sources of information, time span, file size, restrictions and conditions, and available search aids. Corresponds to *Database Directory* and *Database Alert*.

Language: English

Coverage: Primarily U.S. and Canada, with some international coverage

Time Span: Current information

Updating: Monthly

THE DATA INFORMER

Type: Reference (Referral); Source (Full Text)

Subject: Information Systems & Services; Information Systems & Services-Directories

Producer: Information USA, Inc.

Online Service: NewsNet, Inc.

Conditions: Monthly subscription to NewsNet required

Content: Contains full text of *The Data Informer*, a newsletter providing information of interest to current and potential users of databases. Contains announcements and descriptions of new commercially available databases, free or low-cost government-produced databases, and additional sources of free or low-cost information. Also provides information on available publications, consultants, and software for designing, building, and managing databases.

Language: English

Coverage: International

Time Span: March 1984 to date

Updating: Monthly

DATABASE OF DATABASES

Type: Reference (Referral)

Subject: Information Systems & Services-Directories

Producer: M.E. Williams, Inc., in collaboration with the University of Illinois at Urbana-Champaign, Coordinated Science Laboratory, Information Retrieval Research Laboratory

Online Service: DIALOG Information Services, Inc.

Content: Contains descriptions of about 2800 databases accessible through online and batch-processing systems or available on computer-readable media (e.g., tape, diskette, CD-ROM) for in-house use. Covers bibliographic, full-text, and numeric databases, as well as database modeling systems. Each record contains database name, synonyms, and acronyms; file size, frequency of updating, and time span; language of database and of source material; listing of data elements (e.g., accession number, source title, abstract); producer and vendor; and brief content description. Corresponds to *Computer-Readable Databases: A Directory and Data Sourcebook-Science, Technology, Medicine* and *Computer-Readable Databases: A Directory and Data Sourcebook-Business, Law, Social Science, Humanities*.

Language: English

Coverage: International

Time Span: Current information

Updating: Quarterly

DATABASE OF DATABASES

Type: Reference (Referral)

Subject: Information Systems & Services-Directories

Producer: University of Tsukuba

Online Service: University of Tsukuba

Content: Contains about 800 descriptions of databases currently available worldwide, online or in computer-readable form. Each description includes database name, subject areas, frequency of update, time span, growth rate, languages, size, publication types covered, producer names and addresses, distributor name, and online vendors.

Language: English

Coverage: International

Time Span: Current information

Updating: Every 2 years

DATABASE OF OFF-SITE WASTE MANAGEMENT (DOWM)

Type: Reference (Referral)

Subject: Environment

Producer: Public Data Access, Inc.

Online Service: Chemical Information Systems, Inc., a subsidiary of Fein-Marquart Associates (CIS)

Conditions: Annual subscription fee of $300 to CIS required but fee is waived for educational institutions and non-profit public libraries worldwide

Content: Contains information on 365 commercial hazardous waste disposal facilities, including those operated by 8 of the largest waste disposal firms in the U.S. For each site, provides Environmental Protection Agency (EPA) identification number; name of owning company; facility name, address, county, and EPA region; facility type (e.g., transportation, solid waste disposal); wastes handled and processing capacity; permit status (e.g., operating, closed); dates of violations, enforcement actions, and penalties; spill reports; and data from ground water monitoring equipment. Corresponds to *Hazardous Waste Management: Reducing the Risk*, by the Council on Economic Priorities.

Language: English
Coverage: U.S.
Time Span: Current information

DATAPRO PC-SOFTWARE

Type: Reference (Referral)
Subject: Computers & Software
Producer: Datapro
Online Service: DATA-STAR
Content: Contains about 6700 descriptions of personal computer (PC) software available from about 800 vendors. Includes product name, application, hardware requirements, source language, price, available documentation, summary of capabilities and features, and vendor name, address, and telephone number. Corresponds to *Datapro Software Reports*.
Language: English
Coverage: U.S.
Time Span: 1985 to date
Updating: About 250 products a month

DataStat®

Type: Source (Textual-Numeric)
Subject: Pharmaceuticals & Pharmaceutical Industry
Producer: National Data Corporation, Health Care Data Services Division
Online Service: National Data Corporation, Health Care Data Services Division
Conditions: Monthly subscription fee required
Content: Contains descriptions of drug interactions at the ingredient level for individual drugs and therapeutic classes of drugs. Each interaction is classified according to its level of seriousness to the patient. Also includes drug packaging and pricing data. Sources of data include manufacturers' catalogs and standard pharmaceutical reference works.
Language: English
Coverage: Primarily U.S.
Updating: Weekly

DE HAEN DRUG DATA

Type: Source (Textual-Numeric)
Subject: Pharmaceuticals & Pharmaceutical Industry
Producer: Paul de Haen International, Inc.
Online Service: DIALOG Information Services, Inc.
Content: Contains about 80,000 specially prepared reports on drugs that summarize information from the worldwide biomedical literature, including over 1200 journals, newsletters, and conference papers. Each report provides generic and trade name of drug, manufacturer, country of manufacture, usage status (e.g., investigational), type (e.g., efficacy), description, purpose, and results and conclusions of study. Reports are organized into 4 groups, which can be searched individually or simultaneously.
Drugs in Use (DIU). Covers commercially available and investigational drugs used in clinical studies.
Drugs in Research (DIR). Covers investigational drugs involved in pre-clinical and clinical studies.
ADRIS (Adverse Drug Reactions & Interactions System). Covers adverse reactions and interactions of commercially available and investigational drugs.
Drugs in Prospect (DIP). Covers newly synthesized compounds exhibiting pharmacological activity.

Language: English
Coverage: International
Time Span: 1980 to date
Updating: About 2500 records every 2 months

DEA (ANSA'S ELECTRONIC DOCUMENTATION)

Type: Reference (Bibliographic); Source (Full Text)
Subject: News
Producer: Agenzia ANSA
Online Service: Agenzia ANSA
Conditions: Subscription and monthly minimum required
Content: Contains over 1.2 million citations, with some abstracts, to news items originating at Agenzia ANSA and, through cooperative agreements, at Agence France Presse, Reuters, United Press International, and approximately 50 national news agencies worldwide. Includes full text of selected items since January 1982. Corresponds in part to ANSA's domestic news service.
Language: Italian
Coverage: Primarily Italy, with some international news
Time Span: 1975 to date
Updating: Over 400 records a day

DECHEMA (DECHEMA Chemical Engineering and Biotechnology Abstracts Data Bank)

Type: Reference (Bibliographic)
Subject: Biotechnology
Producer: DECHEMA Deutsche Gesellschaft fuer Chemisches Apparatewesen Chemische Technik und Biotechnologie e.V.; FIZ Chemie GmbH
Online Service: FIZ Technik; STN International
Content: Contains about 85,000 citations, with abstracts, to the worldwide literature in all areas of chemical engineering, biotechnology, chemical equipment manufacturing, chemical manufacturing, plant design and construction, computer-aided design, mathematical models and methods, laboratory techniques, analytical chemistry, safety engineering, hazardous materials, pollution control, environmental protection, energy and raw materials supply and conservation, chemical reaction engineering, catalysis, unit operations, process dynamics and control, measurement, instruments, materials of construction, corrosion and corrosion protection, and operating materials. Corresponds in part to *Literaturkurzberichte Chemische Technik und Biotechnologie* (*Dechema Chemical Engineering and Biotechnology Abstracts*) and *Biotechnologie, Verfahren-Anlagen-Apparate* (*Biotechnology, Processes-Plant-Equipment*).
Language: Titles in English and German, with abstracts primarily in German
Coverage: International
Time Span: 1975 to date
Updating: About 830 records a month

DELTAbank (Drug Effects on Laboratory Tests: Attention)

Type: Reference (Bibliographic); Source (Full Text)
Subject: Biomedicine
Producer: Worldwide Medical Information Ltd., Databank on Drug-Diagnostic Test Interactions

Online Service: DATA-STAR

Content: Contains critically evaluated information on how drugs and other factors (e.g., pregnancy, posture, exercise) can influence the interpretation of medical tests. Abstracts, prepared by biochemists, provide clinical information on patients, treatment details, quantitative reports of test results, summary of authors' conclusions, critical commentary, and references to other articles that confirm or contradict the findings. Citations to original articles include summaries of the type of test, drugs or other factors influencing test results, method used, specimen analyzed, and results. Covers thyroid function, 5HIAA, catecholamines, and TDM drugs. Other tests, including glucose, creatinine, metabolites, therapeutic drugs, uric acid, and liver function will be added. Information is extracted from articles in 35 key journals, supplemented by a review of relevant articles identified in MEDLINE *(see)* searches.

Language: English
Coverage: International
Time Span: 1970 to date
Updating: Quarterly

DEQUIP (DECHEMA Equipment Suppliers Databank)

Type: Reference (Referral)
Subject: Biotechnology
Producer: DECHEMA Deutsche Gesellschaft fuer Chemisches Apparatewesen Chemische Technik und Biotechnologie e.V.; FIZ Chemie GmbH
Online Service: STN International

Content: Contains descriptions of about 10,000 products available in the Federal Republic of Germany for the chemical engineering and biotechnology industries from about 2800 companies worldwide. Covers product categories for computer-aided engineering hardware and software; general and specialized analysis and testing equipment; laboratory instruments and chemicals; pumps, compressors, valves, and fittings; process instrumentation, control, and automation equipment; and equipment for use in mechanical and thermal processes, nuclear and radiochemical applications, materials handling and storage, and safety engineering. Includes manufacturer's name, address, and products. Corresponds in part to *ACHEMA Yearbook (Vol. 3), 1985.*

Language: English, French, and German
Coverage: International
Time Span: Current information
Updating: Periodically, as new data become available

DERMAL ABSORPTION DATA BASE

Type: Reference (Bibliographic); Source (Textual-Numeric)
Subject: Toxicology
Producer: U.S. Environmental Protection Agency (EPA), Office of Pesticides and Toxic Substances
Online Service: Chemical Information Systems, Inc., a subsidiary of Fein-Marquart Associates (CIS); Information Consultants, Inc. (ICI) (as part of The Integrated Chemical Information System)
Conditions: Annual subscription fee of $300 to CIS required but fee is waived for educational institutions and non-profit public libraries worldwide; differential charges for subscribers and non-subscribers to ICI.

Content: Contains about 2900 records of information on the qualitative and quantitative health effects of approximately 575 chemical substances administered to humans and test animals via the dermal route. Each record covers a single experiment and includes chemical identification and characteristics; study protocol; description of test organism; summary results; dosage results; detailed absorption, metabolism, distribution, and excretion data; and bibliographic reference.

Language: English
Coverage: International
Time Span: 1970 to date
Updating: Periodically, as new data become available

DETEQ (Dechema Environmental Technology Equipment Databank)

Type: Reference (Referral)
Subject: Environment
Producer: DECHEMA Deutsche Gesellschaft fuer Chemisches Apparatewesen Chemische Technik und Biotechnologie e.V.; FIZ Chemie GmbH
Online Service: STN International

Content: Contains descriptions of about 2000 environmental technology products from 550 companies that are available in the Federal Republic of Germany. Product categories include computer hardware and software; process instrumentation, control, and automation equipment; laboratory instruments and chemicals; and safety engineering equipment. Includes manufacturer's name and address, as well as distributor information. Corresponds in part to *ACHEMA Handbook Pollution Control*, with additional information online.

Language: English, French, and German
Coverage: International
Time Span: Current information
Updating: Periodically, as new data become available

DETROIT FREE PRESS

Type: Source (Full Text)
Subject: News
Producer: Detroit Free Press, Inc.
Online Service: VU/TEXT Information Services, Inc.
Conditions: Subscription to VU/TEXT required

Content: Contains full text of news items and feature articles from the *Detroit Free Press* (Michigan) newspaper. Regional coverage emphasizes the automobile industry and labor issues.

Language: English
Coverage: U.S. (primarily Michigan)
Time Span: March 1982 to date
Updating: Daily

DEUTSCHE PRESSE AGENTUR

Type: Source (Full Text)
Subject: News
Producer: Deutsche Presse-Agentur GmbH
Online Service: DATA-STAR (EUROPADIENST DATENBANK); Dialcom, Inc.
Conditions: Monthly minimum of $100 to Dialcom, Inc. required

Content: Contains full text of the European, Latin American, and North American sections of the Deutsche Presse-Agentur wire service. Covers current affairs and economic and business news of specific interest to each region.

Language: European newswire, German; Latin American newswire, Spanish; North American newswire, English.
Coverage: DATA-STAR, Europe; BT Dialcom, Latin America and North America.

Time Span: DATA-STAR, September 1984 to date; Dialcom, Inc., current information.

Updating: Continuously, throughout the day; about 500 items a week.

DHSS-DATA

Type: Reference (Bibliographic)

Subject: Health Care; Library Holdings-Catalogs; Social Services

Producer: Department of Health and Social Security (DHSS)

Online Service: DATA-STAR; Scicon Limited

Content: Contains approximately 50,000 citations, some with abstracts, to the holdings of the DHSS library, covering health services, social welfare, and social security. Includes books, pamphlets, reports, articles from over 1500 journals, and government publications originating primarily in the U.K., the U.S., and with the World Health Organization. Covers hospital administration; equipment, planning, design, and construction of health service buildings; housing; nursing and primary health care; social policy and social services administration; social services for children, families, the elderly, and handicapped; and social security and occupational pensions. Currently focuses on new holdings; references to older holdings are to be added in the future.

Language: Primarily English

Coverage: Primarily U.K., with some international coverage

Time Span: Most materials, October 1983 to date; earliest data from 1961.

Updating: About 250 records a week

DIACK NEWSLETTER™

Type: Source (Full Text)

Subject: Health Care

Producer: Diack, Inc.

Online Service: NewsNet, Inc.

Conditions: Monthly subscription to NewsNet required

Content: Contains full text of the *Diack Newsletter*, covering recent developments in the field of medical device sterilization and infection control in surgical and hospital environments. Includes feature articles, summaries of research findings, reviews of recent publications, and news of important professional meetings.

Language: English

Coverage: International

Time Span: April 1983 to date

Updating: Every 2 months

DIANE GUIDE

Type: Reference (Referral)

Subject: Information Systems & Services-Directories

Producer: European Information Market Development Group

Online Service: ECHO Service

Content: Contains descriptions of more than 650 databases available through the Euronet-DIANE network. Also contains references to database producers and online services.

Language: English, French, German, and Italian

Updating: Periodically, as new data become available

DIGITAL VILLAGE℠

Type: Reference (Referral); Source (Full Text, Software)

Subject: Flight Schedules; Computers & Software; News

Producer: Global Villages, Incorporated

Online Service: Global Villages, Incorporated

Content: Provides news, information, and services for users of Digital Equipment Corporation (DEC) personal computers. Includes general and financial news *(see AP NEWS)*, airline schedules and fares *(see OAG-EE and AMERICAN AIRLINES EAASY SABRE)*, and listings of DEC equipment and software for sale. Also provides special interest group forums, an electronic mail service, and software that can be downloaded.

Language: English and Spanish

Coverage: International

Time Span: Current information

Updating: Periodically, as new data become available

DIOGENES℠

Type: Reference (Bibliographic); Source (Full Text)

Subject: Biomedicine; Health Care; Pharmaceuticals & Pharmaceutical Industry

Producer: FOI Services, Inc.; Washington Business Information, Inc.

Online Service: BRS

Content: Contains citations to over 25,000 unpublished Food and Drug Administration (FDA) regulatory documents covering prescription and over-the-counter drugs and medical devices (e.g., sunlamps, pacemakers). Also contains full text of FDA and industry press releases, reports, and newsletters covering the medical, pharmaceutical, and health care industries. Sources include the *FDA Enforcement Report, FDA Drug and Device Product Approvals, Federal Register, Washington Drug Letter, Devices and Diagnostics Letter, GMP Letter, Food and Drug Letter*, and *Washington Health Costs Letter*.

Language: English

Coverage: U.S.

Time Span: Varies by source, with earliest data from 1964

Updating: Weekly

DIRECT-NET℠

Type: Reference (Referral); Source (Software)

Subject: Computers & Software

Producer: Pacific Computer Clearinghouse; PC World Communications, Inc.

Online Service: Direct-Net

Conditions: Annual membership fee of $50 to Direct-Net required

Content: Contains reviews and descriptions of more than 5000 IBM PC-compatible software and hardware products, including compatible microcomputers and peripheral devices. Descriptions include product name, category, manufacturer, and price. Also includes demonstration software that users can download. Users can submit requests for further product information from vendors online. Corresponds to PC World's *Annual Software Review* and *Annual Hardware Review*, with additional data available online.

Language: English

Coverage: U.S.

Time Span: Current information

Updating: Daily

DIRECTORY OF ASSOCIATIONS IN CANADA

Type: Reference (Referral)
Subject: Associations & Foundations-Directories
Producer: Micromedia Limited
Online Service: CISTI, Canadian Online Enquiry Service (CAN/OLE)
Conditions: CISTI accessible only in Canada
Content: Contains information on more than 12,000 international, foreign, national, interprovincial, and provincial associations in Canada. Includes name, address, telephone number, chief officer's name, founding date, number of paid employees, number of members, publications, and schedule of meetings. Corresponds to *Directory of Associations in Canada*, 6th edition, 1985.
Language: English and French
Coverage: Canada
Time Span: Current information
Updating: Quarterly

DIRECTORY OF GRADUATE RESEARCH

Type: Reference (Referral)
Subject: Biographies; Chemistry; Education & Educational Institutions-Directories
Producer: American Chemical Society (ACS)
Online Service: BRS; BRS After Dark; BRS/BRKTHRU; BRS/Colleague; TECH DATA
Content: Contains information on U.S. colleges and universities offering advanced degrees in chemistry and related subjects. Covers institution name and address, administrative officers, relevant department names, general and specialized fields of study, degrees offered, and interdisciplinary programs. Also covers biographical information on faculty members of the degree programs, including name, rank, degrees held, major appointments, publications, and areas of research. Corresponds to *ACS Directory of Graduate Research*.
Language: English
Coverage: U.S. and Canada
Time Span: Current information
Updating: Every 2 years

DIRLINE (Directory of Information Resources Online)

Type: Reference (Referral)
Subject: Information Systems & Services-Directories
Producer: National Library of Medicine, Toxicology Information Program
Online Service: National Library of Medicine (NLM)
Content: Contains references to about 15,000 organizations that provide information in their areas of specialization. Each record contains the organization name, address, telephone number (s) , descriptions of broad and specific subject areas covered, holdings (e.g., databases or document collections) , list of representative publications, types of information services provided, and any fees or restrictions on use. Covers library and information centers, professional societies, university research bureaus and institutions, federal and state agencies, hobby groups, testing stations, citizens' organizations, and industrial laboratories. Corresponds to the NATIONAL REFERRAL CENTER DATA BASE *(see)*, with additional information from the National Health Information Clearinghouse (NHIC) on about 800 health-related organizations.

Language: English
Coverage: Primarily U.S., with some coverage of non-U.S. organizations
Time Span: Current information
Updating: Quarterly, with each NRC entry reviewed every 2 years and each NHIC entry reviewed annually

DISCOVER®

Type: Source (Full Text)
Subject: General Interest; Science & Technology
Producer: Time Inc.
Online Service: Mead Data Central, Inc. (as part of NEXIS MAGAZINES *(see)*) ; VU/TEXT Information Services, Inc. (to be available in 1987)
Conditions: Subscription to Mead Data Central required; subscription to VU/TEXT required.
Content: Contains full text of *Discover*, a general-interest magazine covering scientific and technical trends and developments and their social implications. Includes reviews of science-related books, exhibitions, movies, and television programs.
Language: English
Coverage: International
Time Span: Mead Data Central, October 1980 to date; VU/TEXT, 1985 to date.
Updating: Monthly

DISSERTATION ABSTRACTS ONLINE

Type: Reference (Bibliographic)
Subject: Dissertations
Producer: University Microfilms International
Online Service: BRS; BRS After Dark; BRS/BRKTHRU; BRS/Colleague; DIALOG Information Services, Inc.; TECH DATA; University of Tsukuba
Content: Contains citations, with abstracts (since 1980) , to all dissertations accepted for doctoral degrees by accredited U.S. educational institutions and over 200 non-U.S. institutions. Corresponds to the coverage in *Dissertation Abstracts International* (DAI) , *American Doctoral Dissertations* (ADD) , and *Comprehensive Dissertation Index*. On DIALOG and BRS, the database also contains citations to masters' theses corresponding to the coverage in *Masters Abstracts* (MA) .
Language: English
Coverage: International
Time Span: DAI and ADD, 1861 to date; MA, 1962 to date.
Updating: About 2500 DAI records a month and 3000 ADD records a year; 600 MA records added quarterly.

DITR

Type: Reference (Bibliographic)
Subject: Standards & Specifications
Producer: Deutsches Institut fuer Normung e.V., Deutsches Informationszentrum fuer technische Regeln
Online Service: Deutsches Institut fuer Normung e.V. (DIN) , Deutsches Informationszentrum fuer technische Regeln (DITR) ; FIZ Technik
Content: Contains about 40,000 citations, most with abstracts, to German technical rules and standards currently valid in the Federal Republic of Germany. Corresponds to *DIN Catalogue of Technical Rules*.
Language: English and German

Coverage: Federal Republic of Germany
Time Span: Current information
Updating: DIN, monthly; FIZ Technik, quarterly.

DOBIS

Type: Reference (Bibliographic)
Subject: Library Holdings-Catalogs
Producer: National Library of Canada
Online Service: National Library of Canada, Library Systems Centre
Conditions: Accessible only in Canada; monthly subscription required. Non-library institutions have search-only access.
Content: Contains about 4 million bibliographic records of books, monographs, serials, theses, federal and provincial documents, microfiche, music, and other publications or media available in over 300 Canadian libraries. The system provides shared-cataloging access for Canadian libraries and search services only for non-library institutions. All users can search by names, titles, subjects, and various classifications, including Library of Congress (LC) numbers. Sources include the National Library of Canada, CISTI, the Library of Parliament, and several federal libraries, including those of Public Works Canada, Statistics Canada, and the Finance/Treasury Board. Corresponds entirely or in part to several print, microfiche, or other online databases, described below.

Canadiana. Includes cataloging records for monographs, serials, and federal and provincial documents on Canada-related topics. Corresponds to all records in the printed version (from 1951 to date) and microfiche version (from 1973 to date for monographs, 1975 to date for serials and government documents). Excludes pre-1981 pamphlets.

Canadian Theses Microfiche and **Canadian Theses-Printed Version.** Includes citations to all Canadian masters and doctoral theses microfilmed, published, and cataloged by the National Library of Canada since 1981, all theses accepted by Canadian universities not participating in the microfilm program, and all theses of Canadian authorship or association accepted by universities outside Canada and cataloged by the National Library. The print version, which ceased with the introduction of the microfiche format, covers from 1963 to date.

CONSER Microfiche. Includes CONSER records authenticated by the National Library of Canada, ISDS Canada, the Library of Congress, the National Serials Data Program, and the U.S. Government Printing Office.

Canadiana Authorities (Microfiche) (formerly CAN/MARC Authorities). Covers all Anglo-American Cataloguing Rules (AACR2) authorities, including name and uniform (constructed) headings used in *Canadiana*, all name headings authenticated by the National Library of Canada for the Library of Congress since 1976, names from the Canadian Institute for Historical Microreproductions, and names from the National Map Collection of the Public Archives of Canada.

LC MARC Fiche. Includes all Library of Congress records for English-language books published since 1965, "popular" titles published since 1900, and records for monographs in over 35 Roman-alphabet languages.

Union List of Serials in the Social Sciences and Humanities Held by Canadian Libraries. Includes citations to more than 44,000 serials in the social sciences and humanities. Excludes newspapers, law reports, city directories, telephone directories, and unnumbered series.

Union List of Scientific Serials in Canadian Libraries. Contains over 65,000 titles of serials covering scientific, technical, and medical subjects.

Canadian Locations of Journals Indexed for MEDLINE. (*see MEDLINE*)

Cataloguing in Publication (CIP). Includes Canadian and U.S. cataloging data on books in the process of publication. Coverage is limited to quality paperbacks, textbooks, reference books, children's books, art books, monographic loose-leaf services, and monographs published by some government agencies.

Union Catalogue of Library Materials for the Handicapped (CANUC:H) and **Registry of Canadian Works in Progress (CANWIP).** Includes records of special media materials, as well as materials planned for production, for use by the handicapped.

Subsets of this database are available separately through CISTI, Canadian Online Enquiry Service.
Language: English and French
Coverage: Libraries in Canada
Updating: Weekly; about 400,000 records a year.

DOW JONES TEXT-SEARCH SERVICES℠

Type: Source (Full Text)
Subject: News
Producer: Dow Jones & Company, Inc.
Online Service: DATA-STAR; Dow Jones & Company, Inc.
Conditions: Annual minimum of $12 or monthly minimum of $3 to Dow Jones required
Content: Consists of 4 files of business and financial news. Covers over 6000 U.S. companies, 700 Canadian companies, and 50 industries. Users can search by company name and personal names, corporate stock symbol, industry and government codes, and miscellaneous codes (e.g., for ticker news, current-day earnings, economic news, foreign news).

THE BUSINESS LIBRARY. Contains full text of *American Banker, Financial World, Forbes, Inc.*, and *PR Newswire (see)*.

DOW JONES NEWS. Contains selected articles and news stories from *The Wall Street Journal, Barron's*, and Dow Jones News Service ("Broadtape").

THE WALL STREET JOURNAL. Contains full text of news articles from every edition of *The Wall Street Journal*. Does not include Digest of Earnings tables, Dividends Reported and Futures Prices, stock tables, and advertisements.

THE WASHINGTON POST. *(see THE ELECTRONIC WASHINGTON POST LIBRARY)*

Language: English
Coverage: Primarily U.S. and Canada, with some international news
Time Span: DOW JONES NEWS, June 1979 to date; THE WALL STREET JOURNAL, 1984 to date; THE WASHINGTON POST, 1984 to date; THE BUSINESS LIBRARY, 1985 to date.
Updating: DOW JONES NEWS, THE WALL STREET JOURNAL, and THE WASHINGTON POST, daily; THE BUSINESS LIBRARY, monthly.

DRUG INFORMATION FULLTEXT℠

Type: Reference (Bibliographic); Source (Full Text)
Subject: Pharmaceuticals & Pharmaceutical Industry
Producer: American Society of Hospital Pharmacists
Online Service: BRS; BRS After Dark; BRS/BRKTHRU; BRS/Colleague; DIALOG Information Services, Inc.; Knowledge Index; Mead Data Central, Inc. (as a MEDIS database (*see*)); TECH DATA
Conditions: Subscription to Mead Data Central required
Content: Contains full text of about 1200 monographs covering about 50,000 commercially available and experimental drugs in the U.S. Covers uses, interactions, pharmacokinetics, dosage, administration, chemistry, stability, adverse reactions, and preparation information. Also includes Chemical

Abstracts Service Registry Numbers, trade names, manufacturers, and references to journal articles. Corresponds to *American Hospital Formulary Service Drug Information* and *Handbook on Injectable Drugs*; references are available only online.

Language: English
Coverage: U.S.
Time Span: Current information
Updating: Quarterly

DRUGINFO and ALCOHOL USE/ABUSE

Type: Reference (Bibliographic)
Subject: Health Care; Psychology
Producer: University of Minnesota, Drug Information Services
Online Service: BRS; BRS/BRKTHRU; BRS/Colleague; TECH DATA
Content: Contains 2 files on alcohol and drug use/abuse that may be searched together or separately.

DRUGINFO. Contains citations, with abstracts, to monographs, journals, conference papers, instructional guides, and other materials that deal with the educational, sociological, medical, and psychological aspects of alcohol and drug use/abuse. Beginning in 1980 this file also covers research and problems of alcohol use/abuse.

ALCOHOL USE/ABUSE. Contains citations, with abstracts, to journal articles, reprints, unpublished papers, and chapters from books that deal with research in the area of chemical dependency. Includes coverage of the evaluation of treatments, family therapy, use of the Minnesota Multiphasic Personality Inventory (MMPI), and selected materials dealing with alcohol use/abuse problems of adolescents and the elderly.

Language: English
Coverage: International
Time Span: DRUGINFO, 1968 to date; ALCOHOL USE/ABUSE, 1968 to 1978.
Updating: Quarterly

DRUGLINE

Type: Reference (Referral); Source (Full Text)
Subject: Pharmaceuticals & Pharmaceutical Industry
Producer: Huddinge Hospital, Drug Information Center, in cooperation with MIC-KIBIC
Online Service: MIC-KIBIC
Conditions: Contract with Drug Information Center required
Content: Contains over 2000 questions received and answers prepared by clinical pharmacologists at the Drug Information Center. Topics are indexed by Medical Subject Headings (MeSH).
Language: Primarily Swedish, with some items and all indexing in English
Coverage: Scandinavia
Time Span: 1982 to date
Updating: About 200 items a quarter

DUNDIS (Directory of United Nations Databases and Information Systems)

Type: Reference (Referral)
Subject: Information Systems & Services-Directories
Producer: United Nations, Advisory Committee for the Co-ordination of Information Systems (ACCIS)

Online Service: Battelle, Centre de Recherches; ECHO Service; International Computing Centre
Content: Contains descriptions of 700 computerized and non-computerized databases and information services available within the United Nations network.
Language: English, French, and Spanish
Coverage: International
Time Span: Current information
Updating: Periodically, as new data become available

EABS (Euroabstracts)

Type: Reference (Bibliographic)
Subject: Science & Technology
Producer: Commission of the European Communities (CEC)
Online Service: ECHO Service
Content: Contains over 40,000 citations, with abstracts (since 1984), to reports of research results from projects funded (or partially funded) by the European Economic Community and to proceedings of conferences sponsored by the CEC, the European Coal and Steel Community, and Euratom. Covers research in nuclear science and technology, new energy sources, environment, medicine, biology, agriculture, and coal and steel technology. Coverage relates to *Euro-Abstracts, Sections I and II*.
Language: English, French, and German
Coverage: Europe
Time Span: 1968 to date; Euratom records, 1966 to date.
Updating: About 200 records a month

EAST EUROPEAN CHEMICAL AND PHARMACEUTICAL DATABASE

Type: Reference (Bibliographic); Source (Full Text)
Subject: Pharmaceuticals & Pharmaceutical Industry
Producer: Business International S/A
Online Service: DATA-STAR (to be available in 1987)
Content: Contains citations, with abstracts, and some full-text translations of eastern European periodical literature on the pharmaceutical and chemical industries. Covers organic, inorganic, and base chemicals, as well as the related fields of agrochemicals, plastics and rubber, chemical fibers, cosmetics, paints and dyes, photochemicals, and petrochemicals. Primary sources are 85 cyrillic-language news sources, including newspapers (e.g., *Pravda, Izvestiya, Ekonomicheskaya Gazeta* from the Soviet Union; *Malrocznik Ftatystyczny* from Poland; *Plaste und Kautschuk* from the Democratic Republic of Germany; *Rude Pravo* from Czechoslovakia) and news agencies (e.g., TASS, from the Soviet Union; Tanjug, from Yugoslavia; PAP, from Poland; CTK, from Czechoslovakia). Corresponds to *East European Monitor: The Chemical Industry, a Monthly Report on Chemicals and Related Industries in Eastern Europe*.
Language: English
Coverage: Soviet-bloc countries and Yugoslavia
Time Span: 1984 to date
Updating: Monthly

ECDIN (Environmental Chemicals Data and Information Network)

Type: Reference (Bibliographic); Source (Textual-Numeric)
Subject: Chemistry-Properties; Chemistry-Structure & Nomenclature; Environment; Toxicology

Producer: Commission of the European Communities (CEC), Joint Research Centre
Online Service: Datacentralen
Content: Contains information on chemical substances in the environment, providing chemical identification data on approximately 63,000 chemical compounds, acute toxicity data on approximately 20,000 compounds, and additional data for about 2000 chemical substances. Is divided into the following files: Chemical Substances (Registry Numbers), including ECDIN Registry Name and Number, Chemical Abstracts Service Registry Number, European Customs Union Number, and Registry of Toxic Effects of Chemical Substances *(see RTECS)* Number; International Registry of Potential Toxic Chemicals (IRPTC) -Legal; Chemical Synonyms (Names); Physico-Chemical Properties; Chemical Structures, including Wiswesser Line Notation and chemical structure diagram; Chemical Processes; Uses; Production and Trade Statistics; Occupational Safety and Health, covering hazard information, general recommendations for human safety, personal protection, and medical and biological surveillance; Occupational Exposure Limits; Directive 67/548/EEC (Dangerous Substances-Hazard Classification); Classical Toxicity, including organism, exposure, effects, test conditions, and bibliographic data; Aquatic Toxicity, including organism, exposure, effects, test conditions, and bibliographic data; Effects on Microorganisms, including organism, exposure, effects, test conditions, and bibliographic data; Odor and Taste Threshold Concentrations; Analytical Methods; Carcinogenicity; Mutagenicity; Concentration in Human Media, including range and mean concentration values, biological media, pathology, and morphology; Concentration in Animal Media; Concentration in Environmental Matrices; Metabolism in Soil; and Chemical Producers.
Language: English, with chemical names, safety risks, and warning data also in Danish, Dutch, French, German, and Italian
Coverage: International
Updating: Periodically, as new data become available

ECOTHEK

Type: Reference (Bibliographic)
Subject: Environment
Producer: Institut d'Amenagement et d'Urbanisme de la Region d'Ile-de-France (IAURIF)
Online Service: Telesystemes-Questel
Content: Contains over 30,000 citations, with abstracts, to French literature on urban and regional planning and the local ecology of France. Covers oceans, air, water, climate, geography, subsoil, topography, agriculture, forests, flora and fauna, ecology, pollution, transportation, and development. Cited documents include journal articles, reports, books, maps and atlases, theses, conference proceedings, and pamphlets.
Language: French
Coverage: France
Time Span: 1970 to date, with earliest documents from 1882
Updating: Monthly

EDICLINE INFO

Type: Source (Full Text)
Subject: Information Systems & Services
Producer: EDICLINE
Online Service: EDICLINE
Content: Contains information of interest to users of EDICLINE databases. Includes database prices, conditions of access, announcements of user group meetings, and reports on user problems and system changes.

Language: English and German
Time Span: Current information
Updating: Weekly

EDMARS (Educational Document Management and Retrieval System)

Type: Reference (Bibliographic)
Subject: Education & Educational Institutions
Producer: University of Gifu; University of Osaka; Kyoto University of Education; National Institute for Educational Research; University of Tsukuba
Online Service: University of Tsukuba
Content: Contains approximately 95,000 citations, with abstracts, to Japanese journal literature on education.
Language: Japanese
Coverage: Japan
Time Span: 1933 to date
Updating: Periodically, as new data become available

EDUCATION DAILY ONLINE

Type: Source (Full Text)
Subject: Education & Educational Institutions
Producer: Capitol Publications, Inc.
Online Service: SpecialNet (as a SpecialNet database *(see)*)
Conditions: Annual subscription of $425 to Capitol Publications required
Content: Contains full text of *Education Daily*, covering state and federal policies, legislation, and funding of education programs. Also contains news of court cases, civil rights issues, special education, research, and administration.
Language: English
Coverage: U.S.
Time Span: Most current 3 weeks
Updating: Daily

EDUCATION INDEX^{SM}

Type: Reference (Bibliographic)
Subject: Education & Educational Institutions
Producer: The H.W. Wilson Company
Online Service: WILSONLINE
Content: Contains about 50,000 citations to articles, interviews, selected editorials and letters to the editor, and reviews of books, educational films, and software from approximately 350 English-language periodicals, monographs, and yearbooks in the field of education. Covers school administration; pre-school, elementary, secondary, higher, and adult education; counseling and personnel services; teacher and vocational education; and teaching methods. Also covers a wide variety of individual curriculum areas, including the arts, comparative and international education, health and physical education, language and linguistics, library and information science, multi-cultural and ethnic education, psychology and mental health, religious education, science and mathematics, social studies, special education and rehabilitation, and educational research. Corresponds to *Education Index.*
Language: English
Coverage: International
Time Span: September 1983 to date
Updating: Twice a week; about 3000 records a month.

EDUCATIONAL RESEARCH FORUM (Ed R & D)

Type: Source (Full Text)

Subject: Education & Educational Institutions

Producer: American Educational Research Association

Online Service: CompuServe Information Service

Content: Contains news and information on educational research, teaching, counseling, and school administration. Covers such areas as curriculum and instruction, learning and cognition, teacher and professional education, postsecondary education, statistics and research methodology, counseling, the history and sociology of education, and education in non-school professions. Includes summaries of articles published by the American Educational Research Association, news of government policies as they affect educational research, and listings of job opportunities. Users can submit messages, questions, and comments through an electronic bulletin board.

Language: English

Coverage: U.S.

Time Span: October 1982 to date

Updating: Periodically, as new data become available

EDUQ

Type: Reference (Bibliographic, Referral)

Subject: Education & Educational Institutions

Producer: Ministere de l'Education du Quebec

Online Service: IST-Informatheque Inc.

Content: Contains about 4000 citations, with abstracts, to monographs, serials, films, magnetic tapes, and disks related to education in Quebec, Canada. Covers preschool, primary, secondary, post-secondary, and adult education. Includes items on school administration (statistics, personnel, and policy); educational activities; educational psychology and philosophy; parents and community activities; pedagogical developments; and innovations in curriculum.

Language: English and French

Coverage: Canada (Quebec)

Time Span: 1960 to date

Updating: About 500 records twice a year

EdVENT

Type: Reference (Referral)

Subject: Conferences & Meetings; Education & Educational Institutions

Producer: Timeplace, Inc.

Online Service: CompuServe Information Service; Timeplace, Inc.

Conditions: Annual subscription of $1250 to Timeplace, Inc. required

Content: Contains descriptions of approximately 120,000 seminars, conferences, workshops, and other continuing-education courses offered by about 5000 organizations in the U.S. Includes course title and summary, prerequisites (if any), target audiences, cost, dates, location, duration, instructor, credits granted, and sponsor information. Users can request additional information from sponsors or register for courses online.

Language: English

Coverage: Primarily U.S. and Canada, with some international coverage

Time Span: Current information

Updating: Every 2 weeks

Ei ENGINEERING MEETINGS®

Type: Reference (Bibliographic)

Subject: Conferences & Meetings; Bioengineering

Producer: Engineering Information, Inc.

Online Service: Centre de Documentation de l'Armement (CEDOCAR) (Ei ENGINEERING MEETINGS); CISTI, Canadian Online Enquiry Service (CAN/OLE) (EiM); DATA-STAR (EiEM); DIALOG Information Services, Inc. (Ei ENGINEERING MEETINGS); ORBIT Information Technologies Corporation; STN International (MEET)

Conditions: CISTI accessible only in Canada

Content: Contains over 380,000 citations, with abstracts (since January 1985), to published proceedings from approximately 2000 engineering and technical conferences, symposia, meetings, and colloquia held worldwide. Each meeting is referenced in a main record; all papers are referenced individually. Each record includes a complete bibliographic reference, conference sponsor and location, language, date held, and assigned index terms. Covers a wide variety of engineering disciplines including civil, environmental, geological, bioengineering, electrical and electronics, mechanical, nuclear, agricultural and food, metals and mining, industrial management, petroleum and fuel, control devices and principles, communication engineering, applied mathematics and physics, information science, automotive, and aerospace. Beginning in July 1982, review abstracts of conferences are also contained in COMPENDEX (see). Corresponds to *Engineering Conference Index*.

Language: Primarily English

Coverage: International

Time Span: July 1982 to date, with selected coverage of meetings from 1979 to June 1982

Updating: About 9000 records a month; total of about 2000 meetings a year.

THE ELECTRIC PAGES

Type: Reference (Bibliographic, Referral); Source (Full Text)

Subject: News

Producer: The Electric Pages and others, including Sports On-Line, Inc. and the Texas Computer Education Association

Online Service: The Electric Pages

Conditions: Initiation fee of $40 required

Content: Contains a variety of information sources and services, with an emphasis on education and general information of interest in the Austin (Texas) region.

EDUCATIONAL MICRO REVIEW. Contains citations, with abstracts, to selected articles from 26 computer-related periodicals. Covers items related to software for educational administration and instruction and announcements and reviews of business software.

REALLY IMPORTANT COMMUNITY KNOWLEDGE & INFORMATION. Contains information on community volunteer, rape crisis, and child abuse prevention centers.

SPORTS ON-LINE. Contains local sports scores, news, and statistics; ticket information for local events; and scores and highlights of major national sports events. Produced by Sports On-Line, Inc.

TEXAS COMPUTER EDUCATION ASSOCIATION ELECTRONIC RESOURCE CENTER. Contains news of noteworthy developments in various teaching specialties (e.g., history, health) in Texas public schools. Includes descriptions of instructional programs, profiles of teachers, and relevant software. Produced by the Texas Computer Education Association.

TEXAS PARKS & WILDLIFE ONLINE. Contains information

on outdoor recreation (e.g., hunting, fishing, boating) in Texas. Includes reports (e.g., weekly fishing conditions), maps, and directories (e.g., state park wildlife management areas, hunter and boater education courses).

THE ELECTRIC PAGES MAGAZINE. Contains stories on various topics, including general interest (e.g., "Starting a Read-Aloud Program With Your Children"), computer-related topics, business, and education. Also contains book, movie, and entertainment reviews.

NOTE: Also contains numerous user-submitted "columns" and bulletin boards. An electronic mail service is also available.

Language: English
Coverage: U.S. (primarily Austin, Texas area)
Time Span: Current information
Updating: Daily

ELECTRIC POWER INDUSTRY ABSTRACTS

Type: Reference (Bibliographic)
Subject: Environment
Producer: Utility Data Institute for the Edison Electric Institute
Online Service: ORBIT Information Technologies Corporation (EPIA)
Content: Contains citations, with abstracts, to literature on the environmental aspects of new power plants and related facilities. Major topics covered include environmental effects of electric power plants that use nuclear, oil, coal, gas, hydroelectric, geothermal, or solar energy and associated transmission lines; power plant siting methodologies; fuel transportation, storage, and use; licensing and permit data; monitoring programs; land use studies; coastal zone management plans; waste disposal facilities; and safety and risk assessment. Covers technical reports and studies prepared by the electric utilities and their consultants, as well as reports prepared by such federal agencies as the Nuclear Regulatory Commission, U.S. Department of Energy, Bureau of Land Management, U.S. Environmental Protection Agency, Bureau of Reclamation, U.S. Army Corps of Engineers, U.S. Forest Service, U.S. Fish and Wildlife Service, and Rural Electrification Administration. Coverage also includes reports by state agencies, siting commissions and control boards, as well as selected journal articles, conference proceedings, and testimony from Congressional hearings.
Language: English
Coverage: U.S.
Time Span: 1975 to 1984
Updating: Not updated

ELECTRONIC DIRECTORY OF EDUCATION®

Type: Reference (Referral)
Subject: Education & Educational Institutions-Directories
Producer: Market Data Retrieval, Inc.
Online Service: DIALOG Information Services, Inc.
Content: Contains information about educational institutions in the U.S. Covers 3200 colleges and universities, 100,000 schools, 15,000 districts and dioceses, 50 state departments of education, and 15,000 main-branch public libraries. Each record includes institution name, address, and telephone number; names of administrators; enrollment and budget data; and lists of special facilities and services (e.g., special education, vocational education, microcomputer instruction).

Language: English
Coverage: U.S.
Time Span: Current information
Updating: Twice a year

THE ELECTRONIC MAGAZINE

Type: Source (Full Text)
Subject: Computers & Software; Information Systems & Services-Directories
Producer: Learned Information Ltd.
Online Service: ESA-IRS
Content: Contains full text of short articles, news items, product reviews, and book reviews on computers, software, and related technologies. Emphasis is on electronic publishing, online retrieval, library systems, and other information industry applications. Includes authors, titles, and keywords, as well as products, services, and organizations mentioned in each item. Also includes full text of the *Eusidic Database Guide*, which covers over 1750 databases worldwide.
Language: English
Coverage: International
Time Span: August 1984 to date
Updating: Weekly

THE ELECTRONIC WASHINGTON POST LIBRARY℠

Type: Source (Full Text)
Subject: News
Producer: The Washington Post Company
Online Service: Datasolve Limited (as a WORLD REPORTER database *(see)*); DIALOG Information Services, Inc. (WASHINGTON POST ELECTRONIC EDITION); Dow Jones & Company, Inc. (as a DOW JONES TEXT-SEARCH SERVICES database *(see)*); Mead Data Central, Inc. (WPOST) (as part of NEXIS NEWSPAPERS *(see)*); VU/TEXT Information Services, Inc.
Conditions: Annual minimum of $12 or monthly minimum of $3 to Dow Jones required; subscription to Mead Data Central required; subscription to VU/TEXT required.
Content: Contains full text of staff-written news items and feature stories from *The Washington Post* (District of Columbia) newspaper. For each article, includes day and date, edition, section, page, headline, byline, and length.
Language: English
Coverage: Primarily U.S., with some international coverage
Time Span: Mead Data Central, January 17, 1977 to date; DIALOG, April 1983 to date; VU/TEXT, April 16, 1983 to date; Dow Jones, 1984 to date; Datasolve, January 12, 1984 to date.
Updating: Daily

THE ELECTRONIC WASHINGTON POST NEWSLETTER℠

Type: Source (Full Text)
Subject: News
Producer: The Washington Post Company
Online Service: CompuServe Information Service; LEGI-SLATE, Inc.; THE SOURCE
Conditions: Monthly minimum of $10 to THE SOURCE required, with $9 credited toward online usage charges
Content: Contains full text, with brief summaries, of stories selected from the current day's edition of *The Washington Post*. Covers the following areas, with an emphasis on the federal government: the administration, Congress, business and economy, science and technology, the courts and the law, politics, the world and the nation, editorials and commentary, and news summaries and calendars.

Language: English
Coverage: Primarily U.S., with some international coverage
Time Span: THE SOURCE, current five days; CompuServe, current day; LEGI-SLATE, September 1984 to current day.
Updating: About 40 to 80 stories a day

ELEPHANT WALK COMPUTERS
Type: Reference (Referral)
Subject: Computers & Software
Producer: Elephant Walk Computers, Inc.
Online Service: THE SOURCE
Conditions: Monthly minimum of $10 to THE SOURCE required, with $9 credited toward online usage charges
Content: Contains descriptions of microcomputer products that may be ordered online from the producer of the database. Covers products for Apple and IBM computers, including printers, disk drives, modems, and software.
Language: English
Coverage: U.S.
Time Span: 1983 to date
Updating: Periodically, as new data become available

ELFIS (Ernahrungs-, Land- und Forstwissenschaftliches Informationssystem)
Type: Reference (Bibliographic)
Subject: Agriculture; Food Sciences & Nutrition; Veterinary Sciences
Producer: Zentralstelle fuer Agrardokumentation und -information (ZADI)
Online Service: DIMDI
Content: Contains over 23,000 citations to journals, research reports, conference proceedings, and other literature on agriculture, veterinary science, and food sciences and technology. Covers microbiology, biotechnology, grasslands farming, forage growing, plant breeding, timber industry, viticulture, phytomedicine, sugar technology, horticulture, veterinary science, animal production, cereal processing, brewing industry, food processing and packaging, labor management, conservation, and landscape management.
Language: German
Coverage: Federal Republic of Germany
Time Span: 1984 to date
Updating: About 1500 records a month

ELIAS (Environment Libraries Automated System)
Type: Reference (Bibliographic)
Subject: Environment; Library Holdings-Catalogs
Producer: Environment Canada, Departmental Library Branch
Online Service: CISTI, Canadian Online Enquiry Service (CAN/OLE)
Conditions: CISTI accessible only in Canada
Content: Contains citations to the holdings of approximately 65 participating libraries. Covers fully cataloged records for serials, monographs, conferences, proceedings, and technical reports. Subjects covered include conservation and natural resources, environmental impact analysis, environmental management, forestry, land use, meteorology and climatology, pollution, water resources, wildlife, national parks and reserves, historical sites, history, outdoor recreation, archaeology, tourism, architecture, and restoration.

Language: English and French
Coverage: Canada
Time Span: 1976 to date
Updating: About 1200 records a quarter

ELSA
Type: Source (Full Text)
Subject: News
Producer: Schweizerische Depeschenagentur AG
Online Service: DATA-STAR
Content: Contains full text of stories from the news wires of the producer, the Swiss National News Agency (SNA). Covers political, economic, and social news.
ATSA. Contains approximately 110,000 stories in French.
SDAA. Contains approximately 170,000 stories in German.
Language: ATSA, French; SDAA, German.
Coverage: International, with emphasis on Switzerland and Western Europe
Time Span: ATSA, 1984 to date; SDAA, 1983 to date.
Updating: About 400 stories a day

ELSS® (Electronic Legislative Search System)
Type: Reference (Referral)
Subject: Legislative Tracking
Producer: Commerce Clearing House, Inc. (CCH)
Online Service: General Electric Information Services Company (GEISCO)
Conditions: Initiation fee and annual usage minimum to CCH required
Content: A legislative bill tracking service that contains histories of business and tax bills and resolutions introduced during the current regular and special legislative sessions in all 50 states and the U.S. Congress. Information on each item includes jurisdiction (federal or state); bill number, title, and abstract; sponsor; date of introduction; history, from committee activities through executive action; and public act numbers and effective dates for enacted legislation. Vote counts for federal legislation are also available.
Language: English
Coverage: U.S. federal and all 50 states
Time Span: Current legislative session
Updating: Daily

EMBASE℠
Type: Reference (Bibliographic)
Subject: Bioengineering; Biomedicine; Biotechnology; Environment; Health Care; Pharmaceuticals & Pharmaceutical Industry; Toxicology
Producer: Elsevier Science Publishers b.v.
Online Service: BRS; BRS/BRKTHRU; BRS/Colleague; DATA-STAR; DIALOG Information Services, Inc.; DIMDI; TECH DATA; The Japan Information Center of Science and Technology (JICST); University of Tsukuba
Content: Contains over 2.9 million citations, with abstracts, to the worldwide biomedical literature on human medicine and areas of biological sciences related to human medicine. Covers anatomy, anthropology, anesthesiology, biochemistry, bioengineering, cancer, dermatology, developmental biology, drug adverse reactions, drug dependence, drug effects, endocrinology, environmental health and pollution control, forensic science, genetics, gerontology and geriatrics, health econom-

ics, hematology, hospital management, immunology, internal medicine, microbiology, neurology, nuclear medicine, obstetrics and gynecology, occupational health and industrial medicine, ophthalmology, otorhinolaryngology, pathology, pediatrics, pharmacology, physiology, psychiatry, public health, radiology, rehabilitation, surgery, toxicology, and urology. Approximately 40% of the citations added to the database each year do not appear in the corresponding printed abstract journals and indexes.

Language: English

Coverage: International

Time Span: Most services, 1974 to date; BRS, BRS/Colleague, and JICST, 1980 to date.

Updating: Most services, 20,000 records a month; BRS, BRS/Colleague, and DIALOG, 10,000 records twice a month; DATA-STAR, weekly.

EMBL NUCLEOTIDE SEQUENCE DATA LIBRARY

Type: Reference (Bibliographic); Source (Textual-Numeric)

Subject: Biotechnology

Producer: European Molecular Biology Laboratory (EMBL)

Online Service: Bionet; IntelliGenetics, Inc., An IntelliCorp Company; Protein Identification Resource (PIR), National Biomedical Research Foundation (NBRF)

Conditions: To access through Bionet, users must be qualified principal investigators employed by a non-profit organization

Content: Contains nucleotide sequences for over 1500 genes in approximately 3 million bases. Information for each sequence includes title, species, nucleotide composition, length, promoter and gene regions, topology, nucleic acid sequence, and literature references. Sequences are from eukaryote, prokaryote, virus, bacteriophage genetic DNA or RNA, MRNA, and functional RNA molecules.

Language: English

Coverage: International

Time Span: Current information

Updating: IntelliGenetics, Inc., twice a year; all others, annually.

EMCANCER®

Type: Reference (Bibliographic)

Subject: Biomedicine

Producer: Elsevier Science Publishers b.v.

Online Service: DIMDI

Content: Contains citations, with abstracts, to the worldwide literature on cancer. Corresponds to the "Cancer" section of *Excerpta Medica* and to citations from this section contained in EMBASE *(see)*.

Language: English

Coverage: International

Time Span: 1974 to date

Updating: About 2300 records a month

EMDRUGS®

Type: Reference (Bibliographic)

Subject: Biomedicine; Pharmaceuticals & Pharmaceutical Industry

Producer: Elsevier Science Publishers b.v.

Online Service: DIMDI

Content: Contains citations, with abstracts, to the worldwide literature on drugs. Corresponds to the "Pharmacology," "Drug Literature Index," and "Adverse Reactions Titles" sections of *Excerpta Medica* and to citations from those sections contained in EMBASE *(see)*.

Language: English

Coverage: International

Time Span: 1974 to date

Updating: About 9000 records a month

EMFORENSIC®

Type: Reference (Bibliographic)

Subject: Biomedicine; Forensic Sciences & Services

Producer: Elsevier Science Publishers b.v.

Online Service: DIMDI

Content: Contains citations, with abstracts, to the worldwide literature on forensic sciences. Corresponds to the "Forensic Sciences Abstracts" section of *Excerpta Medica* and to the citations from that section contained in EMBASE *(see)*.

Language: English

Coverage: International

Time Span: 1974 to date

Updating: About 300 records a month

EMHEALTH®

Type: Reference (Bibliographic)

Subject: Biomedicine; Health Care

Producer: Elsevier Science Publishers b.v.

Online Service: DIMDI

Content: Contains citations, with abstracts, to the worldwide literature on public health. Corresponds to the "Public Health, Social Medicine, and Hygiene," "Occupational Health and Industrial Medicine," and "Environmental Health and Pollution Control" sections of *Excerpta Medica* and to the citations from those sections contained in EMBASE *(see)*.

Language: English

Coverage: International

Time Span: 1974 to date

Updating: About 2500 records a month

EMTOX®

Type: Reference (Bibliographic)

Subject: Toxicology

Producer: Elsevier Science Publishers b.v.

Online Service: DIMDI

Content: Contains citations, with abstracts, to the worldwide literature on drug toxicity and environmental toxicology. Corresponds to the "Toxicology" and "Pharmacology and Toxicology" sections of *Excerpta Medica* and to the citations from those sections contained in EMBASE *(see)*.

Language: English

Coverage: International

Time Span: 1974 to date

Updating: About 1000 records a month

ENCYCLOPAEDIA BRITANNICA

Type: Source (Full Text)

Subject: Encyclopedias

Producer: Encyclopaedia Britannica, Inc.

Online Service: Mead Data Central, Inc. (EB) (as a NEXIS database)

Conditions: Subscription to Mead Data Central required

Content: Contains the full text of the *Encyclopaedia Britannica*, revised as of 1982. Covers the 10-volume *Micropaedia*, which contains important facts in capsule form; the 19-volume *Macropaedia*, which provides comprehensive information on a wide range of subjects; and the *Encyclopaedia Britannica Book of the Year*, *Science and the Future*, and the *Medical and Health Annual*.

Language: English

ENCYCLOPEDIA OF ASSOCIATIONS

Type: Reference (Referral)

Subject: Associations & Foundations-Directories

Producer: Gale Research Company

Online Service: DIALOG Information Services, Inc.

Content: Provides information on over 19,000 U.S. associations and organizations with voluntary members. Each record contains an organization's name, acronym, address, telephone number, chief officer's name, and a descriptive paragraph providing membership and staff statistics, founding date, statement of purposes and subjects of interest, committee and division names, publications, and convention plans. Corresponds to *Encyclopedia of Associations*.

Language: English

Coverage: U.S.

Time Span: Current year

Updating: Completely revised annually

ENDOC

Type: Reference (Referral)

Subject: Environment

Producer: Commission of the European Communities (CEC), in collaboration with environmental information centers of member countries

Online Service: ECHO Service

Content: Contains descriptions of over 500 environmental information centers in European Economic Community countries.

Language: Danish, Dutch, English, French, German, and Italian

Coverage: Europe

Updating: Annually

ENREP

Type: Reference (Referral)

Subject: Environment; Research in Progress

Producer: Commission of the European Communities (CEC), in collaboration with environmental research organizations of member countries

Online Service: ECHO Service

Content: Contains descriptions of over 25,000 research studies on the environment being conducted in European Economic Community (EEC) countries. Information about each research study includes original title and, when available, English-language title; project description and subjects covered; names of participating staff members; names of sponsors and cooperating organizations; status of the research; and citations to publications resulting from the research. Information about each research organization includes name of organization and parent organization; name of contact person; address; geographical areas covered by the organization; general description of the organization; list of languages in which information is provided; and cross references to the research studies.

Language: English

Coverage: European Economic Community (Belgium, Denmark, Federal Republic of Germany, France, Greece, Ireland, Italy, Luxembourg, The Netherlands, Portugal, Spain, and U.K.)

Updating: Annually

ENSC

Type: Reference (Bibliographic)

Subject: Environment

Producer: Asian Institute of Technology, Environmental Sanitation Information Center

Online Service: Asian Institute of Technology

Content: Contains approximately 4800 citations to the worldwide literature on environmental sanitation. Covers water supply and conservation, recycling and re-use of waste, waste treatment and disposal, and health-related aspects. Sources include journals, monographs, unpublished manuscripts, technical reports, and conference proceedings. Corresponds to *Environmental Sanitation Abstracts*.

Language: English

Coverage: International

Time Span: April 1979 to date

Updating: About 200 items every 4 months

ENVIRODOQ℠

Type: Reference (Bibliographic)

Subject: Environment

Producer: Environnement Quebec

Online Service: IST-Informatheque Inc.

Content: Contains about 7500 citations, with abstracts, to literature on all environmental aspects of the Canadian province of Quebec. Major topics include water resources, geology, forestry, land use, meteorology, air pollution, wildlife, and conservation. Covers technical reports, environmental and socioeconomic impact studies, and studies prepared by the governments of Quebec and Canada and their consultants.

Language: French

Coverage: Canada (Quebec)

Time Span: 1970 to date

Updating: About 250 items a quarter

ENVIROLINE®

Type: Reference (Bibliographic)

Subject: Environment

Producer: EIC/Intelligence Inc.

Online Service: DIALOG Information Services, Inc.; DIMDI; ESA-IRS; ORBIT Information Technologies Corporation

Content: Contains citations (with abstracts, from 1975) to a broad range of issues and topics related to the environment and the management and use of natural resources. Major topic areas included are air, water, and noise pollution; management of renewable and non-renewable resources of the land and water; environmental impact of drugs, chemicals, and biological and radiological contaminants; weather modification; and population planning and control. Covers all types of printed literature, including conference papers, research reports, government documents, and journal articles. Corresponds to *Environment Abstracts* and *Environment Index*.

Language: English

Coverage: International

Time Span: Most services, 1971 to date; DIMDI, 1981 to date.

Updating: About 500 records a month

ENVIRONMENT REPORTER

Type: Source (Full Text)

Subject: Environment

Producer: The Bureau of National Affairs, Inc. (BNA)

Online Service: Mead Data Central, Inc. (as part of LEXIS ENERGY LIBRARY and LEXIS ENVIRONMENTAL LIBRARY); West Publishing Company (to be available in 1987)

Conditions: Subscription to Mead Data Central required; subscription to West Publishing Company required.

Content: Contains full text of the current developments section of *Environment Reporter*, covering state and federal legislative, regulatory, and judicial activities related to pollution control and the environment. Includes air and water pollution, hazardous wastes, solid wastes, mining, land use, and sewage treatment.

Language: English

Coverage: U.S.

Time Span: 1982 to date

Updating: Weekly

ENVIRONMENTAL BIBLIOGRAPHY

Type: Reference (Bibliographic)

Subject: Environment

Producer: Environmental Studies Institute

Online Service: DIALOG Information Services, Inc.

Content: Contains citations to literature on the environment, including water, air, soil, and noise pollution, solid waste management, health hazards, urban planning and other related topics. Corresponds to *Environmental Periodicals Bibliography*.

Language: English

Coverage: International

Time Span: 1973 to date

Updating: About 4000 records every 2 months

ENVIRONMENTAL COMPLIANCE UPDATE

Type: Source (Full Text)

Subject: Environment

Producer: High Tech Publishing Company

Online Service: NewsNet, Inc.

Conditions: Monthly subscription to NewsNet required; differential charges for subscribers and non-subscribers to *Environmental Compliance Update*.

Content: Contains full text of *Environmental Compliance Update*, a newsletter covering legal, economic, and technological developments affecting compliance by business with environmental standards requirements. Includes news and analyses of legislative, regulatory, and judicial activity, as well as assessments of the economic effects of compliance on business.

Language: English

Coverage: U.S.

Time Span: October 1985 to date

Updating: Monthly

ENVIRONMENTAL FATE

Type: Source (Textual-Numeric)

Subject: Chemistry-Properties; Environment

Producer: U.S. Environmental Protection Agency (EPA), Office of Pesticides and Toxic Substances

Online Service: Chemical Information Systems, Inc., a subsidiary of Fein-Marquart Associates (CIS); Information Consultants, Inc. (ICI) (as part of The Integrated Chemical Information System)

Conditions: Annual subscription fee of $300 to CIS required but fee is waived for educational institutions and non-profit public libraries worldwide; differential charges for subscribers and non-subscribers to ICI.

Content: Contains more than 8000 records of information on the environmental fate or behavior (i.e., transport and degradation) of about 450 chemicals released into the environment. Chemicals selected for inclusion are produced in quantities exceeding 1 million pounds per year. Data, extracted from published literature, include environmental transformation rates (e.g., biodegradation, oxidation, hydrolysis) and physical and chemical properties (e.g., water solubility, vapor pressure). The database may contain multiple records, each representing an individual test or observation, for a given chemical.

Language: English

Coverage: International

Time Span: 1970 to date

Updating: Periodically, as new data become available

ENVIRONMENTAL FATE DATA BASES

Type: Reference (Bibliographic); Source (Numeric, Textual-Numeric)

Subject: Chemistry-Properties; Environment; Toxicology

Producer: Syracuse Research Corporation

Online Service: Syracuse Research Corporation

Conditions: Initiation fee of $25 required

Content: Consists of 3 interrelated files of information on the fate (i.e., transport and degradation) of organic chemicals (including hydrocarbons and halogen-, nitrogen- and sulfur-containing compounds) released in the environment.

DATALOG. Contains over 59,000 records covering over 5300 organic chemicals and metals. Each record provides the chemical name, molecular formula, Chemical Abstracts Service (CAS) Registry Number, and one or more of 18 data items relevant to the environmental fate of the chemical (i.e., water solubility, octanol/water partition coefficient, vapor pressure, ultraviolet spectra, dissociation constant, soil adsorption, bioconcentration, evaporation from water, Henry's Law constant, biodegradation, hydrolysis, photooxidation, ecosystems, field studies, and effluent, food, and occupational monitoring data). Each record also contains an abbreviated reference to the source article.

CHEMFATE. Contains actual data derived from the literature pertinent to the fate of over 465 representative chemicals listed in DATALOG. Categories of data include chemical identification information (e.g., molecular formula, molecular weight, chemical name, synonyms); chemodynamic properties (e.g., log octanol/water partition coefficient, log acid dissociation constant, soil adsorption, ultra-violet absorption, vapor pressure, solubility in water); transport properties (e.g., bioconcentration, evaporation from water, Henry's Law constant, soil column transport); laboratory degradation data (e.g., ecosystems, hydrolysis, microbial degradation, degradation in natural systems, oxidation and other reactions, photolysis); and environmental measurements (e.g., air, biota, water and soil monitoring, and data from field studies). Each record also includes the CAS Registry Number, data type, reference to the source article, and a summary of experimental design, methods, and results.

BIOLOG. Contains over 23,000 citations to literature on microbial degradation and toxicity. Records are organized by CAS Registry Number and by 6 categories (i.e., biodegradation/toxicity; oxygen condition (anaerobic/aerobic); culture type (pure enzyme, pure culture, mixed culture, cell-free extract); source (soil, sediment, sewage, fresh water, marine water, other); mechanism reported; and data source).

Language: English

Coverage: International

Updating: Periodically, as new data become available

ENVIRONMENTAL HEALTH NEWS®

Type: Source (Full Text)

Subject: Environment; Occupational Safety & Health

Producer: Occupational Health Services, Inc. (OHS)

Online Service: Executive Telecom System, Inc., Human Resource Information Network; Occupational Health Services, Inc.

Conditions: Annual subscription to Executive Telecom System required

Content: Contains full text of news stories relating to environmental and occupational health. Covers regulatory news from the Occupational Safety and Health Administration (OSHA), the National Institute of Occupational Safety and Health (NIOSH), the U.S. Environmental Protection Agency (EPA) on the Toxic Substances Control Act (TSCA), as well as guidelines from other organizations and related court decisions. Also contains industry news (e.g., chemical spills, personnel changes). Users can review headlines only or complete stories, which are usually not more than 10 lines long.

Language: English

Coverage: U.S.

Time Span: December 1981 to date

Updating: Periodically, as new data become available

ENVIRONMENTAL MUTAGENS

Type: Reference (Bibliographic)

Subject: Biomedicine; Toxicology

Producer: Oak Ridge National Laboratory, Environmental Mutagen Information Center

Online Service: National Library of Medicine (NLM) (as a TOXLINE database (see))

Content: Contains approximately 53,000 citations to the worldwide literature on the testing for mutagenicity and genetic toxicology of chemicals, biological agents, and selected physical agents. Covers only selected studies dealing with the mutagenicity of ionizing or ultraviolet radiation. Also includes some general references on test methods, systems, and organisms. Records also contain Chemical Abstracts Service Registry Numbers.

Language: English

Coverage: International

Time Span: 1969 to date, with some earlier materials

Updating: 3 to 4 times a year

ENVIRONMENTAL RESEARCH IN THE NETHERLANDS

Type: Reference (Bibliographic, Referral)

Subject: Environment; Research in Progress

Producer: Study and Information Centre TNO on Environmental Research

Online Service: TNO Institute for Mathematics, Data Processing, and Statistics

Conditions: Subscription to Study and Information Center TNO required

Content: Contains descriptions of over 4400 current research studies on the environment being conducted in The Netherlands. These descriptions comprise the Dutch contribution to the ENREP database (see). Each record contains organization name and address; project leader; title (in English and Dutch); summary (in Dutch); start and completion dates; and citations to publications resulting from the research. Also contains about 12,000 citations to literature on environmental research. Corresponds to *Onderzoek naar milieu en natuur in Nederland.*

Language: Dutch, with titles also in English

Coverage: The Netherlands

Time Span: 1974 to date

Updating: Annually

ENVIRONMENTAL TERATOLOGY

Type: Reference (Bibliographic)

Subject: Biomedicine; Toxicology

Producer: Oak Ridge National Laboratory, Environmental Teratology Information Center

Online Service: National Library of Medicine (NLM) (as a TOXLINE database (see))

Content: Contains approximately 35,000 citations to the worldwide literature on teratology-the science dealing with causes, mechanisms, and manifestations of structural or functional alterations in animal development. Covers the testing and evaluation for teratogenic activity of chemical, biological, and physical agents and of dietary deficiencies in warm-blooded animals. Primary emphasis is on literature that covers the administration of an agent to pregnant animals and examination of offspring at or near birth for structural or functional anomalies. Records also contain Chemical Abstracts Service Registry Numbers.

Language: English

Coverage: International

Time Span: 1975 to date, with earliest materials from 1912

Updating: Quarterly

EPIDEMIOLOGY INFORMATION SYSTEM

Type: Reference (Bibliographic)

Subject: Toxicology

Producer: Oak Ridge National Laboratory, Toxicology Information Response Center

Online Service: To be announced

Content: Contains approximately 8800 citations to literature that includes analyses of food contaminants and their effects on health. Emphasis is on unavoidable contaminants and natural toxicants in foods. Covers published and unpublished documents in the collection of the Epidemiology Unit of the Food and Drug Administration's Bureau of Foods and other documents identified through literature searches.

Language: English

Coverage: U.S.

Time Span: 1960 to date, with some earlier support documents

Updating: Monthly

ERIC® (Educational Resources Information Center)

Type: Reference (Bibliographic)

Subject: Education & Educational Institutions

Producer: U.S. Department of Education, Office of Educational Research and Improvement

Online Service: BRS; BRS After Dark; BRS/BRKTHRU; BRS/Colleague; DIALOG Information Services, Inc.; Knowledge Index; ORBIT Information Technologies Corporation; TECH DATA; University of Tsukuba

Content: Contains citations, with abstracts, to both the journal and report literature in the field of education and education-related areas. Journal literature corresponds to *Current Index to Journals in Education* (CIJE). Report literature covering significant research and funded projects in education corresponds to *Resources in Education* (RIE). Subjects covered include career, adult, vocational, technical, and teacher education; education of the handicapped, disadvantaged, and the gifted; early childhood education; junior colleges and higher education; reading and communication skills; language and linguistics; education management; counseling and personnel services; information resources; urban education; rural education and small schools; science, mathematics and environment; social studies and social sciences; and tests, measurement, and evaluation.

Language: English

Coverage: Primarily U.S.

Time Span: RIE, 1966 to date; CIJE, 1969 to date.

Updating: About 1200 RIE and 1400 CIJE records a month

ESPECIALIDADES CONSUMIDAS POR LA SEGURIDAD SOCIAL

Type: Source (Numeric)

Subject: Pharmaceuticals & Pharmaceutical Industry

Producer: Ministerio de Sanidad y Consumo, Centro Institucional de Informacion de Medicamentos (CINIME)

Online Service: ENTEL, S.A.

Content: Contains data on about 16,000 drugs distributed under authority of the Social Security system of Spain. Includes quantities and prices. Data are aggregated by province.

Coverage: Spain

Time Span: 1980 to date

Updating: Annually

ESPECIALIDADES FARMACEUTICAS DE ESPANA

Type: Source (Textual-Numeric)

Subject: Pharmaceuticals & Pharmaceutical Industry

Producer: Consejo General de Colegios Oficiales de Farmaceuticos de Espana

Online Service: Consejo General de Colegios Oficiales de Farmaceuticos de Espana

Content: Contains data on about 22,000 drugs marketed in Spain, including repealed and discontinued drugs. Provides trade name, manufacturer code, therapeutic category as defined in GRUPOS TERAPEUTICOS *(see)*, dosage forms and prices, posological data, cautions, pharmacological actions, indications, contraindications, interactions, and side effects. Sources include the pharmaceuticals register of the Ministerio de Sanidad y Consumo, international scientific literature, and technical documentation from pharmaceutical manufacturers.

Language: Spanish

Coverage: Spain

Time Span: 1972 to date

Updating: Periodically, as new data become available

ESPECIALIDADES FARMACEUTICAS ESPANOLAS

Type: Source (Textual-Numeric)

Subject: Pharmaceuticals & Pharmaceutical Industry

Producer: Ministerio de Sanidad y Consumo, Centro Institucional de Informacion de Medicamentos (CINIME)

Online Service: ENTEL, S.A.

Content: Contains descriptions of the approximately 16,000 drugs registered for use in Spain. Includes trade name, form and size, definition, active and excipient ingredients, usage, dosage and administration, manufacturer, and price.

Language: Spanish

Coverage: Spain

Time Span: 1979 to date

Updating: Periodically, as new data become available

EUDISED (European Documentation and Information System for Education)

Type: Reference (Referral)

Subject: Education & Educational Institutions

Producer: Council of Europe, Directorate of Education, Culture and Sport

Online Service: ESA-IRS

Content: Contains approximately 6000 references, with summaries, to recently completed and ongoing educational research in 19 European countries. Covers educational institutions, curricula, management, and personnel; teaching methods and aids, student work, and the teaching profession; psychology, sociology, and philosophy of education; physiology and health; buildings and equipment; economics, public administration and planning; and education documentation and information. Each reference contains the date, researcher name and institution; a summary of study objectives, methods, research sample; results (for completed research projects); and publications resulting from the research. Corresponds to *EUDISED R&D Bulletin.*

Language: Titles in original language and either English or French; abstracts in English, French, or German; descriptors in English, French, German, Dutch, Spanish, Italian, Danish, Greek, and Portuguese.

Coverage: Western Europe, including Yugoslavia

Time Span: 1975 to date

Updating: About 250 records a quarter

EURODICAUTOM

Type: Reference (Referral)

Subject: Terminology & Translations

Producer: Commission of the European Communities (CEC)

Online Service: ECHO Service

Content: Contains translations of more than 370,000 terms and phrases, and more than 90,000 abbreviations in all subject fields, as well as terminology used in European Economic Community (EEC) regulations. Contains for most terms or expressions a sentence or partial sentence in which it occurs; a definition, when available; reference to the source of the item; linguistic or technical explanatory notes; subject field; and a reliability code.

Language: All official languages of the EEC countries except Greek

Coverage: European Economic Community (Belgium, Denmark, Federal Republic of Germany, France, Greece, Ireland, Italy, Luxembourg, The Netherlands, Portugal, Spain, and U.K.)

Updating: About 2000 items a month

EUROPEAN PATENTS REGISTER; INPI-2

Type: Reference (Bibliographic)

Subject: Patents

Producer: European Patent Office (EPO); Institut National de la Propriete Industrielle (INPI)

Online Service: European Patent Office (EUROPEAN PATENTS REGISTER); Telesystemes-Questel (INPI-2)

Conditions: Subscription fee of 250 DM to the European Patent Office required for access through EPO

Content: Contains bibliographic and legal status information on over 180,000 published European patent applications and 47,000 patents from the start of the European patent procedure (June 1978). Information about each patent includes names of inventor, applicant, and agent; title of invention; country of origin; countries designated; and dates of application and publication, as well as opponents and date of opposition. Corresponds to *European Patent Bulletin*.

Language: English, French, and German

Coverage: Contracting states of the European Patent Convention

Time Span: June 1978 to date

Updating: About 900 records a week, on day of publication

EVERYMAN'S ENCYCLOPEDIA

Type: Source (Full Text)

Subject: Encyclopedias

Producer: J.M. Dent & Sons Ltd.

Online Service: DIALOG Information Services, Inc.

Content: Contains full text of the 6th edition of *Everyman's Encyclopaedia*. Includes more than 60,000 items with an emphasis on people, places, and events in the U.K. Many items include bibliographies and cross references to related subjects.

Language: English

Coverage: International, with emphasis on the U.K.

Time Span: Current edition

Updating: Not updated

EXCEPTIONAL CHILD EDUCATION RESOURCES

Type: Reference (Bibliographic)

Subject: Education & Educational Institutions

Producer: The Council for Exceptional Children

Online Service: BRS; BRS After Dark; BRS/BRKTHRU; BRS/Colleague; DIALOG Information Services, Inc.

Content: Contains citations, with abstracts, to the published and unpublished English-language literature on the education of handicapped and gifted children, including the hearing impaired, visually handicapped, mentally retarded, physically handicapped, socially maladjusted, emotionally disturbed, abused or neglected, speech impaired, learning disabled, autistic, culturally different, and severely or multiply handicapped. Corresponds to *Exceptional Child Education Resources*.

Language: English

Coverage: Primarily U.S., with some international coverage

Time Span: 1966 to date

Updating: About 300 records a month

EXIS

Type: Reference (Referral); Source (Textual-Numeric)

Subject: Chemistry-Properties; Environment; Safety

Producer: Exis Limited

Online Service: Exis Limited

Conditions: Annual minimum of 250 pounds (UK) required

Content: Contains information relating to the transport, storage, and handling of hazardous substances, covering chemical properties, regulations, safety precautions, and emergency response procedures. Substances can be searched by standard international identifiers, chemical names, and commonly used synonyms.

IMO. Contains the English-language version of the *International Maritime Dangerous Goods Code* (IMDG), abstracts of the IMO's *Medical First Aid Guide*, and descriptions of emergency response procedures. IMDG data on each substance include chemical and physical properties, relevant documentation, and instructions on packing, containers, stowage, segregation, and limitation of quantities.

Materials Information. Contains transport classifications and properties data for 2400 regulated substances. Worldwide classifications include IMDG and International Civil Aviation Authority classes and United Nations number, name, class, packing group, and subsidiary risks. European classsifications include European Economic Community, ADR (road transport), RID (rail transport), and ADN (inland waterways transport) classes, Kemler hazard-level codes, and European Chemical Industries Association Tremcard (Transport Emergency Card) data. U.K. classifications include Emergency Action Code and regulation classes from the Department of Transport (maritime transport), Health and Safety Executive (road transport), British Rail *List of Dangerous Goods and Conditions of Acceptance*, and the British Waterways Board *Schedule of Dangerous Goods*. U.S. classifications include Department of Transportation class and Response Guide Number, National Fire Protection Association symbol, and Coast Guard Cargo Compatibility Group. Properties data, derived from standard reference works, manufacturers' information, chemical dictionaries, and research papers, include the following: formula, molecular weight, physical description, relative density, melting point, boiling point, flash point, critical temperature, autoignition temperature, flammability range, vapor pressure, viscosity, thermal conductivity, specific heat, coefficient of expansion, behavior in water, threshold limit value, short-term exposure limit, toxicity, and odor threshold.

ADR. Contains references to relevant sections of ADR-European Road Transport regulations for each substance listed in Materials Information.

Chemdata Emergency Response. Contains information of use in responding to chemical emergencies on land, developed by the U.K. National Chemical Emergency Centre. For each substance, provides information on protective clothing and apparatus, physical and physiological hazards, precautions in handling, fire risk, method of decontamination, and a list of chemical companies to contact for further advice.

Hazardous Cargo Contacts. Contains an international list of addresses and telephone numbers for National Competent Authorities, port authorities, training establishments, trade associations, and inspection offices in 114 countries.

Air Transport. Contains full text of dangerous goods regulations of the International Civil Aviation Organization (ICAO) and the International Air Transport Association (IATA).

Language: English, with search terms also in Danish, French, German, and Spanish

Coverage: International, with emphasis on Europe and North America

Time Span: Current information

Updating: Periodically, as new data become available

THE EXPERT AND THE LAW®

Type: Source (Full Text)

Subject: Forensic Sciences & Services

Producer: National Forensic Center

Online Service: Mead Data Central, Inc. (EXPTLW) (as part of NEXIS NEWSLETTERS (see))

Conditions: Subscription to Mead Data Central required

Content: Contains full text of *The Expert and the Law*, a newsletter covering the application of scientific, medical, and technical knowledge to litigation. Includes news about the use of consultants by attorneys and feature articles on the effective use of experts and consultants (e.g., ethical considerations when expert witnesses incur out-of-pocket expenses).

Language: English

Coverage: Primarily U.S., with some international coverage

Time Span: December 7, 1981 to date

Updating: Within 2 weeks after receipt of new materials

EXPERTNET®

Type: Reference (Referral)

Subject: Biographies; Forensic Sciences & Services

Producer: ExpertNet, a division of HealthNet, Ltd.

Online Service: American Bar Association (as an ABA/net database on Dialcom, Inc.); West Publishing Company

Conditions: Subscription to American Bar Association required; subscription to West Publishing Company required.

Content: Contains references to approximately 1000 physicians who can serve as expert witnesses or consultants to attorneys. Covers physicians in all medical specialties. Provides state of residence and first 3 digits of ZIP code, age, present position, professional experience, education, state license, specialty and date of board certification, and hourly fee. Also includes general remarks (e.g., research, publications, awards, medical/legal experience); willingness to consult for plaintiffs, defendants, or either; and any geographic limitations on travel. Name, address, and telephone number are available upon request.

Language: English

Coverage: U.S.

Time Span: Current information

Updating: Monthly

ExVENT

Type: Reference (Referral)

Subject: Conferences & Meetings

Producer: Timeplace, Inc.

Online Service: Timeplace, Inc.

Conditions: Annual subscription of $1250 to Timeplace, Inc. required

Content: Contains descriptions of approximately 250,000 conferences, conventions, trade shows, exhibitions, and other events of interest to businesspeople. For each event, includes date, time, city, site, sponsor, expected attendance, and space requirements.

Language: English

Coverage: Primarily U.S. and Canada, with some international coverage

Time Span: Current information

Updating: Weekly

EYENET©

Type: Reference (Bibliographic, Referral); Source (Full Text)

Subject: Biomedicine; Conferences & Meetings; Pharmaceuticals & Pharmaceutical Industry

Producer: American Society of Contemporary Ophthalmology (ASCO)

Online Service: General Electric Information Services Company (GEISCO)

Conditions: Access limited to ophthalmologists, physicians, and the ophthalmic industry; monthly maintenance fee to ASCO required.

Content: Contains 5 files of information for ophthalmologists and physicians on eye disorders and their treatment.

ELECTRONIC EYE JOURNAL MONTHLY. Contains full text of selected articles, book reviews, editorials, letters to the editor, and classified advertisements to be published in *Annals of Ophthalmology, Glaucoma,* and *Journal of Ocular Therapy and Surgery.* Also contains news bulletins, product announcements and warnings, and a calendar of conferences and meetings. Updated monthly; bulletins and product news updated daily.

EYE DISORDERS. Contains information on disorders of the eye (e.g., of the eyelid, cornea, optic nerve) and preferred and alternate treatments.

PHARMACEUTICALS. Provides information on drugs by brand name. Includes manufacturer, form of application (e.g., ointment), and concentration.

INSTRUMENTS. Provides descriptions of about 3000 instruments, lenses, and other equipment used in the practice of ophthalmology. Descriptions include manufacturer and price.

LITERATURE SEARCH. Provides citations from Excerpta Medica to the worldwide literature in the field of ophthalmology (see EMBASE). Updated weekly.

Language: English

Coverage: International

Time Span: Current information; Literature Search, 1983 to date.

Updating: Varies by file (see Content)

FAIRBASE®

Type: Reference (Referral)

Subject: Conferences & Meetings

Producer: INTAG

Online Service: DATA-STAR; GENIOS Wirtschaftsdatenbanken

Content: Contains references, with some abstracts and statistics, to about 8500 upcoming trade fairs, exhibitions, conferences, and meetings in over 90 countries. Covers events in all industries, including aerospace, electronics, computers, manufacturing technology, mining and oil drilling, construction, electrical engineering, printing and publishing, broadcasting, telecommunications, travel and tourism, transportation, agriculture, and food technology. Includes name and address of sponsoring organization, dates, location, exhibitors, registration price, and data on numbers of visitors, exhibitors, and exhibition space.

Language: English

Coverage: International
Time Span: Current information
Updating: About 500 records a month

FAIREC℠ (Fruits Agro-Industrie Regions Chaudes)

Type: Reference (Bibliographic)
Subject: Agriculture
Producer: Institut de Recherches sur les Fruits et Agrumes (IRFA)
Online Service: Serveur Universitaire National de l'Information Scientifique et Technique (SUNIST)
Content: Contains citations to the literature on fruits and citrus in tropical and sub-tropical regions, agronomy, economics, and technology.
Language: French
Coverage: Tropical areas of Africa, Americas, Asia, and Oceania, and Mediterranean countries
Time Span: 1970 to date
Updating: About 230 records a month

FAMILY RESOURCES©

Type: Reference (Bibliographic, Referral)
Subject: Biographies; Families & Family Life; Health Care & Social Services-Directories; Research in Progress; Social Services
Producer: National Council on Family Relations (NCFR)
Online Service: BRS; BRS After Dark; BRS/BRKTHRU; BRS/Colleague; DIALOG Information Services, Inc.; Executive Telecom System, Inc., Human Resource Information Network
Conditions: Annual subscription to Executive Telecom System required
Content: Provides more than 80,000 citations covering literature and other resources on marriage and the family. Subjects covered include trends and changes in marriage and family; organizations and services to families; family relationships and dynamics; mate selection; marriage and divorce; issues related to reproduction; sexual attitudes and behavior; families with special problems (e.g., violence, drug abuse, child abuse, learning disabilities, alcoholism); family counseling and education; minority groups; and aids for theory and research.

Inventory of Marriage and Family Literature (IMFL). Contains citations, with abstracts, to family-related articles in over 1000 journals. Corresponds to the printed index of the same name from 1973 to 1985. From 1985 to date, all journal articles are indexed at NCFR.

Family Resource and Referral Center (FR&RC). Contains citations, many with abstracts, to such non-journal literature as monographs, government publications, reports, audiovisual materials, and instructional materials. Also includes references to such non-print resources as family study centers, programs, organizations, community resource centers, and databases identified by the FR & RC.

Human Resources Bank. Contains biographical summaries and references to qualified professionals who can be contacted by the general public. Includes psychologists, sociologists, researchers, family life educators, and marriage and family therapists.

Idea Bank. Contains references to work in progress, work planned, and new ideas. Abstracts are submitted by individuals in family-related programs, research, service agencies, and educational institutions.
Language: English

Coverage: International
Time Span: 1970 to date, with some earlier data; journals, 1973 to date.
Updating: DIALOG and Executive Telecom System, monthly; BRS, BRS After Dark, BRS/BRKTHRU, and BRS/Colleague, quarterly.

FAMILY: Australian Family Studies Database

Type: Reference (Bibliographic)
Subject: Families & Family Life
Producer: Institute of Family Studies
Online Service: ACI Computer Services
Conditions: Monthly minimum to ACI required; fees vary depending on service selected.
Content: Contains about 3500 citations, with abstracts, to Australian literature on family life and families. Covers such topics as economics and the family, family relationships and dynamics, sexual attitudes and behavior, fertility and infertility, counseling and education for marriage and parenthood, family law, and social services. Includes books, journal articles, research reports, conference papers, government documents, statistical publications, and unpublished reports.
Language: English
Coverage: Australia
Time Span: 1980 to date
Updating: Monthly, with about 2000 records a year

FAR On-line℗ (Federal Acquisition Regulation)

Type: Source (Full Text)
Subject: Government-U.S. Federal
Producer: Compusearch Corporation
Online Service: Compusearch Corporation
Conditions: Initiation fee of $100 plus $100 monthly minimum per account and $25 initiation fee plus $10 monthly minimum per user ID required; users affiliated with U.S. government agencies or educational institutions receive discounts; option available for no monthly minimum.
Content: Provides access to several files of acquisition, procurement, and contracting regulations covering the provision of goods and services to the U.S. federal government. Contains full text of *Code of Federal Regulations*, Title 48, Volume I, Parts 1-51 (Prescriptions) and Volume II, Part 52 (Clauses and Provisions). Also contains proposed changes, historical data on changes made, and full text of unpublished military FAR Supplements.

Includes the full text of these agency regulations: Agency for International Development (AID), Chapter 7; Air Force Supplement (which has no corresponding printed product); *Air Force Systems Command Procurement Manual*; Army Supplement (which has no corresponding printed product); Department of Defense (DFAR), Chapter 2, including changes 1 through 12; Department of Energy (DOE), Chapter 9; Department of Health and Human Services (HHS), Chapter 3; Department of Housing and Urban Development (HUD), Chapter 24; Department of the Interior (DOI), Chapter 14; Department of Justice (JAR), Chapter 28; Department of Transportation (DOT), Chapter 12; Federal Emergency Management Administration (FEMA), Chapter 44; General Services Administration (GSA), Chapter 5; National Aeronautics and Space Administration (NASA), Chapter 18; Navy Supplement (which has no corresponding printed product); Small Business Administration (SBA), Chapter 22; and

Veterans Administration Supplement (VAR), Chapter 8. Also includes full text of these supplementary materials: Cost Accounting Standards, Chapter 3; Defense Contract Audit Agency Contract Auditor Manual, including all audit procedures, directives, and allowable costs (i.e., direct labor and materials, general and administrative costs, overhead) that are applicable to defense contracts; Federal Information Resources Management Regulation (FIRMR) (chapter number still to be assigned); Federal Acquistion Regulation (FAR), Chapter 1, including changes 1 through 11; FAR On-line Archives, covering the original version and all subsequent changes to altered provisions or clauses in regulations or supplements; FAR On-line Proposed, covering proposed and pending changes to regulations and supplements; and Defense Acquisition Regulations (DAR), covering procurement and contract clauses and provisions referenced in all Department of Defense (DOD) contracts issued to April 1984. Comptroller General Decisions, Boards of Contract Appeals Decisions, and full text of Department of Commerce (DOC) Export Administration regulations will be added.

Language: English

Coverage: U.S.

Time Span: DAR, August 1976 to April 1984; FAR, September 1984 to date.

Updating: Daily

FDA ELECTRONIC BULLETIN BOARD

Type: Reference (Bibliographic, Referral); Source (Full Text)

Subject: Biomedicine; Pharmaceuticals & Pharmaceutical Industry; Conferences & Meetings; Government-U.S. Federal

Producer: Food and Drug Administration (FDA)

Online Service: Dialcom, Inc. (as a FEDNEWS database)

Content: Contains full text of reports, press releases, articles, speeches, and other items issued by the FDA. Includes the weekly enforcement report of FDA-regulated products under recall; citations to articles and full text of selected articles from the monthly *FDA Consumer* magazine; the monthly list of drug and device product approvals; citations to FDA *Federal Register* announcements; newsletters of interest to physicians and other health professionals; news releases translated into Spanish; prepared speeches delivered by the FDA Commissioner and Deputy Commissioner; prepared statements delivered by FDA officials at congressional oversight hearings; and a schedule of upcoming FDA-sponsored meetings and conferences.

Language: English

Coverage: U.S.

Time Span: Current month

Updating: Daily

FEDERAL INDEX©

Type: Reference (Bibliographic)

Subject: Government-U.S. Federal; Legislative Tracking

Producer: National Standards Association

Online Service: DIALOG Information Services, Inc.

Content: Contains citations to the *Congressional Record, Federal Register, and Weekly Compilation of Presidential Documents*. Also includes pertinent citations from CONGRESSIONAL RECORD ABSTRACTS and FEDERAL REGISTER ABSTRACTS *(see)*. Corresponds to *CSI Federal Index*.

Language: English

Coverage: U.S.

Time Span: October 1976 to November 1980

Updating: Not updated

FEDERAL REGISTER ABSTRACTS©

Type: Reference (Bibliographic)

Subject: Legislative Tracking

Producer: National Standards Association

Online Service: BRS (to be available in 1987); BRS After Dark (to be available in 1987); BRS/BRKTHRU (to be available in 1987); BRS/Colleague (to be available in 1987); DIALOG Information Services, Inc. (FEDERAL REGISTER ABSTRACTS); ORBIT Information Technologies Corporation (FEDREG)

Content: Contains abstracts of each document published in the *Federal Register* (FR). Covers regulations and proposed rules to the *Code of Federal Regulations* (CFR), legal notices, Public Law notices, hearings, meetings, Executive Orders and other Presidential documents carried in the *Federal Register*. Elements of information in each record also include citations to FR page numbers, CFR titles and parts, docket numbers, and other reference material. All records are tagged to identify the document's status, i.e., rule, proposed, notice, etc. Corresponds to the daily CSI *Federal Register Abstracts*.

Language: English

Coverage: U.S.

Time Span: March 1977 to date

Updating: About 700 records a week

FEDERAL RESEARCH IN PROGRESS

Type: Reference (Referral)

Subject: Research in Progress

Producer: National Technical Information Service

Online Service: DIALOG Information Services, Inc.; Mead Data Central, Inc. (FRIP) (as a Reference Service database)

Conditions: Records from the National Aeronautics and Space Administration and U.S. Department of Energy are available in the U.S. only; subscription to Mead Data Central required.

Content: Contains descriptions of and references to research in progress and recently completed research sponsored primarily by federal government agencies. Covers basic and applied research in all areas of the life, physical, social, behavioral, and engineering sciences. All records include title, principal investigator, performing organization, and sponsoring organization. Contributing agencies include the U.S. Department of Agriculture, U.S. Department of Energy, National Aeronautics and Space Administration, National Bureau of Standards, National Institute of Occupational Safety and Health, National Institutes of Health, U.S. Geological Survey, Veterans Administration, Transportation Research Board (a private organization supported by public and private funds), and the National Science Foundation.

Language: English

Coverage: Primarily U.S.

Time Span: Current information *(see SSIE CURRENT RESEARCH for historical information on many projects)*

Updating: Twice a year

FEDERAL RESEARCH REPORT

Type: Source (Full Text)

Subject: Funding Sources, Contracts & Awards

Producer: Business Publishers, Inc.

Online Service: NewsNet, Inc.

Conditions: Monthly subscription to NewsNet required; differential charges for subscribers to *Federal Research Report*.

Content: Contains full text of the *Federal Research Report*, a newsletter covering U.S. federal research and development funding. Provides announcements of deadlines, contacts, and addresses associated with grant and contract funding opportunities.
Language: English
Coverage: U.S.
Time Span: 1982 to date
Updating: Weekly

FERIAS Y EXPOSICIONES

Type: Reference (Referral)
Subject: Conferences & Meetings
Producer: Instituto de la Pequena y Mediana Empresa Industrial
Online Service: Ministerio de Industria y Energia
Content: Contains references to about 500 Spanish trade fairs and expositions. Includes dates and location, frequency, size of exposition space, expected number of exhibitors, products being exhibited, and organizer address, telephone, and telex.
Language: Spanish
Coverage: Spain
Time Span: Current year
Updating: Monthly

FIESTA®

Type: Reference (Bibliographic)
Subject: Science & Technology
Producer: Centre de Documentation de l'Armement
Online Service: Centre de Documentation de l'Armement (CEDOCAR)
Content: Contains over 400,000 citations, with abstracts, to literature on a wide variety of topics of interest to the defense community. Covers aeronautics and aerodynamics; astronomy and astrophysics; atmospheric sciences; behavioral and social sciences; biological and medical sciences; bioengineering; chemistry; earth sciences; oceanography; electronics and electrical engineering; non-propulsive energy conversion; materials; mathematical sciences; mechanical, industrial, civil, and marine engineering; military sciences; missile technology; navigation; communications; detection and countermeasures; nuclear science and technology; physics; propulsion; fuels; and space technology. Sources covered include books, standards, patents, government publications, and over 200 journals.
Language: French
Coverage: International
Time Span: 1972 to date
Updating: About 1000 records twice a month

FINANCIAL TIMES INDEX

Type: Reference (Bibliographic)
Subject: News
Producer: DataArkiv AB; Financial Times Business Information Limited (FTBI)
Online Service: DataArkiv AB
Conditions: Monthly subscription of $33 to DataArkiv required
Content: Contains citations, with abstracts, to all news and information published in both the London and Frankfurt editions of the *Financial Times*. Users can search by company names, organizations, geographical locations, people, and products.

Language: English
Coverage: International
Time Span: 1981 to date
Updating: About 14,000 records a month

FINE CHEMICALS DIRECTORY

Type: Reference (Referral)
Subject: Chemistry-Structure & Nomenclature
Producer: Pergamon InfoLine Inc.
Online Service: Pergamon InfoLine
Content: Provides the names of suppliers for approximately 80,000 commercially available chemical substances, including organics, inorganics, biochemicals, dyes, and stains. Also covers small suppliers who offer specialized compounds. Each record, representing one substance, contains compound name, catalog number, compound description, synonyms, molecular formula, suppliers of each grade of the compound, and Wiswesser Line Notation or connection table. Data are obtained from supplier catalogs, including Aldrich, Alfa, Apin, Bayer, Carbolabs, Chemalog, Fairfield, Fisons, Fluorochem, Hoechst, K & K, Kodak, Lancaster, May & Baker, Pierce, Pyraspec, Riedel, Sigma, SSF, TCI, Vega, Vickers, Wiley, Wychem, and Yarsley.
Language: English
Coverage: International
Time Span: Current information
Updating: Several times a year, as new data become available

FOODS ADLIBRA

Type: Reference (Bibliographic)
Subject: Food Sciences & Nutrition
Producer: General Mills, Inc., Foods Adlibra Publications
Online Service: DIALOG Information Services, Inc.
Content: Contains about 111,000 citations, with abstracts, to journal literature on research and development in food technology and packaging. Covers nutritional and toxicological information. Each new food product introduced since 1974 is covered and, as well, these areas: products and processes (new ingredient developments, engineering methods, government regulations and guidelines, patents) ; corporate activities (management and marketing news, market research, marketing statistics, company and association news) ; and economics (commodities, world food economics, international marketing) . Corresponds to *FOODS ADLIBRA*.
Language: English
Coverage: U.S.
Time Span: 1974 to date
Updating: About 1200 records a month

FORENSIC SERVICES DIRECTORY©

Type: Reference (Referral)
Subject: Biographies; Forensic Sciences & Services; Science & Technology
Producer: National Forensic Center
Online Service: Mead Data Central, Inc. (EXPERT) (as a LEXIS and Reference Service database); West Publishing Company
Conditions: Subscription to Mead Data Central required; subscription to West Publishing Company required.
Content: Contains the names of thousands of scientific, medical, and technical experts available to serve as expert trial witnesses or consultants to attorneys, corporations, and the

government. Also lists translators, testing laboratories, investigators, and other specialists providing trial support services. Also includes resources available from specialized libraries, organizations, and agencies. Corresponds to *Forensic Services Directory*.
Language: English
Coverage: Primarily U.S. and Canada, with some international coverage
Time Span: Current information
Updating: 3 to 4 times a year

FORT LAUDERDALE NEWS
Type: Source (Full Text)
Subject: News
Producer: News and Sun-Sentinel Company
Online Service: VU/TEXT Information Services, Inc.
Conditions: Subscription to VU/TEXT required
Content: Contains full text of news items and feature articles from the *Fort Lauderdale News* (Florida), the *Sun-Sentinel* (Florida), and the *Fort Lauderdale News/Sun-Sentinel* (Florida) newspapers.
Language: English
Coverage: U.S. (primarily Fort Lauderdale, Florida area)
Time Span: 1985 to date
Updating: *Fort Lauderdale News* and *Sun-Sentinel*, daily; *Fort Lauderdale News/Sun-Sentinel*, weekly.

FoU (FoU-indeks)
Type: Reference (Bibliographic)
Subject: Science & Technology
Producer: Norwegian Centre for Informatics
Online Service: Norwegian Centre for Informatics
Content: Contains about 11,000 citations to Norwegian research and development reports from projects supported by the Royal Norwegian Council for Scientific and Industrial Research in the fields of science and technology. Descriptors for searching are primarily in Norwegian but some are in English. *(See NTNF-PROJECTS for descriptions of research projects.)*
Language: Norwegian
Coverage: Norway
Time Span: 1974 to date
Updating: About 300 records a quarter

FOUNDATIONS
Type: Reference (Referral); Source (Textual-Numeric)
Subject: Associations & Foundations-Directories; Funding Sources, Contracts & Awards
Producer: The Foundation Center
Online Service: DIALOG Information Services, Inc.
Content: Provides information on non-governmental and non-profit foundations and on the grants that they award. Information is gathered from forms submitted voluntarily by the foundations to The Foundation Center or from public information returns filed with the Internal Revenue Service.
FOUNDATION DIRECTORY. Contains descriptions of more than 4000 foundations that have assets of at least $1 million or that make grants of at least $100,000 annually. Corresponds to *The Foundation Directory*.
FOUNDATION GRANTS INDEX. Covers descriptions of grants of $5000 or more awarded by more than 400 major U.S. philanthropic organizations. Corresponds to *Foundation Grants*

Index Bimonthly and the annual *Foundation Grants Index*.
NATIONAL FOUNDATIONS. Contains descriptions of the more than 23,000 currently active grantmaking foundations.
Language: English
Coverage: U.S.
Updating: FOUNDATION DIRECTORY, revised twice a year; FOUNDATION GRANTS INDEX, every 2 months; NATIONAL FOUNDATIONS, annually.

FRANCIS: EMPLOI ET FORMATION
Type: Reference (Bibliographic)
Subject: Education & Educational Institutions
Producer: Centre National de la Recherche Scientifique, Centre de Documentation Sciences Humaines
Online Service: Centre National de la Recherche Scientifique, Centre de Documentation Sciences Humaines (CNRS/CDSH); G.CAM Serveur; Telesystemes-Questel
Content: Contains over 10,000 citations, with abstracts, to selected French literature in the fields of employment and professional training. Covers 6 subject areas: general aspects of employment, training, and social improvement; relationships between training and employment; education; employment qualifications; the job market; and employees' living conditions. Sources include periodicals, books, research papers, and conference proceedings. Corresponds to the quarterly bulletin *EMPLOI et FORMATION*.
Language: French
Coverage: France
Time Span: 1974 to 1985
Updating: Not updated

FRANCIS: RESHUS (Reseau documentaire en Sciences Humaines de la Sante)
Type: Reference (Bibliographic)
Subject: Health Care
Producer: Centre National de la Recherche Scientifique, Centre de Documentation Sciences Humaines; Institut de recherches mediterraniennes, Reseau d'information en sciences humaines de la sante
Online Service: Centre National de la Recherche Scientifique, Centre de Documentation Sciences Humaines (CNRS/CDSH); G.CAM Serveur; Telesystemes-Questel
Content: Contains over 9000 citations, with abstracts, to selected French literature in the field of health sciences, including the areas of research and teaching; illness; childbirth; mortality; health and society; health organizations and politics; status, management and structure of care and prevention units; expenses and financing; and evaluation of health records. Sources include periodicals, books, conference proceedings, and research papers. Corresponds to the quarterly bulletin *RESHUS*.
Language: French
Coverage: France
Time Span: 1978 to date
Updating: About 300 records a quarter

FRANCIS: SCIENCES DE L'EDUCATION
Type: Reference (Bibliographic)
Subject: Education & Educational Institutions
Producer: Centre National de la Recherche Scientifique, Centre de Documentation Sciences Humaines

Online Service: Centre National de la Recherche Scientifique, Centre de Documentation Sciences Humaines (CNRS/CDSH); G.CAM Serveur; Telesystemes-Questel

Content: Contains over 83,000 citations, about half with abstracts, to the worldwide literature on education. Covers history and philosophy of education; education and psychology; sociology of education; planning and economics; educational research; teaching methods; testing and guidance; school life; vocational training; and adult education and employment. Sources include periodicals, reports, dissertations, and monographs. Corresponds to the *Bulletin Signaletique sciences humaines: section sciences de l'education (520)*.

Language: French, with keywords also in English

Coverage: International

Time Span: 1972 to date

Updating: About 1000 records a quarter

FRANCIS: SOCIOLOGIE

Type: Reference (Bibliographic)

Subject: Sociology

Producer: Centre National de la Recherche Scientifique, Centre de Documentation Sciences Humaines

Online Service: Centre National de la Recherche Scientifique, Centre de Documentation Sciences Humaines (CNRS/CDSH); Telesystemes-Questel

Content: Contains over 60,000 citations, most with abstracts, to the worldwide periodical and other literature in the field of sociology. Covers social psychology; social organization and structure; social problems; human ecology; demography; rural and urban sociology; economic and political sociology; sociology of knowledge, religion, education, art, communication, leisure, organizations, health, law, and work; and social work. Corresponds to the *Bulletin Signaletique sciences humaines: section sociologie (520)*.

Language: French, with keywords also in English

Coverage: International

Time Span: 1972 to date

Updating: About 1000 records a quarter

FRESNO BEE

Type: Source (Full Text)

Subject: News

Producer: Advanced Search Concepts

Online Service: VU/TEXT Information Services, Inc.

Conditions: Subscription to VU/TEXT required

Content: Contains full text of news items, feature articles, stories, and editorials from the *Fresno Bee* (California) newspaper. Regional coverage emphasizes government, agriculture, and agribusiness.

Language: English

Coverage: U.S. (primarily San Joaquin Valley, California area)

Time Span: March 1986 to date

Updating: Daily

FROSTI (Food RA Online Scientific and Technical Information)

Type: Reference (Bibliographic)

Subject: Food Sciences & Nutrition

Producer: Leatherhead Food Research Association

Online Service: Leatherhead Food Research Association (LFRA)

Conditions: Various subscription options available

Content: Contains approximately 150,000 citations, about half with abstracts, to the worldwide literature on food science and technology. Covers food and beverages, analytical methods, quality control, manufacturing, microbiology, food processing, health and nutrition, recipes, and additives. Sources include about 600 scientific and technical journals, bulletins, and technical reports. Corresponds in part to *Abstracts Journal*.

Language: English

Coverage: International

Time Span: 1975 to date

Updating: About 250 items a week

FRSS (Federal Register Search System)

Type: Reference (Bibliographic)

Subject: Legislative Tracking

Producer: Developed jointly by the U.S. National Institutes of Health and the U.S. Environmental Protection Agency

Online Service: Information Consultants, Inc. (ICI) (as part of The Integrated Chemical Information System)

Conditions: Differential charges for subscribers and non-subscribers to ICI

Content: Contains more than 162,000 citations to all *Federal Register* notices related to chemicals and materials. Covers proposed, modified, and final federal regulations related to chemical substances. Each citation contains a description of the action as it relates to a chemical substance or substances, the agency or agencies involved, significant dates, and the affected section of the *Code of Federal Regulations* (CFR). Chemical Abstracts Service Registry Numbers are available for most chemicals cited. Various kinds of cross-references are provided to link notices for a given substance with other related notices, e.g., those that pertain to its components and those in which it is a component.

Language: English

Coverage: U.S.

Time Span: 1977 to November 1983

Updating: Not updated

FSTA (Food Science and Technology Abstracts)

Type: Reference (Bibliographic)

Subject: Food Sciences & Nutrition

Producer: International Food Information Service

Online Service: CISTI, Canadian Online Enquiry Service (CAN/OLE); DATA-STAR; DIALOG Information Services, Inc.; DIMDI; ESA-IRS; GID-SfT; The Japan Information Center of Science and Technology (JICST); ORBIT Information Technologies Corporation

Conditions: CISTI accessible only in Canada

Content: Contains about 300,000 citations, with abstracts, to the worldwide literature in food science and technology dealing with all human food commodities and food processing (except for the production of raw foods). Covers composition and properties, engineering and analysis, quality control and legislation, storage and packaging, and the management of food processes and plants. Patents, standards, books, research reports, and reviews are regularly scanned in addition to the journal literature. Corresponds to *Food Science and Technology Abstracts*.

Language: English
Coverage: International
Time Span: Most services, 1969 to date; JICST, 1981 to date.
Updating: About 1700 records a month

FYI NEWS SERVICE

Type: Source (Textual-Numeric, Full Text)
Subject: General Interest; News
Producer: Western Union Telegraph Company (from information provided by Bunker Ramo, United Press International (UPI), and others)
Online Service: Western Union Telegraph Company
Content: Consists of several files of information and news in a variety of business and general interest areas.
Newsline. Contains selected UPI news stories *(see UPI DataBase)*; in-depth reports on current news topics; business-related bulletins; reports on legislation affecting business from the U.S. Chambers of Commerce; personal computing news and information; sports scores, stories, and bulletins; and news of conditions affecting railroad transportation (e.g., weather and track conditions).
Business and Finance. Contains prices for stocks and stock options on the New York and American Stock Exchanges and NASDAQ Over-The-Counter issues; prices for Treasury bond and note futures, Government National Mortgage Association futures, commodities futures, lumber and plywood futures, petroleum futures, spot prices for 22 agricultural products, and London Metal Market prices; domestic money rates, foreign exchange rates, and spot gold prices; news and analyses of foreign exchange market and stock market developments; Latin American currency prices; and stockholder information.
Personal Interest. Contains a variety of information, including passages from the King James Bible, bestseller lists for hardcover and paperback books, horoscopes, film reviews, ski reports (in season) for 25 states, and texts of congratulatory greetings.
Travel. Contains news and information on business travel, cruises, and airline schedules and fares *(see OAG-EE)*.
Products and Services. Provides product analyses produced by Consumers Union, real estate information covering properties in 25 countries, and an online shopping service.
Forecast. Contains 2-day weather forecasts for 25 major U.S. cities and hurricane advisories for the Gulf of Mexico, the Atlantic, and the Caribbean.
Trade. Provides access to INTERNATIONAL BUSINESS CLEARINGHOUSE.
Language: English
Coverage: International
Time Span: Current day
Updating: Varies by service, from daily to continuously, throughout the day, with most services updated 2 to 3 times a day

GAMBIT 2

Type: Reference (Bibliographic, Referral)
Subject: Legislative Tracking
Producer: Computer Research Group, Inc. (CRG)
Online Service: Tymshare, Inc.
Conditions: Annual subscription fee of $5000 to $10,000 to CRG required
Content: A database system that contains citations, with abstracts, of all bills introduced in both houses of the U.S. Congress. Information on each item includes bill number,

subject or issue keyword, votes taken, amendments, measures, sponsor and co-sponsor, public commentaries, chronology, committee and floor actions, related bills and amendments, and enforcement. Also includes abstracts of articles from *The New York Times, The Wall Street Journal, The Washington Post, Business Week*, and *Fortune* that cover selected current issues.
Language: English
Coverage: U.S.
Time Span: 96th Congress to date
Updating: Daily

GARY POST-TRIBUNE

Type: Source (Full Text)
Subject: News
Producer: Gary Post-Tribune Publishing, Inc.
Online Service: VU/TEXT Information Services, Inc.
Conditions: Subscription to VU/TEXT required
Content: Contains full text of news items and feature articles from the *Gary Post-Tribune* (Indiana) newspaper.
Language: English
Coverage: U.S. (primarily Gary, Indiana area)
Time Span: November 1986 to date
Updating: Daily

GASTROINTESTINAL ABSORPTION DATABASE (GIABS)

Type: Reference (Bibliographic)
Subject: Toxicology
Producer: U.S. Environmental Protection Agency (EPA), Office of Pesticides and Toxic Substances
Online Service: Chemical Information Systems, Inc., a subsidiary of Fein-Marquart Associates (CIS)
Conditions: Annual subscription fee of $300 to CIS required but fee is waived for educational institutions and non-profit public libraries worldwide
Content: Contains over 9000 citations to the worldwide literature on experiments in gastrointestinal absorption, distribution, metabolism, and excretion of orally administered chemical substances. Covers reports on test conditions (e.g., substance tested, test animal) in more than 3400 studies involving more than 2400 chemical substances administered to laboratory animals or human subjects. The database was compiled under the auspices of the SPHERE (Scientific Parameters in Health and Environment, Retrieval and Estimation) program, sponsored by the EPA.
Language: English
Coverage: International
Time Span: 1967 to April 1984; new data to be added when EPA funds become available.
Updating: Irregularly

GenBank® (Genetic Sequences Databank)

Type: Source (Textual-Numeric)
Subject: Biotechnology; Life Sciences
Producer: Bolt, Beranek & Newman, Inc.
Online Service: Bolt, Beranek & Newman, Inc. (through a contract with the U.S. National Institutes of Health GenBank System)
Content: Contains more than 8000 citations to journal articles and technical reports in genetic research, as well as descrip-

tions of DNA and RNA sequences with 50 or more nucleotide bases. Includes more than 6000 reported sequences, totalling over 6 million bases. Each record contains 16 data items, including bibliographic data, sequence annotations (including significant features in each sequence), source organism, and starting point of sequence described. Data are compiled by the Theoretical Biology and Biophysics Group at Los Alamos National Laboratory from several sources, including *Nucleic Acids Research, Nature,* and *Proceedings of the National Academy of Sciences (USA)*.
Language: English
Coverage: Primarily U.S. and Europe
Time Span: 1967 to date
Updating: About 100 records a month

The GenBank® Software Clearinghouse
Type: Reference (Referral)
Subject: Biotechnology; Computers & Software; Life Sciences
Producer: Bolt, Beranek & Newman, Inc.
Online Service: Bolt, Beranek & Newman, Inc. (through a contract with the U.S. National Institutes of Health GenBank System)
Conditions: Quarterly subscription of $50 required
Content: Contains references to about 60 software packages for DNA and RNA sequence analysis. Includes program functions and capabilities; hardware requirements; price; author name, address, and telephone number; and, when available, citations to articles describing or evaluating the software.
Language: English
Coverage: International
Time Span: Current information
Updating: Periodically, as new data become available

GENERAL SCIENCE INDEX℠
Type: Reference (Bibliographic)
Subject: Science & Technology
Producer: The H.W. Wilson Company
Online Service: WILSONLINE
Content: Contains citations to articles and book reviews in over 111 English-language periodicals in the general sciences. Covers astronomy, atmospheric science, biology, botany, chemistry, conservation and environment, earth sciences, food and nutrition, genetics, health and medicine, mathematics, microbiology, oceanography, physics, physiology, and zoology. Corresponds to *General Science Index*.
Language: English
Coverage: Primarily U.S., with some international coverage
Time Span: May 1984 to date
Updating: Twice a week

GENETIC TOXICITY
Type: Source (Textual-Numeric)
Subject: Toxicology
Producer: U.S. Environmental Protection Agency (EPA), Office of Pesticides and Toxic Substances
Online Service: Chemical Information Systems, Inc., a subsidiary of Fein-Marquart Associates (CIS); Information Consultants, Inc. (ICI) (as part of The Integrated Chemical Information System)
Conditions: Annual subscription fee of $300 to CIS required but fee is waived for educational institutions and non-profit public libraries worldwide; differential charges for subscribers and non-subscribers to ICI.
Content: Contains mutagenicity information (e.g., chromosome aberration, DNA repair) on 2618 chemicals (e.g., dyes) that were tested against 38 biological systems (e.g., the Ames test). Data are extracted from published literature.

Language: English
Coverage: International
Time Span: 1970 to date
Updating: Periodically, as new data become available

GENEVA CONSULTANTS REGISTRY (GCR)
Type: Reference (Referral)
Subject: Biographies
Producer: Alpha Systems Resource
Online Service: Mead Data Central, Inc. (as a Reference Service database)
Conditions: Subscription to Mead Data Central required
Content: Contains summaries of the qualifications of more than 1700 individuals available as industry and professional consultants. Covers over 300 occupational titles in the fields of aerospace, agriculture, construction, corporate management, education, electronics, engineering, finance, government relations, law, logistics, manufacturing, marketing, medicine, mining, petroleum, physical sciences, public services, telecommunications, transportation, and utilities. Information on consulting fees is also included.
Language: English
Coverage: International
Time Span: Current information
Updating: Periodically, as new data become available

GEnie™ (General Electric Network for Information Exchange)
Type: Source (Full Text)
Subject: Computers & Software; Encyclopedias; General Interest
Producer: General Electric Information Services Company
Online Service: General Electric Information Services Company (GEISCO)
Conditions: Initiation fee of $18 to GEISCO required
Content: Contains a variety of general and special interest files.
General Interest and Entertainment. Provides access to ACADEMIC AMERICAN ENCYCLOPEDIA *(see)*, and movie and book reviews.
Computers. Provides access to COMPUTING TODAY! *(see)* and various other computer-related publications.
Travel. Provides access to AMERICAN AIRLINES EAASY SABRE *(see)*.
Also includes electronic conferencing, mail, games, a simulated CB (citizens band) system, and special interest groups for computer users. Shopping services are scheduled to be added.
Language: English
Coverage: U.S.
Time Span: Varies by file
Updating: Varies by file

THE GILROY DISPATCH
Type: Source (Full Text)
Subject: News
Producer: Advanced Search Concepts
Online Service: VU/TEXT Information Services, Inc.
Conditions: Subscription to VU/TEXT required

Content: Contains full text of news items and feature articles from *The Gilroy Dispatch* (California) newspaper. Regional coverage emphasizes developments in seismology, agriculture, and the food processing industry.
Language: English
Coverage: U.S. (primarily Santa Clara Valley, California area)
Time Span: April 1985 to date
Updating: Daily

GLOBE AND MAIL ONLINE℠

Type: Source (Full Text)
Subject: News
Producer: Info Globe
Online Service: Info Globe
Conditions: Initiation fee of $125 includes user manual and one-half hour of online connect time
Content: Contains full text of news stories, columns, editorials, letters to the editor, features, and selected advertising that have appeared in *The Globe and Mail*, a national newspaper in Canada, since November 14, 1977. Also covers the *Report on Business* section from January 1, 1978. Corresponds to *The Globe and Mail* newspaper.
Language: English
Coverage: Primarily Canada, with some international news
Time Span: November 14, 1977 to date
Updating: Daily, with each day's newspaper available by 5:00 A.M. Toronto time

GPO MONTHLY CATALOG

Type: Reference (Bibliographic)
Subject: Publishers & Distributors-Catalogs
Producer: U.S. Government Printing Office
Online Service: BRS; BRS/BRKTHRU; BRS/Colleague; DIALOG Information Services, Inc.; TECH DATA
Content: Contains approximately 245,000 citations to the publications of U.S. government agencies, including the U.S. Congress. Covers Senate and House hearings on bills and laws, as well as agency-sponsored studies, fact sheets, maps, handbooks, subject bibliographies, and conference proceedings. Subjects covered include agriculture, economics, energy, public affairs, taxation, law, health, consumer issues, and environment. Corresponds to *Monthly Catalog of United States Government Publications*.
Language: English
Coverage: U.S.
Time Span: July 1976 to date
Updating: About 2500 records a month

GPO PUBLICATIONS REFERENCE FILE

Type: Reference (Bibliographic)
Subject: Publishers & Distributors-Catalogs
Producer: U.S. Government Printing Office (GPO), Superintendent of Documents
Online Service: CompuServe Information Service (GOVERNMENT PUBLICATION INFORMATION SERVICE); DIALOG Information Services, Inc.; Knowledge Index
Content: Contains citations to about 24,000 public documents published by the executive, judicial, and legislative branches of the U.S. federal government and currently sold by the Superintendent of Documents. Also covers forthcoming and recently out-of-print publications. Publications from the executive branch include Presidential statements and agency annual reports, general information and operational reports, selected statistical series, technical reports, maps, administrative regulations, treaties, and periodicals. Judicial publications include slip opinions, reports, proceedings, and periodicals. Documents from the legislative branch include bills, hearings reports, committee and subcommittee publications, and laws. Publications from independent agencies and government corporations are also included. Major subject emphases correspond to the executive branch cabinet-level departments. Legislature branch documents cover all topics on which Congressional activity is focused. Records include availability, price, and GPO stock number. Corresponds to the microfiche *GPO Sales Publication Reference File*.
Language: English
Coverage: U.S.
Time Span: 1971 to date
Updating: Every 2 weeks; updates include changes in availability status.

GRADLINE

Type: Reference (Referral)
Subject: Education & Educational Institutions-Directories
Producer: Peterson's Guides, Inc.
Online Service: DIALOG Information Services, Inc.
Content: Contains descriptions of over 28,000 graduate and professional education programs offered by accredited colleges and universities in the U.S. and Canada. Includes program name and description, administrative head, number of faculty and students, entrance and degree requirements, degree concentration, financial aid available, graduate appointments, research budget, and focus of faculty research. Data are obtained from annual surveys of universities and colleges. Corresponds to the 5-volume *Peterson's Annual Guides/Graduate Study*.
Language: English
Coverage: U.S. and Canada
Time Span: Current information
Updating: Annually

GRANTS

Type: Reference (Referral)
Subject: Funding Sources, Contracts & Awards
Producer: The Oryx Press
Online Service: DIALOG Information Services, Inc.
Content: Contains references to grants offered by federal, state, and local governments; commercial organizations; associations; and private foundations. Each record contains grant program description, requirements, restrictions, contact person and address information, funding amounts, and deadline and renewal information. Information is compiled by the editorial staff of the Oryx Press. Corresponds to the annual *Directory of Research Grants*, *Directory of Biomedical and Health Care Grants*, *Directory of Grants in the Humanities*, and *Directory of Grants in the Physical Sciences*.
Language: English
Coverage: International
Time Span: Current information
Updating: Monthly

GRUPOS TERAPEUTICOS

Type: Source (Textual-Numeric)
Subject: Pharmaceuticals & Pharmaceutical Industry
Producer: Consejo General de Colegios Oficiales de Farmaceuticos de Espana
Online Service: Consejo General de Colegios Oficiales de Farmaceuticos de Espana
Content: Contains data on 423 therapeutic categories of drugs available in Spain. Provides trade name, number of dosage forms available, shelf life, conditions of dispensation (e.g., prescription required), and method of administration. Source is the pharmaceuticals register of the Ministerio de Sanidad y Consumo.
Language: Spanish
Coverage: Spain
Time Span: Current information
Updating: Periodically, as new data become available

GUIDE TO MICROFORMS IN PRINT

Type: Reference (Referral)
Subject: Publishers & Distributors-Catalogs
Producer: Meckler Publishing Co.
Online Service: BRS; BRS After Dark; BRS/BRKTHRU
Content: Contains references to about 125,000 publications currently available on microfiche or microfilm. Covers books, monographs, periodicals, and selected other types of documents (e.g., dissertations). Includes microform title, author, type (fiche or film), price (if available), and name and address of microform publisher. Corresponds to *Guide to Microforms in Print* and the accompanying *Subject Guide* and *Supplement to Microforms in Print*.
Language: English, with titles in original languages
Coverage: International
Time Span: Current information
Updating: Monthly

H.W. WILSON JOURNAL AUTHORITY FILE^{SM}

Type: Reference (Bibliographic, Referral)
Subject: Publishers & Distributors-Catalogs
Producer: The H.W. Wilson Company
Online Service: WILSONLINE
Content: Contains information on more than 2800 periodicals cited in databases and publications of The H.W. Wilson Company. Covers source periodicals cited in *Applied Science & Technology Index, Biological & Agricultural Index, Book Review Digest, Business Periodicals Index, Education Index, Readers' Guide to Periodical Literature, Index to Legal Periodicals, Humanities Index, Social Sciences Index, General Science Index, Art Index,* and *Library Literature.* Includes full title, variant titles, subscription address, price, frequency, language, country of publication, and historical notes (e.g., title changes, cessations, mergers). Also includes indicators of the Wilson databases in which each journal is indexed and, for journals in *Readers' Guide to Periodical Literature,* the availability of the journal in braille, on audio cassette, or on magnetic tape for blind and physically handicapped persons.
Language: English
Coverage: International
Time Span: December 1981 to date
Updating: About 30 records twice a week

HANDICAPPED USERS DATABASE

Type: Reference (Referral); Source (Full Text)
Subject: Social Services
Producer: Georgia Griffith
Online Service: CompuServe Information Service
Content: Contains information on products and services available to handicapped persons, with an emphasis on uses of microcomputers and related devices (e.g., Kurzweil readers). Also includes articles of interest to handicapped and non-handicapped (e.g., teachers, parents) persons, information on for-profit and non-profit service organizations, relevant news, and an electronic bulletin board.
Language: English
Coverage: U.S.
Time Span: Current information
Updating: 6 times a month

HAZARDLINE®

Type: Source (Textual-Numeric)
Subject: Chemistry-Properties; Environment; Toxicology
Producer: Occupational Health Services, Inc.
Online Service: BRS; BRS/BRKTHRU; BRS/Colleague; Executive Telecom System, Inc., Human Resource Information Network; Mead Data Central, Inc. (HAZARD) (as a Reference Service database); Occupational Health Services, Inc. (OHS); TECH DATA
Conditions: Annual subscription to Executive Telecom System required; subscription to Mead Data Central required.
Content: Contains regulatory, health, and precautionary data on over 78,000 hazardous chemicals. Includes chemical name; chemical formula; synonyms, including brand and trade names; Chemical Abstracts Service (CAS) Registry Number; identification number from the *Registry of Toxic Effects of Chemical Substances (see RTECS);* U.S. Department of Transportation (DOT) UN/PLACARD number; U.S. Environmental Protection Agency (EPA) hazardous waste number; a physical description of the substance; chemical and physical properties; incompatibility with other chemical substances; standards and recommendations for personal protective clothing and goggles (including information from the American Conference of Governmental Industrial Hygienists (ACGIH) *Guidelines for the Selection of Chemical Protective Clothing,* Vol. 1); emergency procedures in the event of personal contact; respirator requirements; route of entry of the substance into the body; permissible exposure levels, including carcinogenic, mutagenic, and teratogenic data, CERCLA Hazard Ratings, EPA reportable quantities, Food and Drug Administration (FDA) acceptable daily intake and food tolerances; level of danger to life or health (NIOSH-OSHA Immediately Dangerous to Life or Health (IDLH) value or RTECS toxicity value); symptoms upon exposure; first aid, including antidotes and post-antidote regimens; relevant federal regulations and abstracts of state laws on hazardous materials, transportation, storage, recycling, treatment, radioactive materials, and state right-to-know laws; medical examinations and specific tests required by the Occupational Safety and Health Administration (OSHA); fire-fighting recommendations from the Bureau of Explosives; and guidelines and procedures for dealing with hazardous leaks, spills, and waste disposal. Users can retrieve data on specific chemical substances by searching on various criteria, including chemical name, synonym, keyword, chemical formula, CAS Registry Number, RTECS number, DOT UN/PLACARD number, or symptoms of exposure. Sources of data include OSHA and EPA standards and regulations, National Institute of Occupational Safety and

Health (NIOSH) criteria documents, important and relevant court decisions, and selected relevant standards and guidelines from such other organizations as the American National Standards Institute.
NOTE: On Mead Data Central, users can also search the full text of Material Safety Data Sheets *(see OHS MSDS)*.
Language: English
Coverage: U.S.
Time Span: Current information
Updating: OHS, daily; BRS and Executive Telecom System, monthly; Mead Data Central, quarterly.

HAZARDOUS SUBSTANCES DATA BANK

Type: Source (Textual-Numeric)
Subject: Toxicology
Producer: National Library of Medicine, Toxicology Information Program
Online Service: DIMDI; National Library of Medicine (NLM) (as part of TOXNET)
Content: Contains data on more than 4100 chemical substances that are of known or potential toxicity and to which substantial populations are exposed. Includes 144 data elements grouped into 10 classes of information:
Substance Identification Information. Includes Chemical Abstracts Service name and Registry number, synonyms, molecular formula, standard transportation number, and EPA hazardous wastes number.
Manufacturing/Use Information. Includes manufacturers, methods of manufacturing, major uses, and production data.
Chemical and Physical Properties. Includes color, form, odor, corrosivity, and critical temperatures and pressures.
Safety and Handling Information. Includes a summary of hazards, flammable properties, explosive limits and potential, stability and shelf-life, and U.S. Department of Transportation emergency guidelines.
Toxicity/Biomedical Effects. Includes a summary of toxicity, toxic hazard rating, and populations at special risk.
Pharmacology. Includes drug warnings, therapeutic uses, drug tolerance, and maximum drug dose.
Environmental Fate/Exposure Potential Information. Includes a summary of environmental fate/exposure, pollution sources, environmental transformations and transport, environmental and non-human concentrations, and probable routes of human exposure.
Exposure Standards and Regulations. Includes permissible levels of occupational exposure, allowable tolerances, and water, atmospheric, and soil standards.
Monitoring and Analysis Methods. Includes sampling procedures, analytic procedures, and clinical laboratory methods.
Additional references. Includes references to special reports, online databases, in-process test reports, and accident histories.
Language: English
Coverage: International
Time Span: Current information
Updating: Quarterly

HAZARDOUS WASTE NEWS

Type: Source (Full Text)
Subject: Environment
Producer: Business Publishers, Inc.

Online Service: NewsNet, Inc.
Conditions: Monthly subscription to NewsNet required; differential charges for subscribers and non-subscribers to *Hazardous Waste News.*
Content: Contains full text of *Hazardous Waste News,* a newsletter focusing on compliance and enforcement related to the regulation of hazardous wastes.
Language: English
Coverage: U.S.
Time Span: 1982 to date
Updating: Weekly

HDOK

Type: Reference (Bibliographic)
Subject: Social Services
Producer: The Swedish Institute for the Handicapped
Online Service: The Swedish Institute for the Handicapped
Conditions: Subscription to The Swedish Institute for the Handicapped required
Content: Contains approximately 2500 citations to reports on aids for disabled persons. Primary coverage is on these handicaps: speech impairment, visual impairment, incontinence, motor disorders, and mental retardation. Sources include about 400 journals, as well as reports, reviews of research and development, and selected books. Corresponds in part to *Handikappinstitutes Nyfoervaervslista,* with more citations provided in the printed form.
Language: English and Swedish, with titles also in original languages
Coverage: Primarily Europe, Japan, and U.S.
Time Span: 1972 to 1985
Updating: Updating will resume in 1986

HEALTH AUDIOVISUAL ONLINE CATALOG

Type: Reference (Referral)
Subject: Audiovisual Materials-Catalogs; Biomedicine; Library Holdings-Catalogs
Producer: Northeastern Ohio Universities College of Medicine, Basic Medical Sciences Library and other Ohio medical schools
Online Service: BRS; BRS/BRKTHRU; BRS/Colleague; TECH DATA
Content: Contains citations, with abstracts, to the combined audiovisual collections of 7 Ohio medical schools. Covers more than 5300 audiovisual packages in the areas of medicine, nursing, psychology, and allied health fields. Each record includes title, author or producer, bibliographic data, physical description of the item, and holdings information.
Language: English
Coverage: Primarily U.S., with some international coverage
Time Span: 1960 to date
Updating: Twice a year

HEALTH PLANNING AND ADMINISTRATION

Type: Reference (Bibliographic)
Subject: Health Care
Producer: National Library of Medicine
Online Service: Australian Medline Network; BRS (HEALTH CARE AND ADMINISTRATION); BRS After Dark (HEALTH CARE AND ADMINISTRATION); BRS/Colleague (HEALTH CARE AND ADMINISTRATION); DIALOG Information Services, Inc.; DIMDI; National Library of Medicine (NLM)

Content: Covers numerous topics (e.g., budgeting, finance, organization, administration, management, planning, facilities, and personnel resource development) relevant to the provision of health care services. Citations are drawn from 3000 journals covered in MEDLINE *(see)*; journals reviewed for *Hospital Literature Index*; monographs, monograph chapters, theses, and technical reports supplied by the National Health Planning Information Center; and non-journal citations from the "Health Planning Series" of the *Weekly Government Abstracts*, published by the National Technical Information Service.

Language: English

Coverage: International

Time Span: 1975 to date

Updating: About 3000 records a month

HEALTHCARE EVALUATION SYSTEM

Type: Reference (Referral); Source (Textual-Numeric)

Subject: Health Care & Social Services-Directories

Producer: National Planning Data Corporation

Online Service: National Planning Data Corporation

Content: Contains information on health care facilities, including hospitals, nursing homes, home health agencies, health maintenance organizations (HMOs), outpatient and ambulatory care facilities, and freestanding emergency clinics (FECs). Provides facility name and address; number of beds; numbers of patients, including Medicare and Medicaid patients; average length of stay; types of services offered; and the number and types of surgical procedures performed. Also includes information on approval and accreditation and type of control (e.g., non-profit/church-owned, county government, investor-owned). Information can be retrieved for individual facilities and for all facilities by ZIP code or county. Source of data is SMG Marketing Group Inc.

Language: English

Coverage: U.S.

Time Span: December 1982 to date

Updating: Hospital data, quarterly; HMO, FEC, ambulatory care facility, and home health agency data, annually; nursing home data, periodically, as new data become available.

HEALTHCOM MEDICAL INFORMATION SERVICE

Type: Source (Full Text)

Subject: Health Care

Producer: Robert L. Walter Communications

Online Service: CompuServe Information Service

Content: Contains health care information and advice for consumers. Covers diet and nutrition, mental health, sexuality, traditional and alternative therapies, alcohol and drug use, family health care, women's health issues, and dental care. Also provides a forum for exchanges between health care professionals and users, as well as interactive tutorials on subjects of current interest (e.g., Acquired Immune Deficiency Syndrome (AIDS)). Each tutorial is accompanied by references to selected materials from popular and professional journals.

Language: English

Coverage: U.S.

Time Span: Current information

Updating: Continuously, throughout the day; tutorials, monthly.

HEALTHNET

Type: Source (Full Text)

Subject: Health Care

Producer: HealthNet

Online Service: CompuServe Information Service; General Videotex Corporation/DELPHI

Content: Contains health care information for consumers. Covers symptoms and diseases, drugs, medical tests and procedures, first aid, nutrition, sexuality, exercise, sports medicine, preventive medicine, and environmental health. Also includes topical articles (e.g., effects of caffeine consumption, updates on Acquired Immune Deficiency Syndrome (AIDS), lung cancer, nearsightedness), a self-administered health quiz, and a question and answer forum.

Language: English

Coverage: U.S.

Time Span: Current information

Updating: Monthly

HECLINET (Health Care Literature Information Network)

Type: Reference (Bibliographic)

Subject: Health Care

Producer: Technische Universitaet Berlin, Institut fuer Krankenhausbau, Dokumentation Krankenhauswesen, in cooperation with the hospital institutions of Austria, Denmark, Federal Republic of Germany, Sweden, and Switzerland

Online Service: DIMDI

Content: Contains approximately 70,000 citations, with some abstracts, to the worldwide literature on hospital administration; non-clinical aspects of health services, including health policy, education, organization, and regional planning; hospital design, construction, maintenance, financing, hygiene, and insurance; health economics; and laws. Covers journals in the fields of health care, economics, architecture, and operations research, as well as relevant monographs, conference proceedings, and reports. Corresponds in part to *Informationsdienst Krankenhauswesen* (Health Care Information Service).

Language: Titles and abstracts are in original language and in either English or German; index terms are in English and German.

Coverage: International

Time Span: 1969 to date

Updating: About 750 records every 2 months

HEILBRON

Type: Source (Textual-Numeric)

Subject: Chemistry-Properties

Producer: Chapman & Hall Ltd.

Online Service: DIALOG Information Services, Inc.; Knowledge Index

Content: Contains physical and chemical properties data on approximately 175,000 important substances selected by a panel of experts. Includes molecular weight and formula; melting, freezing, and boiling point; solubility; relative density; optical rotation; dissociation constants; uses; reactions; and Chemical Abstracts Service Registry Number, derivative names, synonyms, and variant compounds. Corresponds to *Dictionary of Organic Compounds (5th edition)* and *Dictionary of Organometallic Compounds*.

Language: English

Time Span: Current information
Updating: Twice a year

HERACLES
Type: Reference (Bibliographic, Referral)
Subject: Sports Medicine
Producer: Sportdoc
Online Service: G.CAM Serveur
Content: Contains about 25,000 references, with abstracts, to scientific and practical source materials on sports, recreation, sports medicine, and physical education. Covers periodicals, books, theses, conference proceedings, microfilms, films, and videotapes.
Language: French
Coverage: Primarily France, with some international coverage
Time Span: 1973 to date
Updating: About 400 records a month

HIGH TECH EUROPE
Type: Reference (Referral); Source (Full Text)
Subject: Technology Transfer
Producer: High Technology Verlag GmbH
Online Service: THE SOURCE
Content: Contains news of technological developments and business opportunities in Europe. Provides feature articles on developments in European laboratories and other research sites, employment opportunities, product and service listings, and offers of goods, licenses, and partnerships to U.S. businesses by European companies.
Language: English
Coverage: Europe and U.S., with some coverage of Japan
Time Span: Current information
Updating: Twice a month

HIGH TECH INTERNATIONAL
Type: Source (Full Text)
Subject: Science & Technology
Producer: High Technology Verlag GmbH
Online Service: NewsNet, Inc.
Conditions: Monthly subscription to NewsNet required; differential charges for subscribers and non-subscribers to *High Tech International*.
Content: Contains full text of *High Tech International*, a newsletter on high-technology industries, including international developments of particular interest to the Federal Republic of Germany and U.S. markets. Covers marketing, production, patents and licenses, and venture capital in such areas as medicine, biotechnology, chemistry, electronics, energy, robotics, and space. Also includes news of personnel changes and analyses of long-term trends.
Language: English
Coverage: Primarily Federal Republic of Germany, with some international coverage
Time Span: August 1984 to date
Updating: Monthly

HISTLINE
Type: Reference (Bibliographic)
Subject: Biomedicine
Producer: National Library of Medicine (NLM), History of Medicine Division

Online Service: National Library of Medicine (NLM)
Content: Contains citations to articles, books, conference proceedings and other literature on the history of medicine. Includes works on individuals, institutions, the profession, diseases, drugs, and medical techniques. Primary sources of information include the MEDLINE *(see)* and CATLINE *(see)* databases. Corresponds to NLM's annual *Bibliography of the History of Medicine*.
Language: English
Coverage: International
Time Span: Earliest records from 1964, with most records from 1970
Updating: About 500 records a month

HOSPITAL DATABASE
Type: Reference (Referral); Source (Textual-Numeric)
Subject: Health Care; Health Care & Social Services-Directories
Producer: Urban Decision Systems, Inc. (UDS)
Online Service: STSC, Inc.
Conditions: Monthly minimum of $150 to STSC, Inc. required
Content: Contains information on hospital facilities and their utilization. Provides hospital name, address, and telephone number; manager's name; type of hospital (e.g., medical-surgical, psychiatric); type of control (e.g., investor-owned, county government); and approval and accreditation. Hospital utilization data include admissions and emergency visits, inpatient and outpatient surgical procedures, hospital occupancy rate and average length of stay per patient, beds per ward (e.g., pediatric, cardiology, oncology), and staffed beds versus unstaffed beds. Also provides data on each facility's market-area demographics, including population, age, sex, and income. Corresponds in part to *Hospital Market Atlas*, published by SMG Marketing Group Inc.
Language: English
Coverage: U.S.
Time Span: Current information
Updating: Periodically, as new data become available

HOUSTON POST
Type: Source (Full Text)
Subject: News
Producer: Houston Post Company
Online Service: VU/TEXT Information Services, Inc.
Conditions: Subscription to VU/TEXT required
Content: Contains full text of news items and feature articles from *The Houston Post* (Texas) newspaper. Regional coverage emphasizes energy, petrochemicals, aerospace, and medicine.
Language: English
Coverage: U.S. (primarily Houston, Texas area)
Time Span: 1985 to date
Updating: Daily

HSELiNE
Type: Reference (Bibliographic)
Subject: Occupational Safety & Health
Producer: Health and Safety Executive, Library and Information Services
Online Service: DATA-STAR; ESA-IRS; Pergamon InfoLine
Content: Contains about 85,000 citations, with abstracts, to the worldwide literature on occupational safety and health.

Covers all U.K. Health and Safety Commission and Health and Safety Executive publications as well as a wide range of periodicals, books, conference proceedings, reports, and legislation. Includes all relevant areas of science and technology with particular emphasis on engineering, manufacturing, agriculture, mining, nuclear technology, explosives, production, industrial air pollution, and occupational hygiene. English-language abstracts are provided for non-English materials.

Language: English

Coverage: International

Time Span: 1977 to date, with some citations to earlier publications

Updating: About 1000 records a month

HUMAN SEXUALITY™

Type: Source (Full Text)

Subject: Biomedicine; Sociology; Psychology

Producer: Clinical Communications, Inc.

Online Service: CompuServe Information Service

Content: Contains information and advice on all aspects of human sexuality. Contains articles, interview and discussion transcripts, interactive programs, and answers to commonly asked questions on such topics as contraception, relationships, sexual dysfunction, homosexuality, and sexually transmitted diseases. Covers developments in such related fields as urology, gynecology, psychiatry, pharmacology, and endocrinology. Users can submit comments and questions online.

Language: English

Coverage: U.S.

Time Span: Current information

Updating: Every 1 to 2 weeks

IALINE

Type: Reference (Bibliographic)

Subject: Food Sciences & Nutrition

Producer: Centre de Documentation des Industries Utilisatrices de Produits Agricoles (CDIUPA), in collaboration with the Centre National de la Recherche Scientifique, Centre de Documentation Scientifique et Technique (CNRS/CDST)

Online Service: Telesystemes-Questel

Content: Covers literature on the scientific, technical, and economic aspects of the food industry. Topics covered include composition, quality, and properties of raw materials, ingredients, and manufactured products; processing and engineering methods; industrial uses of agricultural products and by-products; quality control and regulation; food microbiology and fermentation; pollution problems and wastewater treatment; and economic data on yield, consumption, and commercial trade. Corresponds to the *Industries Agro-Alimentaires: Bibliographie Internationale*.

Language: French

Coverage: International

Time Span: 1970 to date

Updating: About 1300 records a month

IBM PC SIG

Type: Source (Full Text, Software)

Subject: Computers & Software

Producer: THE SOURCE

Online Service: THE SOURCE

Conditions: Monthly minimum of $10 to THE SOURCE required, with $9 credited toward online usage charges

Content: Contains news and information for users of IBM personal computers. Provides announcements and reviews of new products, accessories, and services, including notices of discounts available from vendors; reviews of information sources (e.g., books, newsletters, online services); a directory of bulletin boards and user groups; and software available for downloading.

Language: English

Coverage: U.S.

Time Span: Current information

Updating: Daily

ICAR (Inventory of Canadian Agri-Food Research)

Type: Reference (Referral)

Subject: Agriculture; Research in Progress

Producer: Agriculture Canada, Research Branch

Online Service: CISTI, Canadian Online Enquiry Service (CAN/OLE)

Conditions: CISTI accessible only in Canada

Content: Contains approximately 4200 references to current agricultural and food research and development projects conducted by Canadian federal and provincial governments, universities, industry, and other organizations. Corresponds to *Inventory of Canadian Agricultural Research*.

Language: Records are entered in their original language, either in English or French but not both

Coverage: Canada

Time Span: Current research

Updating: Annually

ICIE DATABASE

Type: Reference (Bibliographic)

Subject: Toxicology

Producer: Oak Ridge National Laboratory (ORNL), Toxicology Information Response Center

Online Service: Oak Ridge National Laboratory

Conditions: Available to staff and contractors of the U.S. Department of Energy and most other government agencies and contractors; permission required from ORNL for other users.

Content: Contains approximately 6000 citations, with abstracts, to literature on the metabolism and health effects of radioisotopes. Covers exposure from radiopharmaceuticals, nuclear fallout, and industrial accidents, as well as related mathematical models, reported in journal articles, technical reports, and unpublished reports collected by ORNL, Health Safety and Safety Research Division, Information Center for Internal Exposure. Also covers dose calculations made in U.S. Department of Energy laboratories and reported in unpublished reports and personal communications.

Language: English

Coverage: International

Time Span: 1909 to date

Updating: Periodically, as new data become available

IEC (Directory of Federally Supported Research in Universities)

Type: Reference (Referral)

Subject: Research in Progress

Producer: CISTI, Information Exchange Centre

Online Service: CISTI, Canadian Online Enquiry Service (CAN/OLE)

Conditions: CISTI accessible only in Canada

Content: Contains descriptions of approximately 135,000 university-based research projects sponsored by 36 funding agencies in Canada. This multidisciplinary database covers all individuals who receive Canadian federal grants. Corresponds to *Directory of Federally Supported Research in Universities.*

Language: English and French

Coverage: Canada

Time Span: Fiscal year 1971 to date

Updating: About 10,000 records a year

IMSPACT

Type: Source (Textual-Numeric)

Subject: Pharmaceuticals & Pharmaceutical Industry

Producer: IMS America, Ltd.

Online Service: IMS America, Ltd.

Conditions: Subscription to printed audits required

Content: Contains reports of 7 audits performed by IMS America of the pharmaceutical industry. Covers *Pharmaceutical Markets, Drugstores; Pharmaceutical Markets, Hospitals; National Disease & Therapeutical Index (NDTI); National Prescription Audit; National Journal Audit; National Mail Audit;* and *National Detailing Audit.* Provides monthly sales data, including hospital and drugstore purchases by company, product class, and individual products (at the package level); medical data, including NDTI information on the usage of drugs (by product, form, and strength) per diagnosis; prescription data, including new prescriptions written and new and refill prescriptions dispensed; and promotional data, including number of units and dollars spent on mail and journal advertising. Also provides data on number of kilograms sold of pharmaceutically active chemicals. Product characteristics covered include formula, price, date of introduction, chemical family, medical usage, application form, and corporate structure of the company manufacturing the product.

Language: English

Coverage: U.S.

Time Span: Current 6 years

Updating: Weekly

INDEX CHEMICUS ONLINE℠

Type: Reference (Bibliographic); Source (Textual-Numeric)

Subject: Chemistry-Structure & Nomenclature

Producer: Institute for Scientific Information (ISI)

Online Service: Telesystemes-Questel (as a DARC database *(see)*)

Content: Contains over 350,000 citations to articles in which new organic chemical compounds have been reported, from approximately 110 journals. Special alerts indicate relevant analytical techniques (e.g., column chromatography, nuclear magnetic resonance), new synthetic methods, biological activities, explosive reactions, and level of experimental detail (for data from 1983 to date). Compounds may be retrieved by structure searching using DARC *(see).* Corresponds in part to *Current Abstracts of Chemistry and Index Chemicus.*

Language: English

Coverage: International

Time Span: Structures, 1962 to date; citations, 1960 to date.

Updating: Monthly, with about 16,000 compounds; about 20,000 references a year.

INDEX TO READER'S DIGEST

Type: Reference (Bibliographic)

Subject: General Interest

Producer: Infordata International Incorporated, in cooperation with the Reader's Digest Association, Inc.

Online Service: BRS (to be available in 1987); BRS After Dark (to be available in 1987); BRS/BRKTHRU (to be available in 1987)

Content: Contains citations to all editorial material, articles, short subjects, humor (e.g., anecdotes, cartoons), illustrations, and biographical mentions published in the *Reader's Digest.*

Language: English

Coverage: U.S.

Time Span: Will cover 1922 to date

Updating: About 30 articles and 150 short subjects a month

INDEX TO U.S. GOVERNMENT PERIODICALS

Type: Reference (Bibliographic)

Subject: Government-U.S. Federal; Publishers & Distributors-Catalogs

Producer: Infordata International Incorporated

Online Service: BRS; WILSONLINE

Content: Contains about 76,000 citations to articles in more than 185 periodicals published by the U.S. federal government. Emphasis is on publications of lasting reference or research value. Also includes letters, book reviews, interviews, and press conference and conference proceedings. Corresponds to *Index to U.S. Government Periodicals.*

Language: English

Coverage: U.S.

Time Span: 1980 to date, with some materials from 1979

Updating: About 1100 records a month

INDICE ESPANOL DE CIENCIA Y TECNOLOGIA

Type: Reference (Bibliographic)

Subject: Science & Technology

Producer: Consejo Superior de Investigaciones Cientificas, Instituto de Informacion y Documentacion en Ciencia y Tecnologia

Online Service: Consejo Superior de Investigaciones Cientificas, Instituto de Informacion y Documentacion en Ciencia y Tecnologia; Ministerio de Cultura, Secretaria General Tecnica; Ministerio de Educacion y Ciencia

Content: Contains over 20,000 citations to Spanish literature on science and technology. Covers agronomy, astronomy and astrophysics, chemistry, earth sciences, engineering, life sciences, logic, mathematics, pharmacology, and physics. Sources include journals, monographs, theses, yearbooks, and proceedings.

Language: Spanish

Coverage: Spain

Time Span: 1979 to date

Updating: Monthly

INDICE MEDICO ESPANOL (IME)

Type: Reference (Bibliographic)

Subject: Biomedicine

Producer: Caja de Ahorros de Valencia; Universidad de Valencia CSIC; Universidad de Valencia, Facultad de Medicina, Centro de Documentacion e Informatica Biomedica

Online Service: Universidad de Valencia, Facultad de Medicina, Centro de Documentacion e Informatica Biomedica (CEDIB)

Content: Contains about 100,000 citations to articles in medical journals published in Spain.

Language: Spanish

Coverage: Spain

Time Span: 1971 to date

Updating: Quarterly

INDUSTRIAL HEALTH & HAZARDS UPDATE℠

Type: Reference (Bibliographic); Source (Full Text)

Subject: Occupational Safety & Health

Producer: Merton Allen Associates

Online Service: NewsNet, Inc.

Conditions: Monthly subscription to NewsNet required

Content: Contains full text of *Industrial Health & Hazards Update*, a newsletter providing abstracts of reports and brief news items on legal and technical aspects of industrial safety. Covers regulations and standards, current litigation, product liability, industry surveys, hazard evaluations for specific workplaces, and toxicology research. Sources include government reports, journals, and news items.

Language: English

Coverage: Primarily U.S., with some international coverage

Time Span: May 1984 to date

Updating: Monthly

INDUSTRY DATA SOURCES℠

Type: Reference (Bibliographic)

Subject: Health Care

Producer: Information Access Co.

Online Service: BRS; BRS/BRKTHRU; BRS/Colleague; DATA-STAR; DIALOG Information Services, Inc.; Mead Data Central, Inc. (INDASO) (as a Reference Service database); TECH DATA

Conditions: Subscription to Mead Data Central required

Content: Contains citations, with abstracts, to over 100,000 sources of data on 65 industries. Sources include market research studies, financial investment studies, special issues of trade journals, statistical reports and studies, economic forecasts, numeric databases, monographs, working papers, dissertations, and industry conference reports. Each reference includes title, publication date, publisher, pages, price, periodicity (if applicable), and summary of content and coverage. Industries covered include advertising, agriculture, broadcasting, chemicals, commercial banking, computers, construction, drugs and pharmaceuticals.

Language: English

Coverage: International

Time Span: U.S. and Canada, 1979 to date; Western Europe, July 1981 to date; Japan and South America, 1982 to date.

Updating: About 2000 records a month

INDUSTRY FILE INDEX SYSTEM

Type: Reference (Referral)

Subject: Occupational Safety & Health

Producer: U.S. Environmental Protection Agency (EPA)

Online Service: Chemical Information Systems, Inc., a subsidiary of Fein-Marquart Associates (CIS)

Conditions: Annual subscription fee of $300 to CIS required but fee is waived for educational institutions and non-profit public libraries worldwide

Content: Contains summaries of EPA regulations covering both specific chemicals and the chemical industry. Contains approximately 12,000 records on specific chemicals and chemical products (e.g., dioxin, asbestos, PCBs, fluorocarbons) and 113 records on individual classes of companies (e.g., pesticide manufacturers). Data can be retrieved by chemical, classes of chemical industry companies, and regulation.

Language: English

Coverage: U.S.

Time Span: Current as of June 1985

Updating: Periodically, as new data become available

INFOMAT BUSINESS DATABASE

Type: Reference (Bibliographic)

Subject: Health Care; News

Producer: BIS Infomat

Online Service: DIALOG Information Services, Inc. (to be available in 1987); Pergamon InfoLine

Content: Contains over 275,000 summaries of business news reports from more than 500 publications worldwide. Covers marketing, advertising, and retail sales; leisure, food, and beverages; automobile industry and automotive services; shipping and transportation; science and technology, including electronics and engineering; chemicals, energy resources, and forest products and packaging; construction; health care and pharmaceuticals; and information technology and telecommunications. Sources include daily and weekly newspapers, bank reports, economics and business journals, trade and professional magazines, and Reuters wire service.

Language: English

Coverage: International

Time Span: 1983 to date

Updating: Weekly

INFORMACION TERAPEUTICA A LOS PACIENTES

Type: Source (Full Text)

Subject: Pharmaceuticals & Pharmaceutical Industry

Producer: Consejo General de Colegios Oficiales de Farmaceuticos de Espana

Online Service: Consejo General de Colegios Oficiales de Farmaceuticos de Espana

Content: Contains full text of instructions to patients for over 10,000 prescription drugs available in Spain. Includes correct utilization, possible side effects, precautions, and contraindications.

Language: Spanish

Coverage: Spain

Time Span: Current information

Updating: Periodically, as new data become available

INFORMATION AND TECHNOLOGY TRANSFER DATABASE

Type: Reference (Bibliographic)
Subject: Science & Technology
Producer: International Research & Evaluation
Online Service: International Research & Evaluation
Content: Contains over 3 million citations, with some abstracts, to materials covering a wide variety of subjects: energy, law enforcement and justice, waste management, fiber optics and lasers, transportation, medicine, health, earth sciences, construction, civil engineering, and agriculture. Sources include annual reports, bibliographies, conference papers, corporate filings, curriculum materials, dissertations, essays, evaluation studies, fact sheets, feasibility studies, handbooks, journal articles, legislation, manuals, newsletters, patents, research reports, resource guides, speeches, standards, statistical compilations, syllabi, taxonomies, technical reports, theses, and treatises. Corresponds in part to ENERGY INFORMATION DATABASE, LAW ENFORCEMENT AND CRIMINAL JUSTICE INFORMATION DATABASE, and WASTE MANAGEMENT AND RESOURCE RECOVERY (see).
Language: English
Coverage: International
Time Span: Earliest data from 1892
Updating: Every 2 weeks; about 400,000 records a year.

THE INFORMATION BANK® ABSTRACTS

Type: Reference (Bibliographic)
Subject: News
Producer: The New York Times Company
Online Service: Mead Data Central, Inc. (as a NEXIS and Reference Service database)
Conditions: Subscription to Mead Data Central required
Content: Contains abstracts of all news and editorial matter from the final Late Edition of *The New York Times* newspaper and selected material from approximately 10 other newspapers and 39 magazines published in the U.S., Canada, and Europe. These other sources include general circulation newspapers (e.g., *The Wall Street Journal*, *The Christian Science Monitor*, *Los Angeles Times*, *Chicago Tribune*); publications in business (e.g., *Barron's*, *Financial Times* (Canada and London), *Fortune*, *Harvard Business Review*); international affairs (e.g., *Economist* of London, *Foreign Policy*); science (e.g., *Scientific American*); and some general interest periodicals (e.g., *Consumer Reports*, *Sports Illustrated*, *U.S. News & World Report*). Items covered include general news articles, forecasts, analyses, surveys, biographies, features, columns, and editorials. Maps, charts, photographs, diagrams, and other graphics are noted but captions are excluded.
Language: English
Coverage: International
Time Span: 1969 to date
Updating: Daily, Monday through Friday (usually 24 to 48 hours after publication)

THE INFORMATION REPORT

Type: Reference (Referral); Source (Full Text)
Subject: Information Systems & Services-Directories
Producer: Washington Researchers Publishing
Online Service: NewsNet, Inc.
Conditions: Monthly subscription to NewsNet required; differential charges for subscribers and non-subscribers to *The Information Report*.

Content: Contains full text of *The Information Report*, a newsletter covering sources of free or low-cost business information and assistance. Includes brief descriptions of relevant newsletters, magazines, directories, bibliographies, databases, and other sources of information provided by federal, state, and local government agencies, associations, and trade unions. Also includes advice on gathering competitive intelligence.
Language: English
Coverage: U.S.
Time Span: 1985 to date
Updating: Monthly

INFORMATION USA

Type: Reference (Referral)
Subject: Information Systems & Services-Directories
Producer: Information USA, Inc.
Online Service: CompuServe Information Service
Content: Contains references to information resources within the departments, agencies, and offices of the U.S. federal government. Covers 10,000 offices, 3000 persons, and 3000 free or low-cost publications. Users can submit questions and receive answers online. Corresponds in part to *Information USA*.
Language: English
Coverage: U.S.
Time Span: Current information
Updating: Daily

INFORMAZIONI PER LE INDUSTRIE

Type: Reference (Bibliographic)
Subject: Occupational Safety & Health
Producer: SIRIO
Online Service: SIRIO
Content: Contains about 8000 citations, with abstracts, to articles on industrial accident prevention, occupational diseases, and industrial pollution in Italy. Corresponds to *Informazioni per le industrie*.
Language: Italian
Coverage: Italy
Time Span: 1974 to date
Updating: Annually

INFOSERV

Type: Reference (Bibliographic)
Subject: Publishers & Distributors-Catalogs
Producer: The Faxon Company, Inc.
Online Service: The Faxon Company, Inc.
Content: Contains approximately 40,000 listings of active serial titles published worldwide. Includes title, subject area, publisher, editor, date of first issue, and publisher's description of the scope and character of the publication. Also contains listings of 5000 serials first published or revised since 1982 and listings of serial back volumes available from Alfred Jaeger, Inc. Users can order sample copies and subscriptions and request additional information online.
Language: English
Coverage: International
Time Span: Current 3 years
Updating: About 300 to 400 items a week

INFOTOX

Type: Source (Textual-Numeric)

Subject: Chemistry-Properties; Occupational Safety & Health

Producer: Centre de Documentation, Commission de la Sante et de la Securite du Travail (CSST)

Online Service: IST-Informatheque Inc.

Content: Contains about 5500 safety data sheets on pure and compound chemical and biological products used in industrial and commercial applications in Quebec. Provides information on physico-chemical and toxicological properties, product regulations, and hazard prevention and first-aid measures. Corresponds to *Repertoire Toxicologique*.

Language: Primarily French, with some records also in English

Coverage: Canada (Quebec)

Time Span: Current information

Updating: About 1000 records a quarter

INNOVATOR'S DIGEST®

Type: Reference (Bibliographic); Source (Full Text)

Subject: Science & Technology

Producer: The InfoTeam, Inc.

Online Service: NewsNet, Inc.

Conditions: Monthly subscription to NewsNet required

Content: Contains full text of *Innovator's Digest*, a newsletter that provides citations, with abstracts, to selected reports on technological innovations. Covers products, materials, processes, techniques, and current research in such fields as agriculture, biomedicine, communications, construction, computers, electronics, engineering, energy, and manufacturing. Also covers the "business" of innovating. Sources include journals, news services, and business, university, and government reports.

Language: English

Coverage: International

Time Span: August 1983 to date

Updating: Every 2 weeks

INPADOC

Type: Reference (Bibliographic)

Subject: Patents

Producer: International Patent Documentation Center

Online Service: FIZ Karlsruhe (INPADOC PATSDI); Pergamon InfoLine (INPADOC)

Conditions: Not accessible through Pergamon InfoLine in Japan or through FIZ Karlsruhe in Canada, Japan, Spain, or U.S.

Content: Contains citations to all types of patents issued in 51 countries and by the European Patent Office and the World Intellectual Property Organization (WIPO) under the Patent Cooperation Treaty of 1970. Each record contains standard bibliographic data. Includes patent family information. Searching for patent equivalents in one or more countries is available only through Pergamon Infoline.

Language: Titles in original languages

Coverage: International

Time Span: FIZ, most recent 6 weeks; Pergamon InfoLine, varies by country with earliest data from 1968.

Updating: About 18,000 records a week

INPADOC PATENTE

Type: Reference (Bibliographic)

Subject: Patents

Producer: International Patent Documentation Center

Online Service: FIZ Karlsruhe

Conditions: Not accessible through FIZ Karlsruhe in Japan or Spain

Content: Contains over 878,000 citations to all types of patents issued in Austria, the Federal Republic of Germany, and Switzerland. Each record contains standard bibliographic data.

Language: German

Coverage: Austria, Federal Republic of Germany, and Switzerland

Time Span: 1978 to date

Updating: About 8000 records a month

INPANEW

Type: Reference (Bibliographic)

Subject: Patents

Producer: International Patent Documentation Center

Online Service: Pergamon InfoLine

Conditions: Not accessible in Japan

Content: Contains the most recent 15 weeks of patent citations (approximately 270,000 citations) to be entered in INPADOC *(see)*. Includes patent family information.

Language: English, with titles in original languages

Coverage: International

Time Span: Most recent 15 weeks of published documents

Updating: About 18,000 records a week

INPI-1 (INPI-BREVETS)

Type: Reference (Bibliographic)

Subject: Patents

Producer: Institut National de la Propriete Industrielle (INPI)

Online Service: Telesystemes-Questel

Content: Contains references to over 570,000 patents published in France since 1969. Includes names of inventor, applicant, and agent; title of invention; International Patent Classification System code; country of origin; and dates of application, publication, and lapse. Corresponds to *Bulletin Officiel de la Propriete Industrielle*.

Language: French

Coverage: France

Time Span: 1969 to date

Updating: About 500 records a week, on day of publication

INPI-3

Type: Source (Numeric)

Subject: Patents

Producer: European Patent Office (EPO); Institut National de la Propriete Industrielle (INPI)

Online Service: Telesystemes-Questel

Content: Contains approximately 4.9 million records that provide links among over 12 million patent documents issued by different countries for the same priority application.

Coverage: International

Time Span: 1969 to date, with some earlier patents

Updating: Monthly

INSTITUTIONENVERZEICHNIS FUER INTERNATIONALE ZUSAMMENARBEIT (IVIZ)

Type: Reference (Referral)
Subject: Education & Educational Institutions
Producer: NOMOS Datapool
Online Service: EDICLINE
Conditions: Initiation fee of 60 pounds (U.K.) to EDICLINE required
Content: Contains information on about 3000 organizations worldwide that participate in academic and research exchanges with the Federal Republic of Germany. Provides name, address, management personnel, description of activities, and list of publications. Sources include the Vereinigung fuer internationale Zusammenarbeit, the Deutschen Akademischen Austauschdienst, the Deutsche Stiftung fuer internationale Entwicklung, and the Institut fuer Auslands beziehungen. Corresponds to the series *Handbuch fuer Internationale Zusammenarbeit.*
Language: English and German
Coverage: International
Time Span: Current information
Updating: Quarterly

INTERACCIONES CON ANALISIS CLINICOS

Type: Source (Textual-Numeric)
Subject: Pharmaceuticals & Pharmaceutical Industry
Producer: Consejo General de Colegios Oficiales de Farmaceuticos de Espana
Online Service: Consejo General de Colegios Oficiales de Farmaceuticos de Espana
Content: Contains brief descriptions of the effects of about 150 drugs or their active ingredients on chemicals in the human body, as determined by blood and urine tests for such substances as bilirubin, calcium, cholesterol, corticosteroids, glucose, lactic acid, magnesium, potassium, prolactin, proteins, triglycerides, urea, and uric acid. Sources include the international scientific literature and pharmacology databases.
Language: Spanish
Coverage: Spain
Time Span: Current information
Updating: Periodically, as new data become available

INTERACCIONES ENTRE MEDICAMENTOS

Type: Reference (Bibliographic) ; Source (Textual-Numeric)
Subject: Pharmaceuticals & Pharmaceutical Industry
Producer: Consejo General de Colegios Oficiales de Farmaceuticos de Espana
Online Service: Consejo General de Colegios Oficiales de Farmaceuticos de Espana
Content: Contains descriptions of interactions between about 6700 pairs of drugs or active ingredients available in Spain. Provides names of drugs, mechanism of interaction, clinical effects and frequency of appearance, means for halting or preventing interaction, summaries of relevant published clinical studies, and bibliography. Sources include the international scientific literature and pharmacology databases.
Language: Spanish
Coverage: Spain

Time Span: 1978 to date
Updating: Periodically, as new data become available

INTERNATIONAL CONSUMER REPORTS (ICR)

Type: Reference (Bibliographic)
Subject: General Interest
Producer: Consumers' Association
Online Service: Datasolve Limited
Content: Contains approximately 27,000 citations, with abstracts, to magazines published by members of the International Organization of Consumers' Unions (IOCU) on consumer protection and the evaluation of consumer goods and services. Covers over 2400 different items, services, or processes (e.g., flea collars, meat labeling, pyramid selling, soil testing kits) ; consumer protection laws; and health, safety, and environmental protection issues.
Language: English, with titles in original languages
Coverage: International
Time Span: 1974 to date
Updating: About 900 records a month

INTERNATIONAL HEALTH PHYSICS DATA BASE

Type: Reference (Referral) ; Source (Textual-Numeric)
Subject: Environment; Occupational Safety & Health
Producer: Creative Information Systems, Inc.
Online Service: General Electric Information Services Company (GEISCO)
Conditions: Annual subscription of $15,000 to Creative Information Systems and monthly minimum of $500 to GEISCO required
Content: Contains information on exposure of individual employees in participating industrial organizations to environmental hazards. Is used in verifying compliance with federal exposure limits for permanent and temporary employees and contractors' employees. For each employee, provides only information directly related to employment, including training and employment history, selected medical data, and cumulative exposure information.
Language: English
Coverage: International
Time Span: 1979 to date
Updating: Daily

INTERNATIONAL INDUSTRIAL OPPORTUNITIES

Type: Reference (Referral) ; Source (Full Text)
Subject: Technology Transfer
Producer: High Tech Publishing Company
Online Service: NewsNet, Inc.
Conditions: Monthly subscription to NewsNet required
Content: Contains information on industrial and technical opportunities sought or offered by individuals and organizations worldwide. Covers products, processes, and technologies in various areas, including avionics, chemicals, construction and manufacturing, metallurgy, and packaging. Includes descriptions of required or available resources (e.g., financial assistance, turnkey services, equipment, training) and contact names and addresses. Also contains analyses of developments affecting international industry and technology transfer.

Language: English
Coverage: International
Time Span: July 1986 to date
Updating: Monthly

INTERNATIONAL MEDICAL TRIBUNE SYNDICATE®

Type: Source (Full Text)
Subject: Health Care; News
Producer: International Medical Tribune Syndicate
Online Service: Dialcom, Inc.
Conditions: Monthly minimum of $100 to Dialcom, Inc. required
Content: Contains news items in the medical and health-care area. Includes current news, feature stories, and regular columns for consumers on such topics as fitness and health, pediatrics, new drugs, medical news for international travelers, nutrition, and dentistry.
Language: English
Coverage: Primarily U.S., with some international coverage
Time Span: Current week
Updating: About 10 to 20 records a week

INTERNATIONAL PATENT CLASSIFICATION

Type: Reference (Referral)
Subject: Patents
Producer: Data produced by World Intellectual Property Organization (WIPO) are supplied to Registro de la Propiedad Industrial, to Telesystemes-Questel by Institut National de la Propriete Industrielle (INPI), and to STN International by Deutsches Patentamt.
Online Service: Registro de la Propiedad Industrial (CLINPAT); STN International (FATIPC); Telesystemes-Questel (INPI-4)
Content: Contains subject headings and classification codes for the 59,000 groups and subgroups of the International Patent Classification System, with an online thesaurus and explanations of the subgroups. Classification codes obtained from this database can be used as search terms in INPI-1 *(see)*, INPI-2 *(see EUROPEAN PATENTS REGISTER)*, and other patents databases. Corresponds to the 4th edition of *International Patent Classification*.
Language: English, French, German, and Spanish
Coverage: International
Time Span: Current information
Updating: Every 5 years

INTERNATIONAL PHARMACEUTICAL ABSTRACTS™

Type: Reference (Bibliographic)
Subject: Pharmaceuticals & Pharmaceutical Industry
Producer: American Society of Hospital Pharmacists
Online Service: BRS; BRS After Dark; BRS/BRKTHRU; BRS/Colleague; DIALOG Information Services, Inc.; DIMDI (as part of TOXLINE *(see)*); ESA-IRS; Knowledge Index; Mead Data Central, Inc. (as a MEDIS database *(see)*); National Library of Medicine (NLM) (as part of TOXLINE *(see)*); TECH DATA; University of Tsukuba
Conditions: Subscription to Mead Data Central required

Content: Contains over 120,000 citations, with abstracts, to the literature pertaining to the development and use of drugs and to the clinical, practical, theoretical, scientific, economic, and ethical aspects of professional pharmaceutical practice. Topics covered include pharmaceutical research, development and technology; adverse drug reactions and toxicity; drug evaluations, analyses, and interactions; pharmaceutical chemistry; and information processing for the pharmaceutical industry. Each abstract of clinical studies includes a description of the study design, number of patients involved, and dosage amounts, forms, and schedules. Each record also contains subject index entries. Corresponds to *International Pharmaceutical Abstracts*.
Language: English
Coverage: International
Time Span: 1970 to date
Updating: About 1200 records a month

INTERNATIONAL REVIEW OF PUBLICATIONS IN SOCIOLOGY (IRPS)

Type: Reference (Bibliographic)
Subject: Sociology
Producer: Sociological Abstracts, Inc.
Online Service: BRS (to be available in 1987); BRS After Dark (to be available in 1987); BRS/BRKTHRU (to be available in 1987); BRS/Colleague (to be available in 1987); DIALOG Information Services, Inc. (as a part of SOCIOLOGICAL ABSTRACTS *(see)*)
Content: Contains about 40,000 citations to book reviews appearing in serials abstracted for SOCIOLOGICAL ABSTRACTS *(see)*. Also provides several hundred book abstracts, including an outline of the contents of each chapter.
Language: English
Coverage: International
Time Span: 1980 to date
Updating: About 1500 records 5 times a year

INTRO

Type: Source (Full Text)
Subject: Information Systems & Services
Producer: Dow Jones & Company, Inc.
Online Service: Dow Jones & Company, Inc.
Conditions: Annual minimum of $12 or monthly minimum of $3 to Dow Jones required
Content: Contains information of interest to users of the Dow Jones online database service. Covers system and service enhancements, tutorial materials, current prices and operating hours, and ordering information on available user aids and software.
Language: English
Time Span: Current information
Updating: At least once a month

IRCS® MEDICAL SCIENCE

Type: Source (Full Text)
Subject: Biomedicine
Producer: Elsevier-IRCS Ltd.
Online Service: BRS; BRS After Dark; BRS/BRKTHRU; BRS/Colleague; DATA-STAR; DIMDI; TECH DATA
Content: Contains full text of the publications that comprise *IRCS Medical Science*, a collection of 30 journals with original research papers in the fields of medicine and biomedicine.

Includes the following monthly, bimonthly, and quarterly journals: *Anatomy and Human Biology; Biochemistry; Biomedical Technology; Cancer; Cardiovascular System; Cell and Molecular Biology; Clinical Biochemistry; Clinical Medicine and Surgery; Clinical Pharmacology and Therapeutics; Connective Tissue, Skin and Bone; Dentistry and Oral Biology; Developmental Biology and Medicine; Drug Metabolism and Toxicology; Endocrine System; Environmental and Social Medicine; Experimental Animals; The Eye and Visual System; Gastroenterology; Hematology; Immunology and Allergy; Metabolism and Nutrition; Microbiology, Parasitology and Infectious Diseases; Nephrology and Urology; Nervous System; Pathology; Pharmacology; Physiology; Psychology and Psychiatry; Reproduction, Obstetrics and Gynecology;* and *Respiratory System and Otorhinolaryngology.*

Language: English

Coverage: International

Time Span: BRS, BRS After Dark, BRS/Colleague, and DATA-STAR, 1981 to date; DIMDI, 1982 to date.

Updating: Twice a month

IRRIS (Interagency Rehabilitation Research Information System)

Type: Reference (Referral)

Subject: Education & Educational Institutions; Health Care; Research in Progress

Producer: National Institute of Handicapped Research (NIHR)

Online Service: BRS

Content: Contains about 2500 records on research and demonstration projects sponsored or undertaken by U.S. federal agencies in educational, vocational, medical, psychosocial, and technical aspects of rehabilitation of handicapped individuals. Each record includes project title, funding agency, organization performing the research, award amount and type (e.g., grant, contract, cooperative agreement), principal investigators, and abstract.

Language: English

Coverage: U.S.

Time Span: Fiscal Years 1983 and 1984 (projects funded during FY1985 will be available in 1987)

Updating: Monthly

ISI/ISTP&B® (Index to Scientific & Technical Proceedings & Books)

Type: Reference (Bibliographic)

Subject: Science & Technology

Producer: Institute for Scientific Information (ISI)

Online Service: DIMDI

Content: Contains citations to worldwide proceedings and books from all scientific and technical disciplines. Each item is indexed at the chapter level. Covers approximately 3400 proceedings, 1650 multi-authored books, 20 annual review series, and 13 review journals. The proceedings correspond to those published in *Index to Scientific & Technical Proceedings.*

Language: English

Coverage: International

Time Span: 1978 to date

Updating: About 12,500 records a month

ISIS SOFTWARE DATENBANK

Type: Reference (Referral)

Subject: Computers & Software

Producer: Nomina Gesellschaft fuer Wirtschafts- und Verwaltungsregister mbH

Online Service: FIZ Technik (to be available in 1987)

Content: Consists of 3 databases that contain profiles of commercially available computer programs in Austria, the Federal Republic of Germany, and Switzerland. Includes hardware requirements, prices and vendor information. Corresponds to *ISIS Reports.*

ISIS Software Report. Contains descriptions of about 3300 application and system programs for large and mid-size computers. Includes programs for applications in accounting, finance, government, maintenance, marketing, materials control, personnel, planning, and text processing, and for use in specific industries (e.g., construction, credit, energy, health care, hotel and restaurant management, insurance, manufacturing, publishing, and transportation).

ISIS Personal Computer Report. Contains descriptions of about 1800 application and system programs for microcomputers. Includes programs for applications in accounting, administration, finance, government marketing, materials control, personnel, planning, telecommunications, text processing, and for specific industries (e.g., agriculture, construction, credit, education, handwork trades, health care, insurance, manufacturing, and publishing).

ISIS Engineering Report. Contains descriptions of about 500 programs for technical data processing and graphics applications. Includes programs for use in civil and mechanical engineering, construction, cutting optimization, and factory management, operations research, plant construction, process control, production management, and statistical analyses simulation.

Language: German

Coverage: Austria, Federal Republic of Germany, and Switzerland

Time Span: Current information

ISST (Information en Sante et Securite du Travail)

Type: Reference (Bibliographic, Referral)

Subject: Audiovisual Materials-Catalogs; Occupational Safety & Health

Producer: Centre de Documentation, Commission de la Sante et de la Securite du Travail (CSST)

Online Service: IST-Informatheque Inc.

Content: Contains about 58,000 citations, with abstracts, to documents or audiovisual materials on occupational health and safety. Includes items available at one or more of 32 sites within the CSST network of documentation centers or industry-based associations in Quebec. Covers legislation, prevention, toxicology, safety, industrial medicine, indemnification plans, and ergonomy. Sources include legislation and regulations from Canada, the U.S., and Europe, government publications, industry guides and newsletters, periodicals, reports, conference proceedings, theses, and audiovisual materials.

Language: French, with titles in original languages

Coverage: International

Time Span: 1979 to date

Updating: About 1000 records a month

JANSSEN

Type: Reference (Referral); Source (Textual-Numeric)
Subject: Chemistry-Properties
Producer: Janssen Chimica
Online Service: Telesystemes-Questel (as a DARC database *(see)*)
Content: Contains references to the more than 11,000 chemicals listed in the *Janssen Chimica Catalog*. Each record contains chemical name, shipping code, prices, formula weight, molecular formula, properties, Janssen number, Chemical Abstracts Service (CAS) Registry Number, and cross references to listings for the same chemical in other catalogs (e.g. Aldrich, Beilstein). Users can order chemicals online. Chemicals may be retrieved by structure searching using DARC *(see)*.
Language: English
Time Span: Current information
Updating: Quarterly

JAPAN ECONOMIC DAILY®

Type: Reference (Referral); Source (Full Text)
Subject: News; Conferences & Meetings
Producer: Kyodo News International, Inc.
Online Service: DATA-STAR (KYODO NEWS); Dow Jones & Company, Inc.
Conditions: Annual minimum of $12 or monthly minimum of $3 to Dow Jones required
Content: Contains news on Japanese business, industry, economics, and finance. Covers developments in computers, robotics, biotechnology, and other high technology industries, as well as government policies and decision making. Provides daily summaries of Tokyo Stock Exchange activity (including Dow Jones and Tokyo Stock Exchange indexes, foreign stock closings, and 10 most active stocks), commodity prices, yen/dollar activity, exchange rates, gold prices, and over-the-counter bond quotations. Also contains weekly schedule of meetings, conferences, and government hearings and a monthly compilation of economic indicators.
Language: English
Coverage: Japan
Time Span: Most recent 5 days
Updating: Daily

JAPAN MARC

Type: Reference (Bibliographic)
Subject: Publishers & Distributors-Catalogs
Producer: National Diet Library
Online Service: University of Tsukuba
Content: Contains over 265,000 citations to Japanese government publications and to books published in Japan by Japanese publishers. Corresponds in part to *Nippon Zenkoku Shoshi (shuukanban)*.
Language: Japanese
Coverage: Japan
Time Span: 1979 to date
Updating: About 1300 records a week

JAPAN TECHNOLOGY BULLETIN

Type: Source (Full Text)
Subject: Science & Technology
Producer: High Technology Verlag GmbH
Online Service: NewsNet, Inc.; THE SOURCE
Conditions: Monthly subscription to NewsNet required; differential charges for subscribers and non-subscribers to *Japan Technology Bulletin*; monthly minimum of $10 to THE SOURCE required, with $9 credited toward online usage charges.
Content: Contains full text of *Japan Technology Bulletin*, a newsletter covering research and development projects in Japan, as well as new products available for marketing. Includes products in such industries as computers and electronics, robotics, chemicals and biochemcials, and energy and resources.
Language: English
Coverage: Japan
Time Span: February 1986 to date
Updating: Monthly

JAPIO® (Japanese Patent Abstracts in English)

Type: Reference (Bibliographic)
Subject: Patents
Producer: Japan Patent Information Organization (JAPIO)
Online Service: ORBIT Information Technologies Corporation
Conditions: Not accessible in Japan
Content: Contains citations, with abstracts, to more than 1 million unexamined Japanese patents issued since 1977. Each record includes inventor, patent holder, patent number, application date, publication date, Japanese Classification Number, and International Patent Classification System code. Also includes Derwent patent and priority numbers to facilitate retrieval of equivalent patents from World Patents Index *(see WPI)*. Corresponds to "Published unexamined patent application" (Kokai Tokkyo Koho).
Language: English
Coverage: Japan
Time Span: 1977 to date
Updating: About 18,000 records a month

JICST FILE ON CURRENT SCIENCE AND TECHNOLOGY RESEARCH IN JAPAN

Type: Reference (Referral)
Subject: Research in Progress; Science & Technology
Producer: The Japan Information Center of Science and Technology
Online Service: The Japan Information Center of Science and Technology (JICST)
Content: Contains descriptions of and references to research in progress in Japan. Includes both current and recently completed basic and applied research in the fields of engineering, science, and technology, with primary coverage of research sponsored by government agencies. Sources include surveys of research institutes of national, public, and private universities; public service corporations; and special governmental corporations. Corresponds to *Current Science and Technology Research in Japan*.
Language: Japanese
Coverage: Japan
Time Span: 1979 to date
Updating: Annually

JICST FILE ON GOVERNMENT REPORTS IN JAPAN

Type: Reference (Bibliographic)

Subject: Research in Progress; Science & Technology

Producer: The Japan Information Center of Science and Technology

Online Service: The Japan Information Center of Science and Technology (JICST)

Content: Contains citations, with abstracts, to reports of research and development projects sponsored by the Japanese government. Covers engineering (e.g., chemical, electrical, environmental, mechanical); science (e.g., computer, new material); and technology (e.g., biological, computer, energy, new material).

Language: Japanese

Coverage: Japan

Time Span: April 1983 to date

Updating: About 900 records a quarter

JICST FILE ON MEDICAL SCIENCE IN JAPAN

Type: Reference (Bibliographic)

Subject: Biomedicine

Producer: The Japan Information Center of Science and Technology

Online Service: The Japan Information Center of Science and Technology (JICST)

Content: Contains citations, with abstracts, to Japanese biomedical literature, including journals and conference proceedings, published in Japan. Covers biological sciences (e.g., cytology, immunology, zoology); veterinary science; and medical sciences (e.g., clinical medicine, dentistry, neurology, pharmacology). Corresponds in part to *Current Bibliography on Science and Technology*.

Language: Japanese

Coverage: Japan

Time Span: 1981 to date

Updating: About 5000 records a month

JICST FILE ON SCIENCE AND TECHNOLOGY

Type: Reference (Bibliographic)

Subject: Science & Technology

Producer: The Japan Information Center of Science and Technology

Online Service: The Japan Information Center of Science and Technology (JICST)

Content: Contains citations, with abstracts, to the worldwide literature on chemistry, civil engineering and architecture, electronics and electrical engineering, energy, environmental pollution, life sciences, management science, mechanical engineering, nuclear engineering, pure and applied physics, and systems engineering. Includes journal articles, conference proceedings, and technical reports. Corresponds to *Current Bibliography on Science and Technology*.

Language: Japanese

Coverage: International

Time Span: 1975 to date

Updating: About 38,000 records a month

JICST FILE ON SCIENCE, TECHNOLOGY, AND MEDICINE IN JAPAN

Type: Reference (Bibliographic)

Subject: Biomedicine; Science & Technology

Producer: The Japan Information Center of Science and Technology

Online Service: The Japan Information Center of Science and Technology (JICST)

Content: Contains about 250,000 citations, with abstracts, to scientific, technical, and biomedical literature published in Japan. Covers chemistry, biochemistry, and life sciences; medicine; electrical engineering and electronics; civil engineering and construction; mechanical engineering; metallurgy; physics; and miscellaneous technologies. Sources include 4000 Japanese publications, including periodicals, technical reports, and conference proceedings *(see JICST FILE ON SCIENCE AND TECHNOLOGY* and *JICST FILE ON MEDICAL SCIENCE IN JAPAN)*. Source documents are in Japanese.

Language: English

Coverage: Japan

Time Span: 1985 to date

Updating: About 14,000 records a month

JIJI PRESS TICKER SERVICE

Type: Source (Full Text)

Subject: News

Producer: Jiji Press, Ltd. (JP)

Online Service: Mead Data Central, Inc. (as part of NEXIS WIRE SERVICES *(see)*); NewsNet, Inc.

Conditions: Subscription to Mead Data Central required; monthly subscription to NewsNet required.

Content: Contains full text of items from the Jiji Press newswire service on general, financial, and industry news in Japan. Covers financial and securities markets, including the Tokyo Stock Exchange; commodities spot and futures markets; and money and foreign exchange markets. Also covers international trade, monetary, and fiscal policies.

NOTE: On NewsNet, items are accessible only through the NewsFlash selective dissemination service and are retained 2 weeks for each user.

Language: English

Coverage: Japan

Time Span: Mead Data Central, 1980 to date; NewsNet, most current 2 weeks.

Updating: Continuously, throughout the day

JOB SAFETY AND HEALTH

Type: Source (Full Text)

Subject: Occupational Safety & Health

Producer: The Bureau of National Affairs, Inc. (BNA)

Online Service: Executive Telecom System, Inc., Human Resource Information Network

Conditions: Annual subscription to Executive Telecom System required

Content: Contains full text of *Job Safety and Health*, a newsletter covering trends in industrial safety practices. Provides analyses of difficult safety problems and their solutions, information on setting up and maintaining safety and health programs, explanations of significant changes in the law, court and agency decisions, and important arbitration awards.

Language: English
Coverage: U.S.
Time Span: August 1985 to date
Updating: Every 2 weeks

THE KAYPRO KNEWS
Type: Source (Full Text, Software)
Subject: Computers & Software
Producer: Mike Guffey
Online Service: THE SOURCE
Conditions: Monthly minimum of $10 to THE SOURCE required, with $9 credited toward online usage charges
Content: Contains news and information of interest to users of Kaypro personal computers. Includes technical application notes, software reviews, and information on public domain software. Users may download public domain software.
Language: English
Coverage: Primarily U.S., with some international coverage
Time Span: Current information
Updating: Every 2 months

KIRK-OTHMER/ONLINE
Type: Reference (Bibliographic); Source (Textual-Numeric, Full Text)
Subject: Chemistry; Chemistry-Properties; Science & Technology
Producer: John Wiley & Sons, Inc.
Online Service: BRS; BRS After Dark; BRS/BRKTHRU; BRS/Colleague; DATA-STAR; TECH DATA
Content: Contains 2 files of data on chemical technology and polymer science.
ENCYCLOPEDIA OF CHEMICAL TECHNOLOGY. Contains full text, including citations, tables, and abstracts, of all 1200 articles in the 3rd edition of the Kirk-Othmer *Encyclopedia of Chemical Technology*. Covers chemical technology in the areas of energy, health, safety, and new materials: agricultural chemicals; chemical engineering; coatings and inks; composite materials; drugs, cosmetics, and biomaterials; dyes, pigments, and brighteners; ecology and industrial hygiene; energy conversion and technology; fats and waxes; fermentation and enzyme technology; fibers, textiles, and leather; food and animal nutrition; fossil fuels and derivatives; glass, ceramics, and cement; industrial organic and inorganic chemicals; metals, metallurgy, and metal alloys; plastics and elastomers; semiconductors and electronic materials; surfactants, detergents, and emulsion technology; water supply, purification, and reuse; and wood, paper, and industrial carbohydrates. Also contains articles relevant to the manufacture and distribution of chemicals in these areas: computers, instrumentation, and control; information retrieval; market research and project planning; patents and trademarks; process development and design; product development and technical service; purchasing, materials allocation, and supply; research and operations management; and transportation of chemical products.
ENCYCLOPEDIA OF POLYMER SCIENCE AND ENGINEERING. Contains full text of articles from the first 4 volumes of the 17-volume 2nd edition of the *Encyclopedia of Polymer Science and Engineering*, published by Wiley Interscience. Includes approximately 800 tables, with 12,000 citations to the worldwide literature on synthetic and natural polymers. Covers polymer morphology and compatibility; molecular, physical, mechanical, and biological properties; and equipment and processes (e.g., test methods) used in polymer engineering. Also covers approximately 100 topics on polymers and computers (e.g., robotics and composites, CAD/CAM). All 17 volumes, a supplement, and index will be available by 1989.

Language: English
Coverage: International
Time Span: *Encyclopedia of Chemical Technology*, 1977 to date, with selected older materials; *Encyclopedia of Polymer Science and Engineering*, 1985 to date.
Updating: Periodically, as new data become available

KNICKERBOCKER NEWS
Type: Source (Full Text)
Subject: News
Producer: Hearst Publishing Group, Capitol Newspapers Division
Online Service: VU/TEXT Information Services, Inc.
Conditions: Subscription to VU/TEXT required
Content: Contains full text of news items and feature articles from the *Knickerbocker News* (New York State) newspaper. Regional coverage emphasizes news of the Hudson River Valley.
Language: English
Coverage: U.S. (primarily Albany, New York area)
Time Span: February 1986 to date
Updating: Daily

KNIGHT-NEWS-TRIBUNE NEWS WIRE
Type: Source (Full Text)
Subject: News
Producer: Knight-News-Tribune News Wire
Online Service: VU/TEXT Information Services, Inc.
Conditions: Subscription to VU/TEXT required
Content: Contains full text of U.S. and international news items, business news items, and feature stories from the Knight-News-Tribune wire. Sources include the *Boston Globe*, *Dallas Morning News*, and all newspapers published by Knight-Ridder Newspapers, Inc. and the Tribune Company.
Language: English
Coverage: International
Time Span: 1986 to date
Updating: Continuously, throughout the day

THE KUSSMAUL ENCYCLOPEDIA®
Type: Source (Full Text)
Subject: Encyclopedias
Producer: General Videotex Corporation/DELPHI
Online Service: General Videotex Corporation/DELPHI
Content: An online encyclopedia based on *The Cadillac Modern Encyclopedia* and supplemented by information from the *Encyclopedia of Mathematics* and the *Encyclopedia of Mythology*.
Language: English
Coverage: International

KYODO ENGLISH NEWS SERVICE
Type: Source (Full Text)
Subject: News
Producer: Kyodo News International, Inc.
Online Service: NewsNet, Inc.
Conditions: Monthly subscription to NewsNet required
Content: Contains full text of domestic and international news items and feature stories relating to Japan. Covers Japanese and world political news, Japanese economic news and lifestyle features, and Pacific Basin (e.g., Korea, Taiwan, People's Republic of China) news gathered and written by Kyodo News Service reporters.

Language: English
Coverage: Primarily Japan, with some international news
Time Span: June 9, 1986 to date
Updating: Daily

LABINFO
Type: Reference (Referral)
Subject: Research in Progress; Science & Technology
Producer: Banque des Connaissances et des Techniques (CNRS/ANVAR)
Online Service: Telesystemes-Questel
Content: Contains descriptions of about 9000 public and private French laboratories conducting basic and developmental research in many areas of science and technology. For each organization, includes such information as name and address, name of research director, size of staff, primary activities, current research projects and applications, experimental capabilities, equipment and facilities, and available publications.
Language: French
Coverage: France
Time Span: Current information
Updating: Annually

LABORATORIOS FARMACEUTICOS ESPANOLES
Type: Source (Textual-Numeric)
Subject: Pharmaceuticals & Pharmaceutical Industry
Producer: Consejo General de Colegios Oficiales de Farmaceuticos de Espana
Online Service: Consejo General de Colegios Oficiales de Farmaceuticos de Espana
Content: Contains data on drugs produced by about 550 Spanish pharmaceutical manufacturers active since 1972, including those that have since discontinued business. Provides drug trade name, therapeutic category as defined in GRUPOS TERAPEUTICOS (see), number of dosage forms available, shelf life, conditions of dispensation (e.g., prescription required), and method of administration. Source is the pharmaceuticals register of the Ministerio de Sanidad y Consumo.
Language: Spanish
Coverage: Spain
Time Span: 1972 to date
Updating: Periodically, as new data become available

LABORATORY HAZARDS BULLETIN
Type: Reference (Bibliographic, Referral)
Subject: Life Sciences; Toxicology
Producer: The Royal Society of Chemistry
Online Service: DATA-STAR; ESA-IRS; Pergamon InfoLine
Content: Contains over 3500 citations, with abstracts, to the worldwide literature and other sources on hazards likely to be encountered in chemical and biochemical laboratories. Covers dangerous chemicals and reactions, biological hazards, new safety precautions, U.K. legislation dealing with these issues, and animal studies of possible relevance to humans. Does not cover transportation of chemicals, well-known hazards, or marketed drugs. Sources include approximately 100 occupational health, chemical, biochemical, toxicological, and medical journals, books, reports, non-print materials (e.g., films, posters), and organizations that provide information on hazards.

Language: English
Coverage: International
Time Span: 1981 to date
Updating: Monthly; about 800 records a year.

LC MARC
Type: Reference (Bibliographic)
Subject: Library Holdings-Catalogs
Producer: Library of Congress (LC)
Online Service: BLAISE-LINE; DIALOG Information Services, Inc.; Library of Congress Information System (LOCIS), as LIBRARY OF CONGRESS COMPUTERIZED CATALOG (LCCC) on SCORPIO (see) and as BOOKS on MUMS (see); Universitetsbiblioteket i Oslo (UBO:AUSE and UBO:SDI); University of Tsukuba; WILSONLINE
Conditions: Annual subscription of 49 pounds (UK) for U.K. users or 56 pounds (UK) for other users to BLAISE Online Services required; available through LOCIS only to users on-site at the Library of Congress.
Content: Contains bibliographic information on approximately 1.9 million monographs published worldwide since 1968. Covers books in English since 1968; in French, since 1973; in German, Portuguese, and Spanish, since 1975; in other Roman alphabet languages, since 1976-77; in South Asian and Cyrillic alphabet languages (in romanized form), since 1979; and in Greek (in romanized form), since 1980. Provides basic bibliographic data from LC Machine Readable Cataloging (MARC) records. Data provided in each record vary by online service, but may include LC card number, title, author, series, publisher, publication date, place of publication, International Standard Book Number, call number, language, document type, notes, and subject classification. Also includes some Cataloging in Publication data. Corresponds in part to the *National Union Catalog*.
NOTE: Through Universitetsbiblioteket i Oslo, UBO:AUSE covers 1982 to date (see also UKMARC) and UBO:SDI covers latest 2 weeks.
Language: Primarily English
Coverage: International
Time Span: Most services, 1968 to date; Universitetsbiblioteket i Oslo, 1982 to date.
Updating: About 15,000 records a month

LEATHERHEAD LIBRARY PERIODICALS
Type: Reference (Bibliographic)
Subject: Food Sciences & Nutrition; Library Holdings-Catalogs
Producer: Leatherhead Food Research Association
Online Service: Leatherhead Food Research Association (LFRA)
Conditions: Various subscription options available
Content: Contains approximately 700 citations to the periodical holdings of the LFRA library, covering food and the food industry. Includes title, publisher, country of origin, language, subscription cost, and subscription status.
Language: English
Coverage: International
Time Span: Current information
Updating: Periodically, as new data become available

LEGI-SLATE®

Type: Reference (Referral) ; Source (Textual-Numeric)

Subject: Government-U.S. Federal; Legislative Tracking

Producer: LEGI-SLATE, Inc.

Online Service: LEGI-SLATE, Inc.

Conditions: Annual subscription (includes unlimited usage) required

Content: A database system containing complete descriptions, histories, and updates of Congressional and regulatory activity. The legislative service includes a description and history of all bills and resolutions introduced in the U.S. Congress. Includes major committee and subcommittee actions and all House and Senate Floor actions. Also contains member voting records, complete schedules of committees and subcommittees, and House and Senate calendars. Data are gathered from the *Congressional Record* and House and Senate committees. The regulatory service contains abstracts of each document published in the *Federal Register*. Covers regulations, rules, and proposed additions and amendments to the *Code of Federal Regulations* (CFR), legal notices, Public Law notices, hearings, meetings, Executive Orders, and other Presidential documents carried in the *Federal Register*. Elements of information in each record also include CFR part numbers, docket numbers, issuing agency, public law authority, and other reference materials. The Vote Rating Service permits analysis of voting performance for any member of the U.S. Congress. The News Service provides full text of *The Washington Post* and *National Journal*, an indexed version of the *Congressional Quarterly Weekly Report*, LEGI-SLATE's *Congressional Checkoff*, and full text of daily press briefings at the White House and Departments of State and Defense.

Language: English

Coverage: U.S.

Time Span: Legislative and Vote Rating Services, 1979 to date (from 96th U.S. Congress) ; regulatory service, 1981 to date (full text of *Federal Register*, 1985 to date) ; News Service, 1985 to date.

Updating: Daily, usually by 12:00 P.M. Eastern Time

LEGI-TECH℠

Type: Reference (Referral) ; Source (Textual-Numeric)

Subject: Government-U.S. Federal; Government-U.S. State; Legislative Tracking

Producer: Legi-Tech Corporation

Online Service: Legi-Tech Corporation

Conditions: Subscription required

Content: A legislative tracking service that contains histories of bills introduced during regular and special legislative sessions of the U.S. Congress and the California and New York state legislatures. Also covers member voting records, political contributions, and lobbyist activities. Information provided includes bill numbers, authors, titles, summaries, and actions. Users can produce several types of reports, including those covering contributions, committee votes, and floor votes for all state and federal elected officials. Sources of data include the *Congressional Record*, legislative clerks, state printers, offices of the Secretary of States, and the Federal Elections Commission.

Language: English

Coverage: U.S., California, and New York

Time Span: 1979 to date

Updating: Daily

THE LEXINGTON HERALD-LEADER™

Type: Source (Full Text)

Subject: News

Producer: Lexington Herald-Leader Company

Online Service: VU/TEXT Information Services, Inc.

Conditions: Subscription to VU/TEXT required

Content: Contains full text of news items and feature stories from *The Lexington Herald-Leader* (Kentucky) newspaper. Each article also includes the day and date, byline, headline, section, and photograph caption information (if applicable). Keywords are available for most articles.

Language: English

Coverage: U.S. (primarily Lexington, Kentucky area)

Time Span: 1983 to date

Updating: Daily

LEXPAT®

Type: Source (Full Text)

Subject: Patents

Producer: Mead Data Central, Inc.

Online Service: Mead Data Central, Inc. (as a LEXIS and NEXIS database)

Conditions: Subscription to Mead Data Central required

Content: Contains full text of more than 800,000 U.S. patents, including all utility patents issued since 1975. Includes the complete specification, claims, and abstract, as well as changes resulting from certificates of correction, reclassification, and reassignment. Over 40 segments of information in each patent document are uniquely identified for searching, including patent number, title, inventor, issue date, examiner, filing date, assignee, claims, and the full text of the specification. Patent documents are organized in 4 files: UTIL, containing all utility patents; PLANT, containing all plant patents; DESIGN, containing all design patents; and ALL, containing all utility, plant, and design patents. The following search-aid files are also available: PATENT CLASSIFICATIONS FILE (CLASS), containing classes, subclasses, and patent numbers; MANUAL OF CLASSIFICATION (CLMNL), containing the classification schedule; and INDEX TO CLASSIFICATION (INDEX), containing references, cross-references, and scope notes to classes and subclasses.

Language: English

Coverage: U.S.

Time Span: 1975 to date

Updating: About 1500 patents a week, within 1 week after issuance

LIBROS ESPANOLES EN VENTA

Type: Reference (Bibliographic)

Subject: Publishers & Distributors-Catàlogs

Producer: Ministerio de Cultura, Instituto Nacional del Libro Espanol

Online Service: Ministerio de Cultura, Secretaria General Tecnica

Content: Contains citations to about 367,000 books published in Spain for which an International Standard Book Number (ISBN) has been assigned. Includes ISBN, author, title, publisher, date, physical format, price, and subjects.

Language: Spanish

Coverage: Spain

Time Span: 1965 to date

Updating: Monthly

LICENSABLE TECHNOLOGY

Type: Reference (Referral)
Subject: Technology Transfer
Producer: Dr. Dvorkovitz & Associates
Online Service: Dr. Dvorkovitz & Associates
Conditions: Subscriptions range in price from a minimum of $1500 a year for a single category to $100,000 for access to the full database, over a 2-year period. Fees include printed copies of descriptions and consulting services.
Content: A database system that contains over 30,000 items of technology available for licensing that have been collected from organizations around the world. Items in the database are divided into approximately 100 subject categories in these broad groups: chemicals, biologicals, mechanicals, electronics, and miscellaneous. Each record contains the title of the technology, licensor, technical description, list of main uses and advantages, degree of development and, if applicable, the patent number. Users search by subject category, record identification number, or with Boolean searches on words in the descriptions.
Language: English
Coverage: International
Updating: Periodically, as new data become available

LIFE®

Type: Source (Full Text)
Subject: General Interest
Producer: Time Inc.
Online Service: Mead Data Central, Inc. (as part of NEXIS MAGAZINES *(see)*); VU/TEXT Information Services, Inc. (to be available in 1987)
Conditions: Subscription to Mead Data Central required; subscription to VU/TEXT required.
Content: Contains full text of *Life*, a magazine covering current events and lifestyle trends. Includes interviews with famous or interesting local, national, or international personalities, as well as photographic views of people, places, and events.
Language: English
Coverage: International
Time Span: Mead Data Central, 1982 to date; VU/TEXT, 1985 to date.
Updating: Monthly

LIFE SCIENCES COLLECTION

Type: Reference (Bibliographic)
Subject: Life Sciences
Producer: Cambridge Scientific Abstracts
Online Service: BRS; BRS After Dark; BRS/BRKTHRU; DIALOG Information Services, Inc.
Content: Contains citations, with abstracts, to worldwide life sciences literature. Corresponds to the 17 abstracting journals published by CSA: *Animal Behaviour Abstracts; Biochemistry Abstracts-Amino-acid, Peptide & Protein; Biochemistry Abstracts-Biological Membranes; Biochemistry Abstracts-Nucleic Acids; Calcified Tissue Abstracts; Biotechnology Research Abstracts* (from 1984 to date); *Chemoreception Abstracts; Ecology Abstracts; Endocrinology Abstracts; Entomology Abstracts; Genetics Abstracts; Immunology Abstracts; Microbiology Abstracts-Algology, Mycology & Protozoology; Microbiology Abstracts-Bacteriology; Microbiology Abstracts-Industrial & Applied Microbiology; Neurosciences Abstracts* (from 1983 to date); *Toxicology Abstracts; Virology Abstracts.*

Also includes *Oncology Abstracts* and *Feeding, Weight, and Obesity Abstracts* for the period they were published.
Language: English
Coverage: International
Time Span: 1978 to date
Updating: About 8200 records a month

Life:NET℠

Type: Reference (Referral); Source (Textual-Numeric)
Subject: Biomedicine
Producer: Human Resource Selection Network, Inc.
Online Service: Human Resource Selection Network, Inc.
Conditions: Available by subscription only to non-profit regional organ banks and their associated affiliates
Content: Contains donor and recipient medical information (e.g., blood type, tissue type) to facilitate matching for transplantation surgery. When new donor data are entered, they are automatically matched with recipient criteria already present in the database. Contact information is provided to both donor and recipient organ banks. Also provides automated cross referencing for variations in tissue typing terminology.
Language: English
Coverage: U.S. and Canada
Time Span: Current information
Updating: Daily

LITHIUM CONSULTATION

Type: Source (Full Text)
Subject: Biomedicine
Producer: University of Wisconsin, Department of Psychiatry, Lithium Information Center
Online Service: University of Wisconsin, Department of Psychiatry, Lithium Information Center
Content: Contains information to assist physicians in selecting patients for lithium treatment and managing their treatment. Users input patient data (including disorders and medications taken) and retrieve information on the patient's suitability for lithium treatment, expected responsiveness of disorders to lithium treatment, possible medical contraindications, procedures for initiating lithium therapy and managing side effects, and alternatives to lithium treatment.
Language: English
Coverage: International
Time Span: Current information
Updating: Periodically, as new data become available

LITHIUM INDEX

Type: Reference (Bibliographic); Source (Full Text)
Subject: Biomedicine
Producer: University of Wisconsin, Department of Psychiatry, Lithium Information Center
Online Service: University of Wisconsin, Department of Psychiatry, Lithium Information Center
Content: Contains about 100 analyses of the worldwide literature on the medical uses of lithium, organized by various topics. Covers interactions with other drugs, side effects, medical conditions, and treatment guidelines. Summaries can be retrieved by such clinical topics as pregnancy, teratogenesis, neurological side effects, kidney damage, sexual function and fertility, cardiovascular system, and cutaneous side effects. Analyses include citations to the source documents.

Language: English
Coverage: International
Time Span: Current information
Updating: Periodically, as new data become available

LITHIUM LIBRARY

Type: Reference (Bibliographic)
Subject: Biomedicine
Producer: University of Wisconsin, Department of Psychiatry, Lithium Information Center
Online Service: University of Wisconsin, Department of Psychiatry, Lithium Information Center
Content: Contains more than 13,000 citations to the worldwide literature on the medical and biological uses of lithium. Sources of information include BIOSIS PREVIEWS *(see)*, ASCATOPICS, printed indexes, books, journals, government reports, and meeting abstracts. Records include title, subject headings, author, journal or other source, and date.
Language: English
Coverage: International
Time Span: 1800s to date
Updating: Periodically, with about 1000 records a year

LOGIBASE

Type: Reference (Referral)
Subject: Computers & Software
Producer: Centrale des Bibliotheques
Online Service: IST-Informatheque Inc.
Content: Contains about 1000 descriptions of software packages commercially available in Quebec, Canada for microcomputers, minicomputers, and mainframe computers. Includes general description of capabilities, areas of application, hardware and software requirements, product medium (e.g., magnetic tape, cassette, or disk), and codes for supplier name. Supplier names and addresses are available in PRODIL *(see)*.
Language: French
Coverage: International
Time Span: 1981 to date
Updating: About 40 records a month

LONG BEACH PRESS-TELEGRAM

Type: Source (Full Text)
Subject: News
Producer: Twin Coast Newspapers, Inc.
Online Service: VU/TEXT Information Services, Inc. (to be available in 1987)
Conditions: Subscription to VU/TEXT required
Content: Contains full text of news items and feature articles from the *Long Beach Press-Telegram* (California) newspaper.
Language: English
Coverage: U.S. (primarily Long Beach, California area)
Updating: Daily

LOS ANGELES TIMES

Type: Source (Full Text)
Subject: News
Producer: Times Mirror Company
Online Service: Mead Data Central, Inc. (as part of NEXIS NEWSPAPERS *(see)*); VU/TEXT Information Services, Inc. (to be available in 1987)

Conditions: Subscription to Mead Data Central required; subscription to VU/TEXT required.
Content: Contains full text of news items, feature stories, and editorials from *The Los Angeles Times* (California) newspaper. Regional coverage includes the entertainment industry, high technology industries, and Pacific Rim commerce.
Language: English
Coverage: U.S. (primarily Los Angeles, California area)
Time Span: 1985 to date
Updating: Daily

LYNX

Type: Reference (Bibliographic)
Subject: Library Holdings-Catalogs; Publishers & Distributors-Catalogs
Producer: Idaps Information Services Pty. Ltd.
Online Service: Idaps Information Services Pty. Ltd.
Content: Contains references to over 6 million books, serials, and other library materials cited in national catalogs, book trade catalogs, and Australian library holdings lists. National catalogs include the AUSTRALIAN NATIONAL BIBLIOGRAPHY *(see)*, National Library of Australia film catalog, British National Bibliography *(see UKMARC)*, and the U.S. Library of Congress catalogs of books *(see LC MARC)*, maps, music, serials, and audiovisual materials. Trade catalogs include the Australian Antiquarian Book Service, Baker & Taylor, BOOKS IN PRINT *(see)*, *British Books in Print (see WHITAKER)*, D.A. Books Australia, and *New Australian Titles*. Library holdings lists cover the Australian National University Library, the Network of Educational Libraries, Parliamentary Library, Patents Office Library, the libraries of the Departments of Employment, Foreign Affairs, Housing, Primary Industry, and Social Security, and other city, state, and university libraries. Online acquisitions and cataloging are available through the LION system.
Language: Primarily English
Coverage: International
Time Span: Varies by source, with earliest data from 1968.
Updating: Varies by source; most files, monthly.

MAC+QUIN

Type: Reference (Bibliographic)
Subject: News
Producer: Consult srl; Istituto per gli studi di politica internazionale (Ispi)
Online Service: SIPE Optimation S.p.A.
Content: Contains over 160,000 citations, with abstracts, to newspaper articles on Italian and international politics relating to economics, culture, and society. Includes names of persons and firms mentioned in the article. Sources are 16 major daily Italian newspapers.
Language: Italian
Coverage: International
Time Span: 1981 to date
Updating: About 250 items a day

MACWORLD

Type: Reference (Referral); Source (Full Text)
Subject: Computers & Software
Producer: Computerworld Pty. Limited
Online Service: The Teledata Network (as a TELEDATA COMPUTER COMMUNICATIONS NETWORK database)

Conditions: Initiation fee of $150 (Australian) for commercial organizations or $50 (Australian) for individual subscribers and monthly minimum to The Teledata Network required

Content: Contains listings of software and hardware available in Australia for the Macintosh computer. Software categories include database management systems, games, graphics, music and speech systems, programming languages, spreadsheet programs, utilities, systems for word processing and accounting, and integrated systems. Also provides news and articles on Macintosh computers. Corresponds to *Australian Macworld Magazine*.

Language: English
Coverage: Australia
Time Span: November 1985 to date
Updating: Weekly

MAGAZINE ASAP®

Type: Reference (Bibliographic) ; Source (Full Text)
Subject: General Interest; News
Producer: Information Access Co.
Online Service: BRS; BRS/BRKTHRU; BRS/Colleague; DIALOG Information Services, Inc.; Mead Data Central, Inc. (as a NEXIS database)
Conditions: Subscription to Mead Data Central required
Content: Contains citations, with the full text, to articles from more than 85 general interest periodicals indexed in MAGAZINE INDEX *(see)*.
NOTE: On Mead Data Central, does not duplicate full-text records already contained in NEXIS (e.g., press releases from PR NEWSWIRE) .

Language: English
Coverage: International
Time Span: 1983 to date
Updating: Monthly

MAGAZINE INDEX®

Type: Reference (Bibliographic)
Subject: General Interest; News
Producer: Information Access Co.
Online Service: BRS; BRS After Dark; BRS/BRKTHRU; BRS/Colleague; DIALOG Information Services, Inc.; Knowledge Index; Mead Data Central, Inc. (MAGIND) (as a Reference Service database)
Conditions: Subscription to Mead Data Central required
Content: Provides coverage of over 400 popular magazines published in the United States and Canada. Contains more than 1.6 million citations to feature articles, news reports, editorials, product evaluations, biographical pieces, short stories, poetry, recipes, reviews, and other features. Subjects covered include current affairs, leisure time activities, performing arts, travel, recreation, sports, home-centered arts, business, and general science and technology. Corresponds to the *Magazine Index* on microform. Records are added daily to NEWSEARCH *(see)* and are transferred to this database monthly. Users can display full text of articles from over 85 magazines.

Language: English
Coverage: U.S.
Time Span: DIALOG, 1959 to March 1970 and 1973 to date; all others, 1959 to date.
Updating: About 12,000 records a month

MAGILL BOOK REVIEWS ONLINE

Type: Reference (Bibliographic)
Subject: General Interest
Producer: Salem Press, Inc.
Online Service: Dow Jones & Company, Inc.
Conditions: Annual minimum of $12 or monthly minimum of $3 to Dow Jones required
Content: Contains about 300 reviews of recently published books. Covers fiction, biography, history, business, computers and telecommunications, sports and leisure, and self-help books. Includes title, author, publisher, number of pages, abstract, and brief commentary. Also provides essays on approximately 500 classic literary works, including novels, short stories, poetry, and plays.

Language: English
Coverage: U.S.
Time Span: 1985 to date
Updating: About 10 reviews a week

MARINELINE

Type: Reference (Bibliographic)
Subject: Aquatic Sciences
Producer: Federal Institute for Geosciences and Natural Resources (GEOFIZ)
Online Service: FIZ Karlsruhe
Content: Contains about 17,000 citations, most with abstracts, to the worldwide literature on marine research and technology. Covers oceanography, earth sciences, and environmental protection; desalinization; raw materials and reserves; materials and system technologies; platform construction and diving technology; and maritime law. Sources include journals, reports, dissertations, and conference proceedings.

Language: English and German
Coverage: International
Time Span: 1972 to date
Updating: About 250 records a quarter

MARQUIS WHO'S WHO

Type: Reference (Referral)
Subject: Biographies
Producer: Marquis Who's Who, Inc.
Online Service: DIALOG Information Services, Inc.; Knowledge Index
Content: Contains biographical information for over 100,000 prominent Americans, including businesspeople, athletes, military officers, politicians and government officials, educators, entertainers, musicians, artists, lawyers, physicians, writers, and scientists. Records contain career history, education (e.g., schools attended, degrees, certifications) , creative works and publications, research interests, family background (e.g., birth date, parents names, citizenship, sex) , marriage information (e.g., date, spouse's name, children's names) , current address, civic and political activities, professional activities and affiliation, religion, and special achievements. The source of information is usually the biographee. Corresponds to the latest editions of *Who's Who in America* and *Who's Who in Frontier Scienc̄e and Technology*, plus updates.

Language: English
Coverage: U.S., Canada, and Mexico
Time Span: Persons alive at publication time
Updating: Quarterly

MARTINDALE ONLINE™

Type: Reference (Bibliographic); Source (Textual-Numeric, Full Text)
Subject: Pharmaceuticals & Pharmaceutical Industry
Producer: The Pharmaceutical Society of Great Britain
Online Service: DATA-STAR
Content: Contains information on about 5100 drugs and ancillary substances. Includes evaluative summaries supplemented by over 58,000 citations, with abstracts, to the worldwide scientific literature. Each entry covers drug definition and description, actions and uses, and preparations. Definition information includes drug name, synonyms, codes, chemical names, molecular formula and weight, Chemical Abstracts Service Registry Number, pharmacopoeias that provide standards, description of physical and pharmaceutical properties (e.g., melting point, solubility, stability, incompatibility), and radiopharmaceutical data (e.g., half-life, radiation emitted). Drug actions information includes uses, actions, and dosage and administration; metabolism and excretion; precautions, contraindications, and interactions; adverse effects and their treatment; antimicrobial action; resistance; and dependence and withdrawal. Preparations information includes proprietary names from many countries, U.K. and U.S. official preparation data, U.K. proprietary preparation data and product license numbers, and manufacturers and distributors. Corresponds to *Martindale: The Extra Pharmacopoeia*.
Language: English
Coverage: International
Time Span: Current information
Updating: Twice a year

MASSACHUSETTS HEALTH DATA CONSORTIUM

Type: Source (Textual-Numeric)
Subject: Health Care
Producer: Data Resources, Inc.
Online Service: Data Resources, Inc. (DRI)
Conditions: Subscription to DRI required
Content: Contains information on hospital treatment costs and payment sources for patients released from Massachusetts hospitals. Includes hospital name, patient's residence (town or ZIP Code), age, type of illness by diagnostic-related group (i.e., standardized government treatment/cost classification), length of stay, clinical subspecialty used in treatment (e.g., physical therapy, cardiology), and payor (e.g., private insurance carrier, Medicare). Sources of data are patient discharge records compiled by the Massachusetts Health Data Consortium.
Language: English
Coverage: U.S. (Massachusetts)
Time Span: 1982 to date
Updating: Annually

MCGRAW-HILL BOOKS/SOFTWARE/ VIDEO

Type: Reference (Bibliographic, Referral)
Subject: Publishers & Distributors-Catalogs
Producer: McGraw-Hill Book Company
Online Service: CompuServe Information Service (as part of THE ELECTRONIC MALL); NewsNet, Inc. (MCGRAW-HILL SEMINARS & BUSINESS INFO)
Conditions: Monthly subscription to NewsNet required
Content: Contains references to software, books, films, video, and training materials available from McGraw-Hill Book Company. Users can place credit card orders online.

Language: English
Time Span: 1984 to date
Updating: NewsNet, every 2 weeks; CompuServe, monthly.

MCI INSIGHT℠

Type: Source (Numeric, Textual-Numeric, Full Text)
Subject: Flight Schedules; General Interest; News
Producer: MCI International; NSI, Inc.
Online Service: NSI, Inc.
Content: Consists of several files of business and general interest news and information.

News, Weather & Sports. Contains news and features from major worldwide news services; economic and business developments from the Middle East; U.S. and global weather conditions and forecasts; U.S. sports news, covering horse racing and current scores, matchups, and standings for the National Basketball Association, National Football League, U.S. Football League, American League, and National League; and international soccer news. Also covers U.S. economic news, including foreign exchange rates, key U.S. financial market interest rates, and leading economic indicators (e.g., consumer and wholesale price indexes, personal income).

Securities and Commodities Markets. Contains stock and options prices for the New York, American, and NASDAQ Over-The-Counter exchanges; market activity updates for municipal bonds, U.S. Treasury notes, and Government National Mortgage Association (GNMA) futures; prices for grain, livestock, sugar, gold, and silver futures; and spot prices for gold, silver, farm products, oil, metals, and coins. Includes the Dow Jones and Standard & Poor's Indexes of stock market activity; commodity market overviews and recommendations; investment ratings for 1500 common stocks; recommendations from investment advisory and brokerage services; and analyses and recommendations on currency purchases from Tech-Monitor Data, Ltd. Also provides a discount brokerage service that allows clients of North American Investment Corporation to buy and sell stocks, bonds, and commodity options online.

Travel. Contains international and U.S. airline schedules and fares *(see OAG-EE)*; hotel, restaurant, and special events guides for 100 U.S. cities and 30 cities abroad; and ski guides for New England and New York.

General Interest. Contains a variety of information, including weekly fiction and non-fiction best-seller lists; television and movie news and reviews; movie reviews in Spanish; synopses of popular soap operas; a guide to current Broadway plays; passages from the Bible; astrological horoscopes; international and American recipes and a cooking conversion table; trivia questions and answers; jokes; and graphics and greetings for holidays and personal events.

Language: English; user guides and file descriptions also in French, German, Italian, and Spanish.
Coverage: International
Time Span: News, most recent 30 days; other information, varies by file.
Updating: Varies by service, from continuously, throughout the day to weekly

MEDIC

Type: Reference (Bibliographic)
Subject: Biomedicine
Producer: Central Medical Library
Online Service: Central Medical Library

Conditions: Subscription fee of 1200 FIM (Finnish marks) required

Content: Contains citations to articles from about 60 medical journals published in Finland and to monographs (e.g., reports of universities or research institutions, conference proceedings, dissertations) which are not typically covered in international databases. Corresponds to *Finmed*.

Language: Primarily Finnish, with descriptors in English

Coverage: Finland

Time Span: 1978 to date

Updating: About 2000 records a year

MEDICAL AND PSYCHOLOGICAL PREVIEWS

Type: Reference (Bibliographic)

Subject: Biomedicine; Psychology

Producer: BRS/Colleague

Online Service: BRS; BRS After Dark; BRS/Colleague; DATA-STAR

Content: Contains citations to articles in 125 key medical journals covered by *Abridged Index Medicus* and to articles in 55 major clinical psychology journals that are also included in other databases covering clinical psychology (e.g., *see PsycINFO* and *SOCIAL SCISEARCH*). Records appear in this file within 10 days (BRS) or 2 weeks (DATA-STAR) of the appearance of the journals in major health sciences libraries. Within 5 to 12 weeks, the biomedical articles are represented in MEDLINE *(see)*. Biomedical literature covers such topics as clinical medicine, nursing, and hospital administration.

Language: English

Coverage: Canada, U.K., and U.S.

Time Span: Most recent 3 to 4 months

Updating: About 1000 records a week

MEDICAL RESEARCH DIRECTORY

Type: Reference (Referral)

Subject: Biomedicine; Research in Progress

Producer: John Wiley & Sons, Inc.

Online Service: DATA-STAR

Content: Contains references to current biomedical research projects being performed at academic institutions, hospitals, government agencies, and other organizations in the U.K. Covers 45 subject areas, including anatomy, pediatrics, nursing, and microbiology. For each project, includes research title, subject area, name of department head, and name and address of affiliated institution. Sources include The British Library's *Research in British Universities, Polytechnics, and Colleges*, and information provided by research councils, National Health Service Regional Health Authorities, and charitable trusts supporting biomedical research. Corresponds to Wiley's *Medical Research Directory* .

Language: English

Coverage: U.K.

Time Span: Current information

Updating: Quarterly

MEDICAMENTOS EN EL EMBARAZO

Type: Reference (Bibliographic) ; Source (Full Text)

Subject: Pharmaceuticals & Pharmaceutical Industry

Producer: Consejo General de Colegios Oficiales de Farmaceuticos de Espana

Online Service: Consejo General de Colegios Oficiales de Farmaceuticos de Espana

Content: Contains full text of original articles, with bibliographies, on risks associated with the use of about 350 drugs available in Spain by pregnant women. Includes description, mechanism, and frequency of adverse effects on mother and fetus, relevant research results, and recommendations on usage. Sources include the international scientific literature and pharmacology databases.

Language: Spanish

Coverage: Spain

Time Span: Articles, current information; bibliographies, 1980 to date.

Updating: Periodically, as new data become available

MEDICAMENTOS EN ENFERMEDADES CRONICAS

Type: Source (Full Text)

Subject: Pharmaceuticals & Pharmaceutical Industry

Producer: Consejo General de Colegios Oficiales de Farmaceuticos de Espana

Online Service: Consejo General de Colegios Oficiales de Farmaceuticos de Espana

Content: Contains full text of original articles on risks associated with the use of over 1500 drugs or active ingredients available in Spain by patients with such chronic conditions as allergy to penicillin or salicilate, angina, asthma, depression, diabetes, epilepsy, glaucoma, hypertension, peptic ulcers, or insufficient function of the heart, liver, or kidneys. Covers general actions of each drug, possible effects on patients with chronic conditions, contraindications, and precautions. Sources include the international scientific literature and pharmacology databases.

Language: Spanish

Coverage: Spain

Time Span: Current information

Updating: Periodically, as new data become available

MEDIFAUNE

Type: Source (Textual-Numeric)

Subject: Aquatic Sciences

Producer: Universite de Nice, Laboratoire d'Oceanographie biologique

Online Service: Serveur Universitaire National de l'Information Scientifique et Technique (SUNIST)

Conditions: Permission of Laboratoire d'Oceanographie biologique required

Content: Contains descriptions of about 6000 Mediterranean marine animal species. Includes binomial catalog, first collection date, identification date, worldwide geographic distribution, bathymetric distribution, ecology, biological information, and market value.

Language: French

Coverage: Mediterranean Sea

Time Span: 1758 to date

Updating: Periodically, as new data become available

MEDIS

Type: Source (Full Text)

Subject: Biomedicine; Health Care

Producer: Mead Data Central, Inc., from data provided by publishers

Online Service: Mead Data Central, Inc.

Conditions: Subscription to Mead Data Central required; includes access to NEXIS.

Content: Contains full text of more than 60 publications in the biomedical area. Users can search by publication, by type of publication (i.e., journals, newsletters, textbooks), or across publications, by specialty area (e.g., surgery, rheumatology, psychiatry, pediatrics, cardiology, oncology, hematology, public health, and general and internal medicine).

Journals. Contains the full text of *American Family Physician* since 1982, *American Journal of Cardiology* since June 1982, *American Journal of Diseases in Children* since June 1982, *American Journal of Medicine* since June 1982, *American Journal of Physical Medicine* since February 1984, *American Journal of Surgery* since June 1982, *Annals of Internal Medicine* since 1983, *Annals of Neurology* since 1984, *Annals of Plastic Surgery* since 1984, *Annals of Surgery* since 1983, *Annals of Thoracic Surgery* since 1984, *Archives of Dermatology* since June 1982, *Archives of General Psychiatry* since June 1982, *Archives of Internal Medicine* since June 1982, *Archives of Neurology* since June 1982, *Archives of Ophthalmology* since June 1982, *Archives of Otolaryngology*, since June 1982, *Archives of Pathology & Laboratory Medicine* since 1982, *Archives of Surgery* since June 1982, *Arthritis & Rheumatism* since 1982, *Blood* since 1983, *British Journal of Surgery* since 1985, *Bulletin on the Rheumatic Diseases* since 1982, *Cancer Treatment Reports* since 1985, *Cancer Treatment Symposia*, 1983-1984, *Clinical Orthopaedics & Related Research* since 1984, *Clinical Pediatrics* since June 1984, *Critical Care Medicine* since 1983, *Journal of the American Medical Association* since October 1982, *Journal of Nervous and Mental Disease* since 1983, *Journal of Pediatric Surgery* since February 1984, *Journal of the National Cancer Institute* since 1984, *Medicine* since 1983, *Pediatrics* since 1984, *Progress in Cardiovascular Disease* since 1984, *Public Health Reports* since 1983, *Seminars in Arthritis and Rheumatism* since February 1984, *Seminars in Hematology* since 1983, *Seminars in Oncology* since June 1983, *Sexually Transmitted Diseases* since 1984, and *Surgery, Gynecology & Obstetrics* since June 1982.

Newsletters. Contains the full text of *Back Pain Monitor* since October 1983, *Clinical Laser Monthly* since August 1983, *Contraceptive Technology Update* since 1982, *Employee Health and Fitness* since 1982, *F-D-C Reports: The Blue Sheet* since 1984, *F-D-C Reports: The Pink Sheet* since 1984, *Hospital Admitting Monthly* since July 1982, *Hospital Employee Health* since 1982, *Hospital Infection Control* since 1982, *Hospital Peer Review* since 1982, *Hospital Risk Management* since 1982, *M-D-D-I Reports: The Gray Sheet* since 1984, *Prospective Payment Survival* since July 1983, *The Rose Sheet* since 1984, and *Same Day Surgery* since 1982.

Textbooks. Contains the full text of *Current Emergency Diagnosis & Treatment* (1983), *Current Medical Diagnosis & Treatment* (1984), *Current Obstetrics & Gynecologic Diagnosis & Treatment* (1982), *Current Pediatric Diagnosis & Treatment* (1982), *Current Surgical Diagnosis & Treatment* (1983), and *Primer on Rheumatic Diseases* (1983).

CONSUMER DRUG INFORMATION. *(see)*

DRUG INFORMATION FULLTEXT. *(see)*

INTERNATIONAL PHARMACEUTICAL ABSTRACTS. *(see)*

MEDLINE. *(see)*

PDQ. *(see)*

Administrative Library. Contains the full text of *Hospitals* since July 1984, Accreditation Manual for Hospitals, 1985 edition, *Quality Review Bulletin* since 1984, and *JCAH Perspectives* since 1984.

Language: English
Time Span: Varies by publication *(see Content)*
Updating: Not updated

MEDITEC

Type: Reference (Bibliographic)
Subject: Bioengineering
Producer: FIZ Technik
Online Service: DIMDI; FIZ Technik
Content: Contains about 58,000 citations, with abstracts, to the worldwide literature on biomedical engineering. Covers biological sciences (e.g., biomechanics, biophysics, biochemistry, biocybernetics); biomedical measurements (e.g., recording, processing and evaluation of physiological parameters); medical diagnostics (e.g., electro-diagnostics, X-ray diagnostics, ultrasonic diagnostics, nuclear-medical diagnostics, clinical laboratory technology, optical methods); medical therapeutics (e.g., electro-therapy, ultrasonic therapy, nuclear-medical therapy, radiation therapy); artificial organs and functions (e.g., orthopedics, aids for disabled persons, biomaterials); and clinical engineering.
Language: Titles and search terms in English and German, with abstracts in English (20%) or German (80%)
Coverage: International
Time Span: 1968 to date
Updating: About 600 records a month

MEDLINE

Type: Reference (Bibliographic)
Subject: Biomedicine; Biotechnology; Food Sciences & Nutrition; Health Care; Pharmaceuticals & Pharmaceutical Industry; Toxicology
Producer: National Library of Medicine (NLM)
Online Service: Australian Medline Network; BRS; BRS After Dark; BRS/BRKTHRU; BRS/Colleague; DATA-STAR; DIALOG Information Services, Inc.; DIMDI (MEDLARS); The Japan Information Center of Science and Technology (JICST); Knowledge Index; Mead Data Central, Inc. (as a MEDIS database *(see)*); MIC-KIBIC; National Library of Medicine; PaperChase; TECH DATA
Conditions: Subscription to Mead Data Central required
Content: Provides access to the worldwide biomedical literature, including research, clinical practice, administration, policy issues, and health care services. Contains references to articles from 3200 journals published in the U.S. and about 70 other countries. Also covers chapters and articles from selected monographs through 1981. Author abstracts (from 1975) are available for about 60% of the citations. Corresponds in part to coverage of *Index Medicus, Index to Dental Literature*, and *International Nursing Index*.
Language: English
Coverage: International
Time Span: DIMDI and PaperChase, 1964 to date; Australian Medline Network, BRS, BRS After Dark, BRS/Colleague, DATA-STAR, DIALOG, Knowledge Index, MIC-KIBIC, and NLM, 1966 to date; JICST, 1972 to date.
Updating: About 25,000 records a month

MEDREP

Type: Reference (Referral)
Subject: Biomedicine; Health Care; Research in Progress
Producer: Commission of the European Communities (CEC)

Online Service: ECHO Service
Content: Contains descriptions of current biomedical and health care research projects in European Economic Community (EEC) member countries. Includes project title, research organization, project leaders, and summary of goals and research activities. Corresponds to *Permanent Inventory of Biomedical and Health Care Research Projects*.
Language: Danish, Dutch, English, French, German, Italian, Spanish, and Swedish, with project titles also in English
Coverage: European Economic Community (Belgium, Denmark, Federal Republic of Germany, France, Greece, Ireland, Italy, Luxembourg, The Netherlands, Portugal, Spain, and U.K.)
Time Span: 1972 to date
Updating: Periodically, as new data become available

MEETING AGENDA

Type: Reference (Referral)
Subject: Conferences & Meetings
Producer: Commissariat a l'Energie Atomique (CEA), Centre d'Etudes Nucleaires de Saclay
Online Service: Telesystemes-Questel
Content: Contains announcements of congresses, conferences, meetings, workshops, exhibitions, and fairs worldwide in all areas of science, technology, and social science. Areas covered include aeronautics, agriculture, biology, medicine, chemistry, earth sciences, electronics, electrical engineering, energy materials, mathematics, engineering, equipment, missile technology, navigations, telecommunications, military science, physics, fuels, and space technology. Information is obtained from meeting announcements and programs.
Language: English and French
Coverage: International
Time Span: Forthcoming meetings for the next 2 to 3 years
Updating: Twice a month; about 15,000 records a year.

MENTAL HEALTH ABSTRACTS

Type: Reference (Bibliographic)
Subject: Biomedicine; Psychology
Producer: IFI/Plenum Data Company
Online Service: BRS (NCMH); BRS/BRKTHRU (NCMH); BRS/Colleague (NCMH); DATA-STAR; DIALOG Information Services, Inc. (MENTAL HEALTH ABSTRACTS); Knowledge Index (MENTAL HEALTH ABSTRACTS); TECH DATA
Content: Contains over 495,000 citations, with abstracts, to the worldwide literature on mental health. Covers the biomedical, behavioral, and social aspects of the development and maintenance of "normal" behavior and emotional well-being and the etiology, diagnosis, treatment, prevention, and socio-legal implications of mental illness. Topics covered include aging and geriatrics, alcoholism and drug abuse, behavioral medicine, child psychology, education, ethics, family, genetics, mental health services, mental retardation, motivation, personality, prevention, psychiatry, psychology, psychopharmacology, schizophrenia, sexology, sleep, stress, suicide, treatment and therapy, and violence. Materials are drawn from about 1200 journals and from books, technical reports, workshops and conference proceedings, and symposia. Far Eastern literature and non-print materials are also included.
Language: English
Coverage: International
Time Span: BRS, BRS/BRKTHRU, BRS/Colleague, and DATA-STAR, 1969 to 1981; DIALOG, 1969 to date.
Updating: BRS, BRS/BRKTHRU, BRS/Colleague, and DATA-STAR, not updated; DIALOG, about 2000 records a month.

MENTAL MEASUREMENTS YEARBOOK©

Type: Reference (Referral)
Subject: Education & Educational Institutions; Psychology; Tests & Measurements
Producer: Buros Institute of Mental Measurements
Online Service: BRS; BRS After Dark; BRS/BRKTHRU; BRS/Colleague; TECH DATA
Content: Contains descriptive information and reviews of English-language tests from the *Mental Measurements Yearbook*. Covers over 1850 standardized educational, personality, vocational aptitude, psychological, and related English-language tests. Information provided about each test includes name and classification; author (s); publisher, publication date, and price; time requirements; existence of validity and reliability data; score descriptions, levels, and intended populations; and critical reviews.
Language: English
Coverage: International
Time Span: 1974 to date
Updating: Monthly

.MENU℠-THE INTERNATIONAL SOFTWARE DATABASE

Type: Reference (Referral)
Subject: Computers & Software
Producer: International Software Database Corp.
Online Service: CompuServe Information Service (as part of THE ELECTRONIC MALL); DIALOG Information Services, Inc.; Knowledge Index; Quantum Computer Services, Inc. (as part of QuantumLink *(see)*)
Content: Contains over 75,000 listings of commercially available software for microcomputers, minicomputers, and some mainframes. Each record includes a short description of the software, categories for broad areas of application (e.g., medical, dental, educational, scientific, and systems), codes for compatible minicomputers and microcomputers (e.g., Atari, PET, APPLE, TRS-80, Honeywell, DEC PDP-11), hardware and software requirements, distribution medium, purchase price, and supplier name. Includes software for both computer experts and hobbyists. Users can order software online. Corresponds to the following publications: *The Software Catalog: Business Software, The Software Catalog: Health Professions, The Software Catalog: Microcomputers, The Software Catalog: Minicomputers*, and *The Software Catalog: Science and Engineering.*
Language: English
Coverage: International
Time Span: Current information
Updating: Replaced monthly

THE MERCK INDEX ONLINE

Type: Source (Full Text)
Subject: Pharmaceuticals & Pharmaceutical Industry
Producer: Merck & Company, Inc.
Online Service: BRS; BRS/BRKTHRU; BRS/Colleague; Chemical Information Systems, Inc., a subsidiary of Fein-Marquart Associates (CIS); TECH DATA; Telesystemes-Questel
Conditions: Annual subscription fee of $300 to CIS required but fee is waived for educational institutions and non-profit public libraries worldwide
Content: Contains full text of over 10,000 monographs describing approximately 30,000 chemicals, drugs, biologi-

cals, and veterinary and agricultural products. Includes patent information; chemical, generic, trivial, and trademark names; preparations; molecular formulas and weights for title substances and derivatives; properties; Chemical Abstracts Service Registry Number; principal pharmacological actions; and toxicity of substances. Corresponds to the 10th edition of *The Merck Index*. Includes monographs that have been written or revised since publication of the 10th edition.
Language: English
Coverage: International
Time Span: Current information
Updating: Twice a year

EL MIAMI HERALD
Type: Source (Full Text)
Subject: News
Producer: Miami Herald Publishing Company
Online Service: VU/TEXT Information Services, Inc.
Conditions: Subscription to VU/TEXT required
Content: Contains Spanish-language version of MIAMI HERALD *(see)*. Covers some stories not included in the *Miami Herald*.
Language: Spanish
Coverage: U.S. (primarily Florida), with some international news
Time Span: 1983 to date
Updating: Daily

MIAMI HERALD
Type: Source (Full Text)
Subject: News
Producer: Miami Herald Publishing Company
Online Service: VU/TEXT Information Services, Inc.
Conditions: Subscription to VU/TEXT required
Content: Contains full text of news articles and feature stories from the final and regional editions (Palm Beach, Broward County, Keys, Gulf, and Treasure Coast) of the *Miami Herald* (Florida) newspaper. Covers local, national, and international (especially Latin American) news, as well as business and financial news, social events, and obituaries. Does not include advertisements, comics, and illustrations. Covers some stories not in *El Miami Herald*.
NOTE: Spanish-language version available separately in EL MIAMI HERALD *(see)*.
Language: English
Coverage: U.S. (primarily Florida), with some international news
Time Span: 1983 to date
Updating: Daily

MICRO CITY
Type: Reference (Referral)
Subject: Computers & Software
Producer: Michigan Office Supply
Online Service: THE SOURCE
Conditions: Monthly minimum of $10 to THE SOURCE required, with $9 credited toward online usage charges
Content: Contains descriptions of personal computer software and hardware (including peripherals) that can be purchased through Michigan Office Supply. Includes printers, modems, disk drives, and supplies, as well as educational, business, and game programs. Also contains information of interest (e.g., programming tips and game-playing techniques) to personal computer users.

Language: English
Coverage: U.S.
Time Span: Current information
Updating: Periodically, as new data become available

MICRO MD MEDICAL NETWORK
Type: Reference (Referral); Source (Full Text)
Subject: Computers & Software; Health Care
Producer: MICRO MD
Online Service: CompuServe Information Service; General Videotex Corporation/DELPHI
Conditions: Initiation fee of $49.95 required for access through General Videotex Corporation
Content: Contains full text of *Micro MD Newsletter*, providing information on the use of computers in physicians' offices. Includes reviews of computer products and services, tips on buying, and suggestions for business and clinical applications of microcomputers. On General Videotex Corporation, a catalog of hardware and software products and an electronic bulletin board are also available.
Language: English
Coverage: U.S.
Time Span: May 1984 to date
Updating: Every 2 weeks

MICROCOMPUTER INDEX®
Type: Reference (Bibliographic)
Subject: Computers & Software
Producer: Database Services
Online Service: DIALOG Information Services, Inc.; Knowledge Index
Content: Contains citations, with abstracts, to reviews and commentaries on the use and applications of microcomputers and software packages. Covers over 75 microcomputer journals and popular magazines, including *Byte, Practical Computing, InfoWorld, Personal Computing, MacWorld*, and *PC World*. Includes summaries of general articles about microcomputers, book reviews, software reviews, discussions of applications in various settings, and descriptions of new microcomputer products. Corresponds to the bimonthly *Microcomputer Index*.
Language: English
Coverage: U.S. and U.K.
Time Span: 1981 to date
Updating: Quarterly

MICROCOMPUTER SOFTWARE & HARDWARE GUIDE
Type: Reference (Referral)
Subject: Computers & Software
Producer: R.R. Bowker Company
Online Service: DIALOG Information Services, Inc.
Content: Contains descriptions of over 29,000 microcomputer software programs available in the U.S. from over 3500 publishers. Each description includes compatible hardware, operating system requirements, release date, language, price, and publisher contact information. Corresponds to *Software Encyclopedia*. Descriptions of microcomputer hardware and peripherals are scheduled to be added.
Language: English
Coverage: U.S.
Time Span: Current information
Updating: About 500 records a month

MICROLOG

Type: Reference (Bibliographic)

Subject: Research in Progress; Science & Technology

Producer: Micromedia Limited

Online Service: CISTI, Canadian Online Enquiry Service (CAN/OLE)

Conditions: CISTI accessible only in Canada

Content: Contains citations, with some abstracts, to Canadian research and report literature in all subject fields. Covers monographs, annual reports, and reports in series issued in English or French by the following types of organizations: all levels of government in Canada, research institutions, universities, laboratories, professional societies, corporations, consultants, and associations. Does not include commercially-published books or serials (other than annual reports, statistical reviews, and financial statements). Corresponds to *Microlog Index*.

Language: English and French

Coverage: Canada

Time Span: 1979 to date, with abstracts from 1985 to date

Updating: About 1400 records a quarter

MICROSEARCH™

Type: Reference (Bibliographic, Referral)

Subject: Computers & Software

Producer: Information, Inc.

Online Service: CompuServe Information Service; ORBIT Information Technologies Corporation; THE SOURCE

Conditions: Monthly minimum of $10 to THE SOURCE required, with $9 credited toward online usage charges

Content: Contains over 30,000 citations, with abstracts, to reviews of more than 12,000 microcomputer products from about 200 publications, including *Byte, InfoWorld, Popular Computing*, and *Personal Computing*. Covers hardware, software, peripherals, and accessories. Also contains manufacturers' product descriptions and names and addresses of about 5000 manufacturers and software publishers.

Language: English

Coverage: Primarily U.S.

Time Span: 1981 to date

Updating: About 500 records every 2 weeks

THE MIDNIGHT TURTLE™

Type: Reference (Bibliographic, Referral); Source (Full Text, Software)

Subject: Computers & Software

Producer: Young Peoples' Logo Association

Online Service: Young Peoples' Logo Association (YPLA)

Conditions: Initiation fee of $10 required

Content: Contains information on computer programming, with an emphasis on the Logo programming language. Includes references to articles, books, magazines, and papers, as well as a list of Logo user groups worldwide. Also contains public domain software that may be downloaded and 3 electronic bulletin boards covering such topics as Logo, BASIC, PILOT, "For Kids Only", and ONLINE ADVENTURE GAMES.

Language: English

Coverage: International

Time Span: Varies, with earliest data from 1968

Updating: Daily

MILITARY VETERANS SERVICES

Type: Reference (Referral); Source (Full Text)

Subject: Social Services

Producer: David Aldstadt

Online Service: CompuServe Information Service

Content: Contains information of interest to U.S. veterans, particularly Vietnam War veterans. Provides news of political and legislative developments (e.g., changes in G.I. benefits); information on Agent Orange, covering legal actions, studies conducted by the Centers for Disease Control in Atlanta and the Air Force, reviews of medical literature, and resource contacts; and information from the Department of Defense and National League of Families on prisoners of war and persons missing in action. Also provides a directory of information on each person whose name is inscribed on the Vietnam Veterans Memorial in Washington, D.C., a listing of veterans organizations, and a schedule of events of particular interest to veterans. Available only to military veterans are a forum for the online exchange of ideas and experiences and a national locator service for finding individuals.

Language: English

Coverage: U.S.

Time Span: April 1984 to date

Updating: Daily

MORBIDITY & MORTALITY WEEKLY REPORT

Type: Source (Full Text)

Subject: Biomedicine

Producer: U.S. Department of Health and Human Services, Public Health Service, Centers for Disease Control. Data are supplied to NewsNet by Information Services, Inc.

Online Service: AMA/NET; NewsNet, Inc. (MMWR PLUS)

Conditions: Subscription fee of $50 to AMA/NET required; monthly subscription to NewsNet required with differential charges for subscribers and non-subscribers to *Morbidity & Mortality Weekly Report*.

Content: Contains full text of *Morbidity & Mortality Weekly Report*, providing news, information, and summary data on the incidence and prevalence of infectious diseases, adverse drug and vaccine reactions, toxic exposures, and substance abuse. Does not include graphics.

Language: English

Coverage: International

Time Span: AMA/NET, current week; NewsNet, June 8, 1984 to date.

Updating: Weekly

NARIC© (REHABDATA)

Type: Reference (Bibliographic, Referral)

Subject: Health Care; Social Services

Producer: National Rehabilitation Information Center (NARIC)

Online Service: BRS; BRS After Dark; BRS/BRKTHRU; BRS/Colleague

Content: Contains over 13,000 citations to both print and audiovisual materials relating to the rehabilitation of physically or mentally disabled persons. Groups covered include blind, deaf, developmentally disabled, spinal-cord-injured, and emotionally disturbed persons. Includes reports from projects funded by the National Institute of Handicapped Research (NIHR) and the Rehabilitation Services Administration (RSA), as well as journal articles, audiovisual materials, directories, and commercial publications.

Language: English
Coverage: International
Time Span: 1950 to date
Updating: About 200 records a month

NARIC© ABLEDATA

Type: Reference (Referral)
Subject: Health Care
Producer: National Rehabilitation Information Center
Online Service: BRS; BRS After Dark; BRS/BRKTHRU; BRS/Colleague
Content: Contains over 13,000 product descriptions of rehabilitation aids and equipment for disabled persons. Covers therapeutic, sensory, educational, vocational, transportation, and other types of technical items. Information provided for each product includes generic name, brand name (i.e., trade name and/or model number), manufacturer's name, availability (i.e., major distributor), approximate cost, user comments (e.g., contraindications, limitations) and, if available, formal evaluation data. Also provides address information for each manufacturer in the Manufacturer Address Data Collect File.
Language: English
Coverage: U.S.
Time Span: Current information
Updating: About 200 records a month

NASA

Type: Reference (Bibliographic, Referral)
Subject: Science & Technology
Producer: American Institute of Aeronautics and Astronautics (AIAA), Technical Information Service (TIS); National Aeronautics and Space Administration (NASA), Scientific and Technical Information Branch
Online Service: ESA-IRS (STAR and IAA files, under the name NASA); National Aeronautics and Space Administration, RECON (all files, under listed names)
Conditions: Available through ESA-IRS only in Europe, by tripartite arrangements with ESA-IRS and NASA. Available through NASA, via NASA/RECON, only in the U.S., to NASA Research Centers and contractors, NASA-sponsored Industrial Application Centers, other government agencies and contractors, and universities with scientific and engineering activities that are related to aeronautics and space research.
Content: A family of files with a primary focus on citations and abstracts to the worldwide journal and report literature on aeronautics and astronautics.

STAR. Contains citations, with abstracts, to reports published by NASA in the semimonthly *Scientific and Technical Aerospace Reports*. Covers reports issued by NASA and its contractors, as well as other U.S. government agencies, universities, and private and public research organizations throughout the world. Includes aeronautics, astronautics, chemistry and materials, engineering, geosciences, life sciences, mathematical and computer sciences, physics, social sciences, and space sciences. Covers 1962 to date. Updated twice a month.

IAA. Contains citations, with abstracts, corresponding to *International Aerospace Abstracts*, published by the American Institute of Aeronautics and Astronautics. Covers the open literature (e.g., journals, monographs, theses, conference proceedings) in the same subject areas as STAR. Covers 1962 to date. Updated twice a month.

ASRDI Safety File. Contains about 11,900 citations and abstracts to reports generated by the Aerospace Safety Research and Development Institute (ASRDI). Covers fire technology, cryogenic fluids, and mechanics of structural failure. Covers 1975 and 1976. Not updated.

AEROSPACE MEDICINE AND BIBLIOGRAPHY. Contains about 11,700 selected citations from *Aerospace Medicine and Biology Bibliography*. Covers 1964 to 1969. Not updated.

OLDER SCIENTIFIC AND TECHNICAL AEROSPACE REPORTS EXTENDED. Contains citations to unclassified, unlimited-distribution reports of limited significance within NASA. These reports are not announced in *Scientific and Technical Aerospace Reports* (STAR). Covers 1968 to date. A backfile, covering 1962 to 1967, is available through NASA in the UNCLASSIFIED ALTERNATE DATABASE. Updated twice a month.

RESEARCH AND DEVELOPMENT CONTRACT SEARCH FILE. Contains references to NASA contract and grant awards. Covers 1972 to date. Updated monthly.

RESEARCH AND TECHNOLOGY OBJECTIVES AND PLANS. Contains over 8000 descriptions of NASA-sponsored research in progress. Covers 1971 to date. Updated annually.

Also includes NASA TECH BRIEFS *(see)*, NASA DIRECTORY OF NUMERICAL DATABASES, NASA NALNET BOOKS, and NASA NALNET PERIODICALS.
Language: English
Coverage: Primarily U.S., with some international coverage
Time Span: Varies by file *(see Content)*
Updating: Varies by file *(see Content)*

NASA TECH BRIEFS

Type: Reference (Bibliographic)
Subject: Science & Technology
Producer: National Aeronautics and Space Administration (NASA), Scientific and Technical Information Branch
Online Service: National Aeronautics and Space Administration, RECON
Conditions: Available only in U.S., to NASA Research Centers and contractors, NASA-sponsored Industrial Application Centers, other government agencies and contractors, and universities with scientific and engineering activities that are related to aeronautics and space research.
Content: Contains approximately 10,500 citations, with abstracts, to articles taken from *NASA Tech Briefs*, published quarterly by the NASA Technology Utilization Division. Covers descriptions of new products and processes developed by NASA facilities and contractors. Includes these subjects: electronic components and circuits, electrical systems, fabrication technology, life sciences, machinery, materials, mathematics and information sciences, mechanics, and physical sciences. Emphasis is on current-awareness and problem-solving information in such areas as new and potential products, new industrial processes, advances in basic and applied research, improvements in shop and laboratory techniques, new sources of technical data, and computer software.
Language: English
Coverage: U.S.
Time Span: 1962 to date
Updating: Periodically, as new data become available

NATIONAL EMERGENCY EQUIPMENT LOCATOR SYSTEM

Type: Reference (Referral)
Subject: Environment

Producer: Developed by I.P. Sharp Associates under the direction of Environment Canada, in cooperation with the Ministry of Transport (Canada) and the Petroleum Association for the Conservation of the Canadian Environment (PACE)

Online Service: I.P. Sharp Associates

Conditions: Enrollment with Environment Canada required

Content: Contains information needed to locate the required emergency and protective equipment and materials, including air and water craft, in the event of an environmental emergency such as an oil spill or spill of hazardous material. Includes equipment description, name of owning organization, and telephone number. Also covers how earlier spills were handled and information for identifying and handling hazardous chemicals. Equipment locations are in Canada only.

Language: English

Coverage: Canada

Updating: Irregularly, by users

NATIONAL GROUND WATER INFORMATION CENTER

Type: Reference (Bibliographic)

Subject: Aquatic Sciences

Producer: National Water Well Association

Online Service: National Water Well Association

Conditions: Initiation fee of $100 required

Content: Contains approximately 26,000 citations to the worldwide literature on ground water and hydrogeology. Covers books, journals, technical reports, government publications, conference proceedings, and citations from *Selected Water Resources Abstracts (see WATER RESOURCES ABSTRACTS)*.

Language: English

Coverage: U.S.

Time Span: Earliest data from 1900

Updating: Every 2 weeks

NATIONAL NEWSPAPER INDEX℠

Type: Reference (Bibliographic)

Subject: News

Producer: Information Access Co.

Online Service: BRS; BRS After Dark; BRS/BRKTHRU; BRS/Colleague; DIALOG Information Services, Inc.; Knowledge Index; Mead Data Central, Inc. (NWSIND) (as a Reference Service database)

Conditions: Subscription to Mead Data Central required

Content: Contains citations to articles, news reports, editorials, letters to the editor, obituaries, product evaluations, biographical pieces, poetry, recipes, columns, cartoons, illustrations, and reviews from *The Christian Science Monitor, Los Angeles Times, The New York Times* (Late and National Editions), *The Wall Street Journal* (Eastern and Western Editions), and *The Washington Post* (Final Edition). Covers the full range of subjects found in national newspapers: general interest news, business, life and living, leisure-time activities, home-centered arts, sports, recreation, travel, performing arts, literature, social affairs, science and technology, agriculture, consumer product evaluations, regional news, and environmental issues. Corresponds to the *National Newspaper Index* on microform. Records are added daily to NEWSEARCH *(see)* and are transferred to this database monthly.

Language: English

Coverage: U.S.

Time Span: Most newspapers, 1979 to date; *The Washington Post* and *Los Angeles Times*, 1982 to date.

Updating: About 14,000 records a month

NATIONAL PESTICIDE INFORMATION RETRIEVAL SYSTEM

Type: Source (Textual-Numeric)

Subject: Agriculture

Producer: National Pesticide Information Retrieval System, Purdue University

Online Service: National Pesticide Information Retrieval System, Purdue University (as a database on Planning Research Corporation (PRC))

Conditions: Membership fee of $100 in first year plus $15 monthly minimum required; renewal memberships are $200 a year.

Content: Contains information on about 60,000 pesticide products registered with the U.S. Environmental Protection Agency (EPA) and with U.S. state agencies that have registration programs. Includes product names, names and addresses of manufacturers and other registrants, names and percentages of active ingredients, types of formulations in which the product is marketed (e.g., water-soluble, dust), type of pesticidal activity (e.g., herbicide, insecticide), toxicity signal word that appears on the product label (i.e., caution, danger, warning), sites to which the product is applied (e.g., buildings, animals, crops), pests for each site, use classification (i.e., restricted or general use), tolerances for food crop uses (by ingredient or commodity), and EPA and state registration numbers. Registration standards data tables contain EPA chemical registration requirements, including necessary studies, identification of incomplete study data, and time span for supplying incomplete data. Experimental Use Permits (EUPs) and emergency exemptions (section 18s) are also available. Also covers some pest control products that have been canceled by the EPA and are no longer legally sold or used. Full text of the newsletters of the EPA Office of Pesticide Programs (since 1984) are also available. Also contains EPA fact sheets providing summaries on a chemical-by-chemical basis of active ingredients used in pesticide product formulation.

Language: English

Coverage: U.S.

Time Span: Current information, with some coverage of canceled products

Updating: Weekly

NATIONAL REFERRAL CENTER DATA BASE

Type: Reference (Referral)

Subject: Information Systems & Services-Directories

Producer: Library of Congress

Online Service: Library of Congress Information System (LOCIS), as NATIONAL REFERRAL CENTER MASTER FILE on SCORPIO; National Library of Medicine (NLM) (as part of DIRLINE *(see)*)

Conditions: Available through LOCIS only to users on-site at the Library of Congress and through National Library of Medicine, only to U.S. users.

Content: Provides references to about 14,000 organizations that are qualified and willing to answer questions or provide information in their areas of specialization. Includes organization name, address, telephone number(s), descriptions of broad and specific subject areas covered, holdings (e.g., databases or document collections), list of representative publications, types of information services provided, and fees or restrictions. Corresponds in part to the NRC series *Directory of Information Resources in the United States* and the informal series *Who Knows?*

Language: English
Coverage: Primarily U.S., with some coverage (about 7%) of non-U.S. organizations
Time Span: Most recent data available
Updating: Quarterly, with each entry reviewed every 2 years

NBRF NUCLEIC ACID SEQUENCE DATABASE

Type: Source (Textual-Numeric)
Subject: Biotechnology
Producer: National Biomedical Research Foundation
Online Service: Bionet; IntelliGenetics, Inc., An IntelliCorp Company; Protein Identification Resource (PIR), National Biomedical Research Foundation (NBRF)
Conditions: To access through Bionet, users must be qualified principal investigators employed by a non-profit organization
Content: Contains descriptions of approximately 1800 genetic sequences in approximately 3 million bases. Covers all nucleic acid sequences for proteins and some regulatory and promoter sequences. Descriptions include function of sequence, sequence features of biological interest, and source (i.e., DNA or RNA). Sources include scientific books, scientific journals (e.g., *Journal of Biological Chemistry, Proceedings of the National Academy of Science USA, Nature, Nucelic Acids Research, Biochemistry, European Journal of Biochemistry, FEBS Letters*), and private communications. Corresponds in part to *Nucleic Acid Sequence Database*, with additional data available online.
Language: English
Coverage: International
Time Span: 1972 to date
Updating: Quarterly

NBRF-PIR PROTEIN SEQUENCE DATABASE

Type: Reference (Bibliographic); Source (Textual-Numeric)
Subject: Biotechnology
Producer: National Biomedical Research Foundation
Online Service: Bionet; IntelliGenetics, Inc., An IntelliCorp Company; Protein Identification Resource (PIR), National Biomedical Research Foundation (NBRF)
Conditions: To access through Bionet, users must be qualified principal investigators employed by a non-profit organization
Content: Contains descriptions of over 3000 partial and whole protein sequences representing over 770,000 amino acids that were isolated or inferred from the gene sequences. Descriptions include function of protein, taxonomy, sequence features of biological interest, how sequence was experimentally determined, unambiguously determined residues within the sequence, and citations to relevant literature. Sources include scientific books, scientific journals (e.g., *Journal of Biological Chemistry, Proceedings from the National Academy of Science USA, Nature, Nucelic Acids Research, Biochemistry, European Journal of Biochemistry*, and *FEBS Letters*), and private communications. Corresponds to *NBRF Atlas of Protein Sequence and Structure*, with more current information online.

Language: English
Coverage: International
Time Span: 1965 to date
Updating: Quarterly

NDEX (Newspaper Index)

Type: Reference (Bibliographic)
Subject: News
Producer: Bell & Howell
Online Service: ORBIT Information Technologies Corporation
Content: Contains citations to international, national, state, and local news items in these major U.S. newspapers: *Chicago Sun-Times* (from 1979 to 1982), *Chicago Tribune* (from 1976 to 1981), *Washington Post* (from 1976 to 1981), *Denver Post* (from 1979 to date), *Detroit News, Houston Post, Los Angeles Times, New Orleans Times Picayune, San Francisco Chronicle* (from 1976 to date), *St. Louis Post-Dispatch* (from 1980 to date), *USA Today*, and *Boston Globe* (from 1983 to date). Corresponds to the printed *Newspaper Index* series. Also includes these nationally-known Black newspapers from the *Index to Black Newspapers: Amsterdam New York News, Atlanta Daily World, Baltimore Afro-American, Bilalian News* (Chicago) (1979 to 1981), *Chicago Defender, Cleveland Call & Post, Norfolk Journal & Guide, Los Angeles Sentinel, Michigan chronicle, New Pittsburgh Courier* (1979 only), and *St. Louis Argus* (from 1980 to 1982).
Language: English
Coverage: Primarily U.S., with some international news
Time Span: Most newspapers, 1976 to date; most Black newspapers, 1979 to date.
Updating: About 25,000 records a month

THE NEC ADVANCED PERSONAL COMPUTER III SOFTWARE CATALOG

Type: Reference (Referral)
Subject: Computers & Software
Producer: NEC Information Systems
Online Service: THE SOURCE
Conditions: Monthly minimum of $10 to THE SOURCE required, with $9 credited toward online usage charges
Content: Contains descriptions of software packages tested by NEC Information Systems and found to run successfully under the MS-DOS operating system on the NEC Advanced Personal Computer III. Software categories include communications, languages, utilities, database management systems, spreadsheets, word processors, business and accounting, and education. For each product, includes name and description, hardware and software requirements, price, and manufacturer's name, address, and telephone number.
Language: English
Coverage: Primarily U.S.
Time Span: Current information
Updating: Periodically, as new data become available

NEDRES (National Environmental Data Referral Service)

Type: Reference (Bibliographic, Referral)
Subject: Environment
Producer: National Oceanic and Atmospheric Administration, National Environmental Data Referral Service (NOAA/NEDRES)

Online Service: BRS; BRS After Dark; BRS/BRKTHRU; BRS/Colleague

Content: Contains over 13,000 descriptions of sources of publicly available environmental data collected by environmental satellites, oceanographic vessels, weather stations, buoys, and environmental observers. Types of data sources covered include computer-readable data files, printed publications, data file documentation (e.g., manuals, codebooks), and organizations that provide environmental data. Covers climatological, meteorological, oceanographic, geophysical, geological, geographic, hydrological and limnological data. Each record includes title or name of data source; descriptions of purpose and general characteristics of the data; data collection methods; data processing and quality control; time period; geographic area (including named places; Federal Information Processing Standard Country, State, County, and named place codes; U.S. Geological Survey Hydrologic Unit codes; U.S. Forest Service and U.S. Fish and Wildlife Service Ecoregion codes; and latitude/longitude rectangles); names of observed or computed parameters and variables; general descriptors such as chemical compound and biological organism names; availability of data (e.g., contact person or organization and volume, media, and conditions of use); principal investigator(s); program, project name or acronyms, and contract or grant; processing organization (if different from contact); related publications; and discipline, type, and organization codes.

Language: English

Coverage: Primarily U.S. and Canada

Time Span: Varies, with earliest data from the early 1800s

Updating: Quarterly

THE NEW TECH TIMES®

Type: Reference (Referral)

Subject: Science & Technology

Producer: WHA Television, The New Tech Times

Online Service: CompuServe Information Service

Content: Contains information relating to "The New Tech Times," a weekly half-hour television program on new technology (including computers, robotics, music, video, and medical technologies) airing on the Public Broadcasting Service. Includes a list of broadcast times for all cities that carry the program, previews of program content for the next 4 broadcasts, supplementary information on people and products covered in the previous 4 broadcasts, and selected user letters and responses. Users can place online orders for program transcripts and other materials, and can submit suggestions for future programs.

Language: English

Coverage: U.S. and Canada

Time Span: Previous and coming month

Updating: Weekly

NEW YORK DAILY NEWS

Type: Source (Full Text)

Subject: News

Producer: New York News Inc.

Online Service: VU/TEXT Information Services, Inc. (to be available in 1987)

Conditions: Subscription to VU/TEXT required

Content: Contains full text of news items and feature articles from *New York Daily News* (New York) newspaper.

Language: English

Coverage: U.S. (primarily New York metropolitan area)

Updating: Daily

THE NEW YORK TIMES

Type: Source (Full Text)

Subject: News

Producer: The New York Times Company

Online Service: Mead Data Central, Inc. (NYT) (as part of NEXIS NEWSPAPERS *(see)*)

Conditions: Subscription to Mead Data Central required

Content: Contains full text of all news and editorial material in the final Late edition of *The New York Times*, including all sections of the Sunday paper. From June 1, 1980, all items include controlled-vocabulary indexing, full bibliographic information, and descriptions of charts, graphs, tables, photographs, cartoons, and maps that appeared in the original article.

Language: English

Coverage: U.S. and international

Time Span: June 1980 to date

Updating: Daily

NEWS/RETRIEVAL WORLD REPORT℠

Type: Source (Full Text)

Subject: News

Producer: Dow Jones & Company, Inc.

Online Service: Dow Jones & Company, Inc.

Conditions: Annual minimum of $12 or monthly minimum of $3 to Dow Jones required

Content: Covers selected front-page U.S. national and international news stories from United Press International.

Language: English

Coverage: International

Time Span: Most recent 24 hours

Updating: Continuously, throughout the day

NEWSBRK

Type: Source (Full Text)

Subject: Information Systems & Services

Producer: BRS

Online Service: BRS After Dark; BRS/BRKTHRU

Content: Contains full text of *NEWSBRK*, a newsletter for users of the BRS After Dark and BRK/BRKTHRU services. Contains database descriptions, searching tips, and announcements of new features.

Language: English

Time Span: Current information

Updating: Irregularly

NEWSEARCH®

Type: Reference (Bibliographic)

Subject: General Interest; News

Producer: Information Access Co. (IAC)

Online Service: BRS (DAILY); BRS After Dark (DAILY); BRS/BRKTHRU (DAILY); BRS/Colleague (DAILY); DIALOG Information Services, Inc.; Knowledge Index; Mead Data Central, Inc. (as a Reference Service database)

Conditions: Subscription to Mead Data Central required

Content: Contains citations to the current month's magazine, journal, and newspaper literature. Coverage of magazines is identical to that of MAGAZINE INDEX *(see)*, of newspapers is identical to that of NATIONAL NEWSPAPER INDEX *(see)*, of law journals and legal newspapers is identical to that of LEGAL RESOURCE INDEX *(see)*, and of trade and industry journals is identical to that of TRADE AND INDUSTRY INDEX *(see)* and AREA BUSINESS DATABANK *(see)*. Also contains daily additions of records from THE COMPUTER DATABASE *(see)* and MANAGEMENT CONTENTS *(see)* and the full text of press releases from PR NEWSWIRE *(see)*. In the middle of each month, citations through the end of the previous month are transferred to the appropriate main database.

Language: English
Coverage: International
Time Span: Current month
Updating: About 1300 to 1700 records a day

NEWSNET ACTION LETTER

Type: Source (Full Text)
Subject: Information Systems & Services
Producer: NewsNet, Inc.
Online Service: NewsNet, Inc.
Conditions: Monthly subscription to NewsNet required
Content: Contains information for users of the NewsNet online service. Includes announcements of new online newsletters being offered, profiles of newsletters, enhancements to the software, tips on searching techniques, and descriptions of search commands. NewsNet's Online Bulletin is also available, providing current news throughout the week.

Language: English
Coverage: U.S.
Time Span: May 1983 to date
Updating: Monthly

NEXIS® MAGAZINES

Type: Source (Full Text)
Subject: Computers & Software; General Interest; Legislative Tracking; Science & Technology
Producer: Mead Data Central, Inc.
Online Service: Mead Data Central, Inc.
Conditions: Subscription to Mead Data Central required; includes access to the Exchange Service, Reference Service, and MEDIS *(see)*.
Content: Contains full text of these magazines:
ABA Banking Journal (Simmons Boardman Publishing Company), since 1980; *ADWEEK* (A/S/M Communications, Inc.), since 1984; *Aerospace America* (American Institute of Aeronautics and Astronautics, Inc.), since 1984; *Aviation Week & Space Technology* (McGraw-Hill, Inc.), since 1975; *Business Week* (McGraw-Hill, Inc.), since 1975; *BYTE* (McGraw-Hill, Inc.), since 1982; *Chemical Engineering* (McGraw-Hill, Inc.), since 1981; *Chemical Week* (McGraw-Hill, Inc.), since 1975; *Coal Age* (McGraw-Hill, Inc.), since 1981; *Congressional Quarterly Editorial Research Reports* (Congressional Quarterly, Inc.), since 1975; *Congressional Quarterly Weekly Report* (Congressional Quarterly, Inc.), since 1975; *Data Communications* (McGraw-Hill, Inc.), since 1982; *Defense & Foreign Affairs* (The Perth Corporation), since 1981; *Defense Electronics* (EW Communications, Inc.), since 1982; *Discover* (TIME Inc.), since October 1980 *(see)*; *Dun's Business Month* (Dun & Bradstreet Publications Corporation), since 1975; *The Economist* (The Economist Newspaper Limited), since 1975; *ElectronicsWeek* (McGraw-Hill, Inc.), since 1981; *Engineering and Mining Journal* (McGraw-Hill, Inc.), since 1981; *Engineering News-Record* (McGraw-Hill, Inc.), since 1981; *Financial World* (Financial World Partners),

since 1983; *Forbes* (Forbes, Inc.), since 1975; *Foreign Affairs* (Council on Foreign Relations, Inc.), since 1981; *Fortune* (TIME Inc.), since 1977; *Harvard Business Review* (John Wiley & Sons, Inc.), since 1976; *High Technology* (High Technology Publishing Corporation), since September 1981; *Inc.* (Inc. Publishing Corporation), since June 1981; *Industry Week* (Penton/IPC), since 1981; *Interavia Aerospace Review* (Interavia S.A.), since November 1984; *International Defense Review* (Interavia S.A.), since November 1984; *Issues in Bank Regulation* (Bank Administration Institute), since winter 1981; *Journal of Bank Research* (Bank Administration Institute), since winter 1981; *Life* (TIME Inc.), since 1982 *(see)*; *The Magazine of Bank Administration* (Bank Administration Institute), since 1981; *Marine Engineering/Log* (Simmons Boardman Publishing Corporation), since 1983; *Maclean's* (Maclean Hunter Limited), since 1985; *Mechanical Engineering* (The American Society of Mechanical Engineers), since 1982; *Microwave Systems News & Communications Technology* (EW Communications, Inc.), since 1982; *Mining Annual Review* (The Mining Journal, Ltd.), since June 1981; *Mining Journal* (The Mining Journal, Ltd.), since 1981; *Mining Magazine* (The Mining Journal, Ltd.), since 1981; *Money* (TIME Inc.), since 1982; *National Journal* (National Journal Inc.), since 1977; *Newsweek* (Newsweek), since 1975; *Nuclear News* (American Nuclear Society, Inc.), since 1982; *Offshore* (PennWell Publishing Company), since 1980; *Oil & Gas Journal* (PennWell Publishing Company), since 1978; *People* (TIME Inc.), since December 28, 1981 *(see)*; *Public Relations Journal* (Public Relations Society of America), since 1983; *Sports Illustrated* (TIME Inc.), since December 28, 1981; *Time* (TIME Inc.), since 1981 *(see)*; *U.S. News & World Report* (U.S. News & World Report, Inc.), since 1975; *United States Banker* (Kalo Communications, Inc.), since 1983; *The Washington Quarterly* (Strategic and International Studies, Georgetown University), since winter 1982; and *WorldPaper* (World Times Incorporated), since 1983.

Most magazines listed above can be searched individually, as a group (MAGS), and by subject group (BUS for general business and companies; FIN for financial markets and investments; GOVT for government and defense; NEWS for broad news coverage on all subjects; TRDTEC for trade, science, and technology). Profiles (PROFILE) of each magazine, including publisher's name and address, publication date range, frequency, and updating, are also available.

Language: English
Coverage: International
Time Span: Varies by source *(see Content)*
Updating: Generally, weekly magazines updated weekly, one week after publication; monthly magazines updated monthly, 3 weeks after publication.

NEXIS® NEWSLETTERS

Type: Source (Full Text)
Subject: Biotechnology; Health Care
Producer: Mead Data Central, Inc.
Online Service: Mead Data Central, Inc.
Conditions: Subscription to Mead Data Central required; includes access to the Exchange Service, Reference Service, and MEDIS *(see)*.
Content: Contains full text of these newsletters: *Ad Day* (A/S/M Communications, Inc.), since 1982; *Advanced Manufacturing Technology* (Technical Insights, Inc.), since 1982; *Banking Expansion Reporter* (Law & Business, Inc.), since 1982; *Bioprocessing Technology* (Technical Insights, Inc.), since 1982; *ChemWeek Newswire* (McGraw-Hill, Inc.), since July 1983; *Coal Outlook* (Pasha Publications), since October

1975; *Coal Week* (McGraw-Hill, Inc.), since 1981; *Coal Week International* (McGraw-Hill, Inc.), since 1981; *Communications Daily* (Television Digest, Inc.), since 1984; *Corporate EFT Report* (Phillips Publishing, Inc.), since 1985; *Daily Report for Executives* (The Bureau of National Affairs, Inc.), since 1982; *Defense & Foreign Affairs Daily* (The Perth Corporation), since 1981; *Defense & Foreign Affairs Weekly* (The Perth Corporation), since 1981; *Defense Industry Report* (Industry News Service, Inc.), since 1982; *East Asian Executive Reports* (East Asian Executive Reports), since September 1979; *Economic Week* (Citibank, N.A.), since 1981; *EFT Report* (Phillips Publishing, Inc.), since 1985; *Electric Utility Week* (McGraw-Hill, Inc.), since 1981; *Electrical Marketing* (McGraw-Hill, Inc.), since May 1982; *E&MJ Mining Activity Digest* (McGraw-Hill, Inc.), since 1982; *Enhanced Recovery Week* (Pasha Publications), since September 1980; *The Executive Speaker* (The Executive Speaker), since June 1980; *The Expert and The Law* (National Forensic Center), since December 1981; *FEDWATCH* (Money Market Services, Inc.), since March 1984; *Financial Services Week* (Phillips Publishing, Inc.), since 1985; *Foster Natural Gas Report* (Foster Associates, Inc.), since 1981; *Genetic Technology News* (Technical Insights, Inc.), since 1982; *Green Markets* (McGraw-Hill, Inc.), since May 1982; *Health Care Financing* (Prescott, Ball, Turben Inc.), since April 1985; *High-Tech MATERIALS Alert* (Technical Insights, Inc.), since 1984; *Inside Energy/with Federal Lands* (McGraw-Hill, Inc.), since 1981; *Inside F.E.R.C.* (McGraw-Hill, Inc.), since 1981; *Inside N.R.C.* (McGraw-Hill, Inc.), since 1981; *Inside R&D* (Technical Insights, Inc.), since 1982; *Interavia Air Letter* (Interavia S.A.), since November 1984; *International Petrochemical Report* (McGraw-Hill, Inc.), since May 1982; *Keystone News Bulletin* (McGraw-Hill, Inc.), since May 1982; *Latin America Commodities Report* (Latin American Newsletters, Limited), since December 1976; *Latin America Regional Reports* (for the Andean Group, Caribbean, Southern Cone, Mexico, Central America, and Brazil) (Latin American Newsletters, Limited), since November 1971; *Latin America Special Reports* (for Venezuela, Mexico, and Colombia) (Latin American Newsletters, Limited); *Latin America Weekly Report* (Latin American Newsletters, Limited), since October 1979; *McGraw-Hill's Biotechnology Newswatch* (McGraw-Hill, Inc.), since May 1981; *Metals Week* (McGraw-Hill, Inc.), since 1981; *Middle East Executive Reports* (Middle East Executive Reports), since September 1978; *Military Space* (Pasha Publications), since April 1984; *Morgan Economic Quarterly* (Morgan Guaranty Trust Company of New York), since 1982; *NuclearFuel* (McGraw-Hill, Inc.), since 1981; *Nucleonics Week* (McGraw-Hill, Inc.), since 1981; *Platt's Oilgram News* (McGraw-Hill, Inc.), since 1981; *Platt's Oilgram Price Report* (McGraw-Hill, Inc.), since May 1982; *Securities Week* (McGraw-Hill, Inc.), since 1981; *Space Business News* (Pasha Publications Inc.), since July 1983; *The Spang Robinson Report on Artificial Intelligence* (Artificial Intelligence Publications), since 1985 ; *SynFuels* (McGraw-Hill, Inc.), since 1982; *Update/The American States* (Tower Consultants International, Inc.), since 1981; *Washington Financial Reports* (The Bureau of National Affairs, Inc.), since 1982; *Wharton Economic News Perspectives* (Wharton Econometric Forecasting Associates), since 1982; and *World Financial Markets* (Morgan Guaranty Trust Company of New York), since 1982.

Most newsletters listed above can be searched individually, as a group (NWLTRS), and by subject group (BUS for general business and companies; FIN for financial markets and investments; GOVT for government and defense; NEWS for broad news coverage on all subjects; TRDTEC for trade, science, and technology). Each newsletter (or all newsletters) and subject group can be selected and combined at will for searching. Profiles (PROFILE) of each newsletter, including publisher's name and address, publication date range, frequency, and updating are also available.

Language: English
Coverage: International
Time Span: Varies by source *(see Content)*
Updating: Generally, weekly publications updated weekly, one week after publication; monthly publications updated monthly, 3 weeks after publication.

NEXIS® NEWSPAPERS

Type: Source (Full Text)
Subject: Computers & Software; News
Producer: Mead Data Central, Inc.
Online Service: Mead Data Central, Inc.
Conditions: Subscription to Mead Data Central required; includes access to the Exchange Service, Reference Service, and MEDIS *(see)*.
Content: Contains full text of these newspapers: *American Banker* (American Banker, Inc.), since 1979 *(see)*; *BBC Summary of World Broadcasts* and *Monitoring Reports* (The British Broadcasting Corporation-Monitoring Service), since 1979 *(see WORLD REPORTER)*; *The Bond Buyer* (The Bond Buyer), since 1981 *(see)*; *The Christian Science Monitor* (The Christian Science Publishing Society), since 1980; *Computerworld* (CW Communications, Inc.), since 1982 (including *Computerworld on Communications* since May 1983 and *Computerworld Focus* since 1985); *The Current Digest of the Soviet Press* (The Current Digest of the Soviet Press), since June 1983; *DM News* (Mill Hollow Corp.), since February 1985; *Facts on File World News Digest* (Facts on File, Inc.), since 1975 *(see)*; *Financial Times* (The Financial Times Limited), since 1982; *InfoWorld* (Popular Computing, Inc.), since July 1983; *The Japan Economic Journal* (The Nihon Keizai Shimbun, Inc.), since June 1980; *Legal Times* (Law & Business, Inc.), since 1982; *The Los Angeles Times* (Times Mirror Company), since 1985 *(see)*; *The MacNeil/Lehrer NewsHour* (MacNeil-Lehrer-Gannett Productions), since 1982; *Manchester Guardian Weekly* (Guardian Publications Limited), since 1981; *The National Law Journal* (New York Law Publishing Company), since 1983; *The New York Times* (The New York Times Company), since June 1980 *(see)*; *The Washington Post* (The Washington Post Company), since 1977 *(see THE ELECTRONIC WASHINGTON POST LIBRARY)*; and *WorldPaper* (World Times Incorporated), since 1983.

Most newspapers listed above can be searched individually, as a group (PAPERS), and by subject group (BUS for general business and companies; FIN for financial markets and investments; GOVT for government and defense; NEWS for broad news coverage on all subjects; TRDTEC for trade, science, and technology). Profiles (PROFILE) of each newspaper, including publisher's name and address, publication date range, frequency, and updating are also available.

Language: English
Coverage: International
Time Span: Varies by source *(see Content)*
Updating: Varies by source

NEXIS® WIRE SERVICES

Type: Source (Full Text)
Subject: News
Producer: Mead Data Central, Inc.
Online Service: Mead Data Central, Inc.
Conditions: Subscription to Mead Data Central required; includes access to the Exchange Service, Reference Service, and MEDIS *(see)*.

Content: Contains full text of these newswire services: Asahi News Service (Japan) since August 1, 1984; The Associated Press international, national, business, and sports wires since January 1, 1977 *(see AP NEWS)*; Business Wire since September 19, 1983; Central News Agency (Taiwan) since April 2, 1984; Inter Press Service-USA since April 1, 1984; Jiji Press Ticker Service (Japan) since January 4, 1980 *(see)*; Kyodo English News Service (Japan) since March 8, 1980 *(see)*; PR Newswire since January 21, 1980 *(see)*; Reuters General News Reports since April 15, 1979; Reuters North European News Service since December 1, 1981; Southwest Newswire since February 1, 1984; States News Service since August 1, 1984; United Press International international, national, business, and sports wires since September 26, 1980 and state and regional wires since November 1, 1980 *(see UPI DataBase)*; and Xinhua (New China) News Agency (People's Republic of China) since January 1, 1977.

Most wire services listed above can be searched individually, as a group (WIRES), and by subject group (BUS for general business and companies; FIN for financial markets and investments; GOVT for government and defense; NEWS for broad news coverage on all subjects; TRDTEC for trade, science, and technology). Profiles (PROFILE) of each wire service, including publisher's name and address, publication date range, frequency, and updating are also available.

Language: English
Coverage: International
Time Span: Varies by source *(see Content)*
Updating: 12 to 48 hours after stories have appeared on the wires

NIKKEI-File

Type: Reference (Bibliographic)
Subject: News; Science & Technology
Producer: NKS
Online Service: NKS (Nihon Keizai Shimbun) (as a database on Nippon Telegraph and Telephone Public Corporation)
Content: Contains over 600,000 citations, with some abstracts, to articles from 4 daily newspapers *(Japan Economic Daily*, including local editions, *NIKKEI Industrial Daily, NIKKEI Marketing Journal*, and *Chemical Daily News)* and 6 monthly journals *(NIKKEI Business, NIKKEI Computer, NIKKEI Architecture, NIKKEI Electronics, NIKKEI Mechanical*, and *NIKKEI Medical)* published by NKS. Also covers the Japanese-language edition of *Scientific American*.
Language: Japanese
Coverage: Primarily Japan, with some international news
Time Span: Primarily 1979 to date
Updating: Daily, with *Japan Economic Daily, NIKKEI Industrial Daily*, and *Chemical Daily News*, available 3 to 4 days following publication date; other publications available 1 week following publication date.

NIOSHTIC

Type: Reference (Bibliographic)
Subject: Occupational Safety & Health
Producer: U.S. Department of Health and Human Services, Public Health Service, National Institute for Occupational Safety and Health, Priorities and Research Analysis Branch (NIOSH)
Online Service: ARAMIS (a cooperative service of the Swedish Center for Working Life, Swedish National Board of Occupational Safety and Health, and The Swedish National Environmental Protection Board); DIALOG Information Services, Inc. (OCCUPATIONAL SAFETY AND HEALTH); Pergamon InfoLine (NIOSH)

Content: Contains over 130,000 citations, with abstracts, to literature on occupational safety and health from more than 400 journals, monographs, and technical reports. Covers toxicology, epidemiology, pathology and histology, occupational medicine, health physics, injury prevention, ergonomics, biochemistry, physiology and metabolism, industrial hygiene, processes and materials in the work place, behavioral sciences, education and training, and control technology.
Language: English
Coverage: International
Time Span: 1900 to date
Updating: About 3000 records a quarter

NIPSᴹ (Nippan Information Processing System)

Type: Reference (Bibliographic, Referral)
Subject: Publishers & Distributors-Catalogs
Producer: Nippon Shuppan Hanbai Inc.
Online Service: Japan Computer Technology Co. Ltd.
Content: Contains approximately 32,000 citations to Japanese-language books currently available in Japan. Includes title, author, content, mailing address information for publisher, International Standard Book Number (ISBN), Japanese Book Standard Number, Japan Decimal Code, and identification of "best sellers" and literary prize winners.
Language: Japanese
Coverage: Japan
Time Span: April 1975 to date
Updating: Daily

NLM/NIH INFORMATION SERVICE

Type: Reference (Referral); Source (Full Text)
Subject: Biomedicine; Conferences & Meetings
Producer: American Medical Association (AMA), in conjunction with the National Library of Medicine (NLM) and the U.S. National Institutes of Health (NIH)
Online Service: AMA/NET
Conditions: Subscription fee of $50 to AMA/NET required
Content: Contains news and information from the National Institutes of Health (NIH) and the National Library of Medicine (NLM).

News from the NLM. Contains news of upcoming NLM meetings and events (e.g., MEDLINE online training seminars). Also contains information on recent NLM acquisitions.

Computerized Searches from the NLM. Contains descriptions of online searches conducted by NLM on its MEDLINE *(see)* database. Search results are available for purchase.

NIH Meetings of Clinical Interest. Contains a calendar of upcoming NIH-sponsored meetings covering topics of interest to practicing physicians.

NIH Consensus Development Meetings. Contains a calendar of past and upcoming meetings on specific issues in biomedicine. Also provides a summary of findings from each meeting.

Current Clinical Studies at NIH. Contains descriptions of current disease treatment programs. Includes name and location of treatment facilities and patient admission criteria.
Language: English
Coverage: Primarily U.S.
Time Span: Current information
Updating: Monthly

NORDSER

Type: Reference (Bibliographic)
Subject: Biomedicine; Library Holdings-Catalogs
Producer: Karolinska Institute, Library and Information Center (KIBIC)
Online Service: MIC-KIBIC
Content: Contains approximately 27,000 citations to the worldwide literature on biomedicine held by libraries in Denmark, Finland, Iceland, Norway, and Sweden. Sources include the KIBIC union catalog for biomedical serials, Nordic Union Catalogue for Periodicals (NOSP), and SERLINE (see).
Language: English
Coverage: International
Time Span: 1978 to date
Updating: About 200 items a month

NORMEQ

Type: Reference (Bibliographic)
Subject: Standards & Specifications
Producer: Bureau de Normalisation du Quebec
Online Service: IST-Informatheque Inc.
Content: Contains about 1300 citations, with abstracts, to international and Canadian standards published by the Quebec Standards Office. Covers minerals, construction materials, agriculture, transportation, tools, office supplies, textiles, food products, packaging materials, sports and art supplies, and documentation standards. Provides publication title, document type, reference number, date of publication, language, and system of measurement (international or English). Corresponds to *NORMES-Catalogue des normes quebecoises*.
Language: French
Coverage: Canada (Quebec)
Time Span: 1967 to date
Updating: About 50 records twice a year

NPSPEPSY

Type: Reference (Bibliographic)
Subject: Education & Educational Institutions; Psychology
Producer: National Library for Education
Online Service: Norwegian Centre for Informatics
Content: Contains about 5000 citations to Norwegian journal literature on education and psychology. Corresponds to a publication of the same name.
Language: Primarily Norwegian, with all records in original language and keywords in Norwegian
Coverage: Primarily Norway, with some international coverage
Time Span: 1978 to 1982
Updating: Not updated; *see PEPSY for current information (1980 to date)*.

NTIS® (National Technical Information Service)

Type: Reference (Bibliographic)
Subject: Science & Technology
Producer: National Technical Information Service
Online Service: BRS; BRS After Dark; BRS/BRKTHRU; BRS/Colleague; Centre de Documentation de l'Armement (CEDOCAR); CISTI, Canadian Online Enquiry Service (CAN/OLE); DATA-STAR; DIALOG Information Services, Inc.; ESA-IRS; The Japan Information Center of Science and Technology (JICST); Knowledge Index; Mead Data Central, Inc. (as a Reference Service database); ORBIT Information Technologies Corporation; STN International; TECH DATA

Conditions: CISTI accessible only in Canada; subscription to Mead Data Central required.
Content: Contains about 1.2 million citations, most with abstracts, to unrestricted technical reports from U.S. and non-U.S. government-sponsored research, development, and engineering analyses. The unpublished U.S. reports are prepared by federal, state, and local agencies and their contractors or grantees. Major areas covered include the biological, social, and physical sciences, mathematics, engineering, and business information. Includes announcements of computer-readable software and data files, U.S. government-owned inventions, selected reprints, federally sponsored translations, and some non-English-language reports. Corresponds to the biweekly publication *Government Reports Announcements & Index* (GRA & I) and in part to the weekly *Abstract Newsletters*.
Language: English
Coverage: Primarily U.S., with some international coverage
Time Span: BRS, BRS After Dark, BRS/BRKTHRU, BRS/Colleague, CISTI, DATA-STAR, DIALOG, ESA-IRS, Knowledge Index, ORBIT, STN, and TECH DATA, 1964 to date; CEDOCAR and FIZ, 1974 to date; Mead Data Central, 1980 to date; JICST, 1981 to date.
Updating: BRS, BRS After Dark, BRS/BRKTHRU, BRS/Colleague, CISTI, ESA-IRS, FIZ, STN, and TECH DATA, about 5000 records a month; all others, about 2600 records twice a month.

NTNF-PROJECTS (Norges Teknisk-Naturvitenskapelige Forskningsraad)

Type: Reference (Referral)
Subject: Research in Progress; Science & Technology
Producer: Norwegian Centre for Informatics
Online Service: Norwegian Centre for Informatics
Content: Contains descriptions of over 500 current research projects supported by the Royal Norwegian Council for Scientific and Industrial Research. *(See FoU for citations to reports from research projects)*
Language: Norwegian
Coverage: Norway
Time Span: Current information
Updating: Annually

NURSING & ALLIED HEALTH

Type: Reference (Bibliographic)
Subject: Biomedicine; Health Care
Producer: CINAHL
Online Service: BRS; BRS After Dark; BRS/BRKTHRU; BRS/Colleague; DATA-STAR; DIALOG Information Services, Inc.; TECH DATA
Content: Contains about 40,000 citations to articles in more than 340 journals in nursing and the following allied health disciplines: physical therapy, respiratory therapy, cardiopulmonary technology, medical and laboratory technology, occupational therapy, radiologic technology, social services in health care, emergency services, medical records, health sciences librarianship, medical assisting, the physician's assistant, surgical technology, and health education. Also covers relevant articles from MEDLINE *(see)* and from management, psychological, and popular journals. Also lists new books in nursing and allied health fields. Corresponds to *Cumulative Index to Nursing & Allied Health Literature*.
Language: English

Coverage: International
Time Span: 1983 to date
Updating: About 3500 records every 2 months

NUTRITION ANALYSIS SYSTEM

Type: Source (Textual-Numeric)
Subject: Food Sciences & Nutrition
Producer: DATANETWORK, a division of Applied Business Systems, Inc.
Online Service: DATANETWORK, a division of Applied Business Systems, Inc.
Conditions: Monthly minimum of $100 covers analysis of 33 recipes; additional recipes can be analyzed for $3 each.
Content: A database system for the analysis of nutrients in a recipe, meal, or daily dietary intake, based on data for about 2500 ingredients developed by the U.S. Department of Agriculture (USDA) and reported in Handbook 456 and other USDA sources. Users enter recipe data by indicating the recipe name, ingredient numbers, and household unit designators (e.g., cups, teaspoons) from the USDA Handbook, and amount of each ingredient required. Reports contain analyses of moisture content, calories, proteins, carbohydrates, fat, unsaturated fat, cholesterol, sodium, potassium. In addition, sodium, potassium. vitamins A and C, thiamin, riboflavin, niacin, calcium, iron, and phosphorus content are shown as percentages of the U.S. Recommended Daily Allowance (USRDA).
Language: English
Updating: Periodically, as new ingredient information is released by the USDA or published and authenticated by the industry

OAG-EE (Official Airline Guide-Electronic Edition)

Type: Source (Numeric)
Subject: Flight Schedules
Producer: Official Airline Guides, Inc.
Online Service: Official Airline Guides, Inc. (OAG-EE)
Conditions: Varies by gateway
Content: Contains passenger flight schedules and fares for over 750 North American and international airlines. Information on each flight (about 150,000 each month) includes origin and destination airports; North American and international fares; airline, equipment, and flight number; service provided; flight departure and arrival times; travel duration; and number of intermediate stops. Provides references for U.S. and European cities without scheduled service to the nearest airports and distances to those airports from the originally requested cities. Also contains information from OAG's *Travel Planner* guides on about 29,000 hotels and motels in North America, the Pacific Basin area, and Europe, including names, addresses, rates, and quality ratings.
Coverage: International
Time Span: Current day and next 364 days
Updating: Fares, daily; schedules, weekly.

OB/GYN SERVICES

Type: Source (Full Text, Software)
Subject: Health Care
Producer: Dr. Frederick R. Jelovsek
Online Service: CompuServe Information Service
Content: Contains obstetrical and gynecological information for health care consumers and medical professionals. Includes a forum on health care concerns (e.g., hypertension and preg-

nancy), with a question and answer section; full text of *Computers in Patient Care Survey*, a newsletter covering computer applications in obstetrics, gynecology, and neonatology; and a library of software programs (e.g., a program for calculating fetal parameters using measurements obtained through ultrasonography) for use in obstetrical and gynecological medical practices.
Language: English
Coverage: Primarily U.S., with some coverage of international meetings and conferences
Time Span: July 1984 to date
Updating: Forum, daily; *Computers in Patient Care Survey*, quarterly.

OCCUPATIONAL SAFETY & HEALTH REPORTER

Type: Source (Full Text)
Subject: Occupational Safety & Health
Producer: The Bureau of National Affairs, Inc. (BNA)
Online Service: Executive Telecom System, Inc., Human Resource Information Network
Conditions: Annual subscription to Executive Telecom System required
Content: Contains full text of *Occupational Safety & Health Reporter*, a newsletter covering legislative, regulatory, and judicial developments involving worker safety and health. Covers proposed and final standards and regulations of the Occupational Safety and Health Administration (OSHA), enforcement activities, legal activities of the courts and the Occupational Safety and Health Review Commission, investigations, congressional hearings, petitions for variances from OSHA standards, announcements of grants or denials, news about worker safety and health conferences, and worker right-to-know laws at the state and federal levels. Includes full text of selected proposed rules, standards, and regulations.
Language: English
Coverage: U.S.
Time Span: March 1985 to date
Updating: Weekly

OCEANIC ABSTRACTS

Type: Reference (Bibliographic)
Subject: Aquatic Sciences
Producer: Cambridge Scientific Abstracts
Online Service: BRS (to be available in 1987); BRS After Dark (to be available in 1987); BRS/BRKTHRU (to be available in 1987); BRS/Colleague (to be available in 1987); DIALOG Information Services, Inc.; ESA-IRS
Content: Contains approximately 167,000 citations to the worldwide literature on oceanography and marine-related aspects of other sciences. Includes biology, geology and geophysics, meteorology, acoustics and optics, desalination, pollution, resources, engineering, mining, ships and shipping, submersibles and buoys, and government laws and regulations. Corresponds to coverage of *Oceanic Abstracts*.
Language: English
Coverage: International
Time Span: 1964 to date
Updating: About 1750 records every 2 months

OCLC

Type: Reference (Bibliographic)

Subject: Library Holdings-Catalogs

Producer: Library of Congress (LC) and participating libraries

Online Service: OCLC Online Computer Library Center, Inc.

Conditions: Three categories of access are available: (1) Participant, for libraries that do all Roman alphabet cataloging online or by tapeload; (2) Special User, for libraries that use the online system but do not qualify as participants (e.g., national libraries, library schools); (3) Partial User, for libraries that elect not to contribute their Roman alphabet cataloging but use any of the non-cataloging subsystems.

Content: A total database system that provides technical support services to libraries for shared cataloging, interlibrary loan, serials check-in, and acquisitions. Subscribers can access the OCLC On-Line Union Catalog, a database of over 14 million Library of Congress MARC records, British Library UKMARC records (since 1985), and member records to identify an existing cataloging record for an item, to change that record for their own use, to input a new record, and to generate catalog cards or magnetic tapes. The database covers cataloging for books, manuscripts, sound recordings, serials, audiovisual materials, maps, and music scores. OCLC is also the host for the CONSER serials database and the U.S. Newspapers Program. Access to the records in the database is provided through several search keys, including LC card number, ISBN, ISSN, CODEN, author, title, and author/title combinations. The database is also used with the Interlibrary Loan Subsystem to enable users to identify libraries that have a particular item in their collections and to order items from the holding libraries.

Language: Primarily English

Coverage: International

Time Span: 2150 BC to date

Updating: Continuously, throughout the day; about 30,000 records a week.

OCLC EASI REFERENCE

Type: Reference (Bibliographic)

Subject: Library Holdings-Catalogs

Producer: OCLC Online Computer Library Center, Inc.

Online Service: BRS; BRS/BRKTHRU; BRS/Colleague

Content: Contains about 1 million bibliographic citations from the OCLC On-Line Union Catalog (see OCLC) for works with publication dates within the most recent 3 years. Covers books, serials, sound recordings, musical scores, maps, manuscripts, audiovisual materials, and software. All major bibliographic elements, except for holdings information, are included.

Language: Primarily English

Coverage: International

Time Span: Most recent 3 years

Updating: About 100,000 records a quarter

OHM-TADS (Oil and Hazardous Materials-Technical Assistance Data System)

Type: Source (Textual-Numeric)

Subject: Environment; Toxicology

Producer: U.S. Environmental Protection Agency (EPA), Emergency Response Division

Online Service: Chemical Information Systems, Inc., a subsidiary of Fein-Marquart Associates (CIS); Information Consultants, Inc. (ICI) (as part of The Integrated Chemical Information System)

Conditions: Annual subscription fee of $300 to CIS required but fee is waived for educational institutions and non-profit public libraries worldwide; differential charges for subscribers and non-subscribers to ICI.

Content: Contains data gathered from published literature on materials that have been designated oil or hazardous materials. Provides technical support for dealing with potential or actual dangers resulting from the discharge of oil or hazardous substances. Up to 126 data fields, some textual and some numeric, may be present for each record (i.e., one material). A record includes identification of the substance (Chemical Abstracts Service Registry Number, common and trade names, and chemical formula), physical properties, uses, toxicity, handling procedures, and suggested methods for disposing of spilled materials.

NOTE: On CIS, the database covers 1402 materials.

Language: English

Updating: Periodically, as new data become available

OHS MSDS (MATERIAL SAFETY DATA SHEETS)

Type: Source (Textual-Numeric)

Subject: Chemistry-Properties; Occupational Safety & Health

Producer: Occupational Health Services, Inc. (OHS)

Online Service: Mead Data Central, Inc. (MSDS) (as a Reference Service database); Occupational Health Services, Inc.

Conditions: Subscription to Mead Data Central required; monthly minimum to OHS required.

Content: Contains identification, handling, and hazard disclosure information on over 75,000 chemical substances that require documentation by chemical manufacturers under the Hazard Communication and Labeling Standard of the Occupational Safety and Health Administration (OSHA). For each chemical, provides substance identification, including chemical name, trade names, and molecular formula; manufacturer's or importer's name, address, and telephone number; physical data, including description, boiling and melting points, specific gravity, evaporation rate, and solubility in water; fire and explosion data, including flash point, upper and lower ignition limits, and firefighting techniques; toxicity and health effects, including first aid and antidotes; reactivity, including incompatibilities (e.g., explosive reaction with hydrogen peroxide), decomposition, and polymerization; handling, storage, or disposal conditions to avoid; and spill and leak procedures, including requirements for protective equipment. Sources include OSHA, the National Institute for Occupational Safety and Health, the U.S. Environmental Protection Agency, and Dreisbach's Handbook of Poisoning.

Language: English

Time Span: Current information

Updating: OHS, daily, about 400 to 500 records a month; Mead Data Central, quarterly.

ONLINE PRODUCT NEWS

Type: Source (Full Text)

Subject: Information Systems & Services

Producer: Worldwide Videotex

Online Service: NewsNet, Inc.

Conditions: Monthly subscription to NewsNet required; differential charges for subscribers and non-subscribers to *Online Product News*.

Content: Contains full text of *Online Product News*, a newsletter on products, services, and developments in the videotex and teletext industry, with emphasis on telecommunications products for personal computers. Covers major videotex services accessible through microcomputers, dedicated terminals, and broadcast and cable television, as well as other electronic information services (e.g., electronic mail, telesoftware).

Language: English

Coverage: International

Time Span: February 1984 to date

Updating: Monthly

ONTARIO EDUCATION RESOURCES INFORMATION SYSTEM

Type: Reference (Bibliographic)

Subject: Education & Educational Institutions

Producer: Ontario Ministry of Education

Online Service: BRS; BRS After Dark; BRS/BRKTHRU; BRS/Colleague; TECH DATA

Content: Contains about 10,000 citations, with abstracts, to educational research reports, curriculum guidelines, policy papers, and related materials prepared or sponsored by the Ministry of Education, the Ministry of Colleges and Universities, school boards, and other educational organizations and agencies in Ontario, Canada. Information provided on each document includes title, material type (e.g., report; correspondence course), language, author, corporate author, publication information, date, educational level, target population, special features and/or components, funding source, contact person, and availability.

Language: English or French, depending on the language of the original document

Coverage: Canada (Ontario)

Time Span: Primarily 1972 to date, with selected coverage of earlier materials

Updating: 3 times a year

OON

Type: Reference (Bibliographic)

Subject: Library Holdings-Catalogs; Science & Technology

Producer: CISTI

Online Service: CISTI, Canadian Online Enquiry Service (CAN/OLE)

Conditions: CISTI accessible only in Canada

Content: Contains citations to the holdings of the CISTI library. Covers monographs, technical reports, and conference proceedings in all areas of science, technology, and medicine.

Language: English

Coverage: International

Time Span: 1978 to date

Updating: About 2100 records every 2 weeks

ORIADOC (Orientation and Access to Information and Documentation Sources in France)

Type: Reference (Referral)

Subject: Information Systems & Services-Directories

Producer: Services du Premier Ministre, Commission de Coordination de la Documentation Administrative (CCDA)

Online Service: G.CAM Serveur; Telesystemes-Questel

Content: Contains references to approximately 2500 public and private libraries and information sources in France. Covers archives, documentation centers, information services, bibliographic databases, and libraries. Each record contains organization name, address, and telephone number; administrative level and description of the governmental unit or agency served; statute under which it was created; brief history and outline of purpose; publications, types of services (e.g., bibliographic research, Selective Dissemination of Information (SDI)), and information networks in which it participates; fields and specific topics covered; characteristics of its manual or automated catalog (e.g., number of items, number of records added yearly, time span covered); types of items collected (e.g., periodicals, monographs, reports, official documents, patents, audiovisual materials); conditions of access to the collection (e.g., open to the public, authorization for use required) and service hours; and access tools (e.g., subject and author indexes).

Language: French

Coverage: France and French territories

Time Span: Current information

Updating: Annually

ORION

Type: Reference (Bibliographic)

Subject: Library Holdings-Catalogs

Producer: University of California, Los Angeles (UCLA), University Research Library

Online Service: University of California, Los Angeles, University Research Library

Conditions: Monthly minimum of $25 required

Content: Contains over 1.3 million cataloging, order, and processing records for books, journals, and other materials acquired by the UCLA library system since 1977.

Language: Primarily English

Coverage: International

Time Span: 1977 to date

Updating: Continuously, throughout the day

THE ORLANDO SENTINEL

Type: Source (Full Text)

Subject: News

Producer: The Orlando Sentinel Communications Company

Online Service: VU/TEXT Information Services, Inc.

Conditions: Subscription to VU/TEXT required

Content: Contains news items and feature articles from *The Orlando Sentinel* (Florida) newspaper. Regional coverage emphasizes tourism, business, and high technology industries.

Language: English

Coverage: U.S. (primarily Orlando, Florida area)

Time Span: April 1985 to date

Updating: Daily

ORTHOBASE℗

Type: Reference (Bibliographic, Referral); Source (Full Text)

Subject: Biomedicine; Conferences & Meetings; Sports Medicine

Producer: Medical Literature Review Inc.

Online Service: Medical Literature Review Inc.

Conditions: Five-year subscription of $250 and monthly minimum of $20 to Medical Literature Review Inc. required; medical residents pay $100 with no minimum fee.

Content: Contains over 45,000 citations, 85% with abstracts or summaries, to the worldwide literature on orthopedics, orthopedic surgery, sports medicine, and related specialties. Covers most articles in 43 orthopedic and related specialty journals and relevant articles in another 200 journals, as well as textbooks, educational aids (e.g., audio cassettes, video-tapes), and newspapers. Corresponds to *Orthopaedic Index.* Also contains monthly summaries of over 50 articles from current literature, with editorial comments provided by noted orthopedic clinicians; summaries of presentations from key conferences and of conference reports in newspapers and newsletters; and full text of *Orthopedics Today* newsletter.

Provides a calendar of conferences, meetings, and special events; descriptions of available products (e.g., immobilization products, implant materials, endoscopic equipment) including references from clinical studies, vendor data and prices; current orthopedic medicine employment opportunities, including academic positions, residencies, and private practice positions; and a directory of orthopedic specialists, manufacturers, hospitals, and professional services. Several electronic services, including mail, classified advertisements, and online booking of airline and hotel reservations are available. Continuing Medical Education credits may be earned from the State University of New York at Stony Brook for completion of online quizzes based on reviews of current orthopedic literature.

Language: English
Coverage: International
Time Span: 1930 to date
Updating: Monthly

PASCAL M

Type: Reference (Bibliographic)
Subject: Science & Technology
Producer: Centre National de la Recherche Scientifique, Centre de Documentation Scientifique et Technique (CNRS/CDST)
Online Service: ESA-IRS; Telesystemes-Questel
Content: Contains over 300,000 citations, with abstracts, to the worldwide literature in science and technology. Covers applied science, biomedicine, chemistry, earth sciences, fundamental and applied biology, marine science, physics, psychology, and space science. Sources include books, theses, reports, conference proceedings, and more than 4200 periodicals. Corresponds to *PASCAL SIGMA 1: Sciences exactes et technologie, PASCAL SIGMA 2: Sciences de la vie I*, and *PASCAL SIGMA 3: Sciences de la vie 11.*

Language: French, with titles and descriptors also in English
Coverage: International
Time Span: 1984 to date
Updating: About 2700 records a month

PASCAL: AGROLINE

Type: Reference (Bibliographic)
Subject: Agriculture
Producer: Centre National de la Recherche Scientifique, Centre de Documentation Scientifique et Technique (CNRS/CDST); Institut National de la Recherche Agronomique (INRA)
Online Service: ESA-IRS; Telesystemes-Questel

Content: Contains about 95,000 citations, with abstracts, to the worldwide literature on agriculture. Covers agricultural bioclimatology, genetics and plant breeding, general agronomy, phytopathology, plant physiology, plant yield, plant protection, soils, and weeds. Sources include books, periodicals, theses, reports, and conference proceedings. Corresponds to *PASCAL THEMA 280: Sciences agronomiques, productions vegetales.*

Language: French, with titles and descriptors also in English
Coverage: International
Time Span: 1980 to date
Updating: About 1800 records a month

PASCAL: BIOTECHNOLOGIES

Type: Reference (Bibliographic)
Subject: Biotechnology
Producer: Centre National de la Recherche Scientifique, Centre de Documentation Scientifique et Technique (CNRS/CDST)
Online Service: ESA-IRS; Telesystemes-Questel
Content: Contains about 20,000 citations, with abstracts, to the worldwide literature on biotechnology. Covers biochemistry, cell biology, microbiology, and applications of cultured micro-organisms and cells in agriculture, energy, food processing, medicine, metallurgy, and pollution control. Sources include books, periodicals, theses, reports, and conference proceedings. Corresponds to *PASCAL THEMA 215: Biotechnologies.*

Language: French, with titles and descriptors also in English
Coverage: International
Time Span: 1982 to date
Updating: About 600 records a month

PASCAL: MEDECINE TROPICALE

Type: Reference (Bibliographic)
Subject: Biomedicine
Producer: Centre National de la Recherche Scientifique, Centre de Documentation Scientifique et Technique (CNRS/CDST)
Online Service: ESA-IRS; Telesystemes-Questel
Content: Contains about 17,000 citations, with abstracts, to the worldwide literature on tropical medicine. Covers human and animal parasites and diseases; the biology and control of vectors, intermediate hosts, and reservoirs; ergonomics; nutrition; physical and social characteristics of populations; public health; and medical issues relating to travelers. Sources include books, periodicals, theses, reports, and conference proceedings. Corresponds to *PASCAL THEMA 235, Medecine tropicale.*

Language: French, with titles and descriptors also in English
Coverage: International
Time Span: 1982 to date
Updating: About 540 records a month

PASCAL: ONCOLOGY

Type: Reference (Bibliographic)
Subject: Biomedicine
Producer: Centre National de la Recherche Scientifique, Centre de Documentation Scientifique et Technique (CNRS/CDST)
Online Service: DIALOG Information Services, Inc. (to be available in 1987); ESA-IRS; Telesystemes-Questel; University of Tsukuba

Content: Contains citations, with abstracts, to the worldwide oncology literature. Covers clinical and experimental carcinology, epidemiology, public health, and the basic sciences (e.g., immunology, virology). Corresponds to *PASCAL THEMA E89: Cancer.*
Language: English and French
Coverage: International
Time Span: 1985 to date *(see CANCERNET for earlier information)*
Updating: Monthly

PASCAL: ZOOLINE

Type: Reference (Bibliographic)
Subject: Agriculture; Aquatic Sciences; Life Sciences
Producer: Centre National de la Recherche Scientifique, Centre de Documentation Scientifique et Technique (CNRS/CDST); Institut National de la Recherche Agronomique
Online Service: ESA-IRS; Telesystemes-Questel
Content: Contains about 100,000 citations, with abstracts, to the worldwide literature on fundamental and applied zoology of land and fresh-water invertebrates. Covers taxonomy, biology, physiology, pathology; invertebrate damage to plants, crops, stored foodstuffs, and other materials; effects of pollution and pesticides on invertebrates; and apiculture and sericulture. Sources include books, periodicals, theses, reports, and conference proceedings. Corresponds to *PASCAL THEMA 260: Zoologie fondamentale et appliques des Invertebres (milieu terrestre, eaux douces)*, with abstracts available only online.
Language: French, with titles and descriptors also in English
Coverage: International (primarily temperate-climate countries)
Time Span: 1979 to date
Updating: About 1300 records a month

PATDATA

Type: Reference (Bibliographic)
Subject: Patents
Producer: BRS
Online Service: BRS; BRS After Dark; BRS/BRKTHRU; BRS/Colleague; TECH DATA
Content: Contains citations, with abstracts, to about 700,000 U.S. utility patents issued since 1971 and all reissue patents and defense publications issued by the U.S. Patent and Trademark Office since 1975. Each record includes patent number, date, title, inventor, inventor address, patent assignee, application data, foreign priority information, and codes of the U.S. and International Patent Classification Systems. Also includes cited references to U.S. and non-U.S. patents.
Language: English
Coverage: Primarily U.S., with some international coverage
Time Span: 1975 to date
Updating: About 1200 records a week

PATDPA (Deutsche Patentdatenbank)

Type: Reference (Bibliographic)
Subject: Patents
Producer: Deutsches Patentamt
Online Service: STN International
Content: Contains about 530,000 citations, with abstracts, to German patents, patent applications, and utility models in the fields of science and technology. Sources include publications of the German Patent Office, the European Patent Office, and the World Intellectual Property Organization.

Language: German
Coverage: Federal Republic of Germany
Time Span: 1981 to date
Updating: About 2000 citations a week

PATENT ABSTRACTS OF CHINA

Type: Reference (Bibliographic)
Subject: Patents
Producer: International Patent Documentation Center with English-language abstracts provided by the Patent Documentation Service Center of The People's Republic of China
Online Service: Pergamon InfoLine
Content: Contains about 2000 citations, with abstracts, to patents issued by the Patent Office of the People's Republic of China. Each record includes standard bibliographic data and patent family information.
Language: English
Coverage: The People's Republic of China
Time Span: April 1985 to date
Updating: Weekly

PATENT FAMILY SERVICE/PATENT REGISTER SERVICE

Type: Reference (Bibliographic)
Subject: Patents
Producer: International Patent Documentation Center
Online Service: International Patent Documentation Center (INPADOC)
Content: Contains priority numbers and bibliographic information on approximately 16,000,000 patent families. Covers patents issued by 51 countries and 2 international organizations. Also includes legal status information for 8 countries.
Language: Original languages of publishing country
Coverage: International
Time Span: Varies by country, with earliest data from 1964
Updating: Daily

PATOS (Patent-Online-System)

Type: Reference (Bibliographic); Source (Full Text)
Subject: Patents
Producer: Bertelsmann InformationsService GmbH; WILA-Verlag KG
Online Service: Bertelsmann InformationsService GmbH; DATA-STAR
Content: Contains about I million citations, with some abstracts, to patents published by the German Patent Office (Deutches Patentamt). Includes names and addresses of inventor, registrant, and legal representative; registration, publication, and international priority dates; types of examinations and findings; and full text of main claim, excluding formulas and illustrations. For patents published between fall 1981 and spring 1984, also includes full text of summary, excluding formulas and illustrations. Corresponds to *Auszuege aus den Offenlegungsschriften.*
Language: German
Coverage: Federal Republic of Germany
Time Span: October 1968 to date
Updating: Weekly

PATSEARCH℠

Type: Reference (Bibliographic)
Subject: Patents
Producer: Pergamon InfoLine Inc.
Online Service: Pergamon InfoLine
Content: Contains citations, with abstracts, to more than 1 million U.S. patents issued since 1970. Covers utility patents, reissue patents since July 1975, defense publications since December 1976, and all PCT (Patent Cooperation Treaty) patent applications. Covers patents in all areas of science and technology. Each record includes inventor, patent holder, dates, foreign priority information, codes of the U.S. and International Patent Classification Systems, and the main claim (from January 1984). Also contains cited references to U.S. and non-U.S. patents. Includes exemplary claims that define the inventions protected by patents from January 1975.
Language: English
Coverage: Primarily U.S., with some international coverage
Time Span: 1970 to date
Updating: About 1400 records a week

PDQ℠ (Physician Data Query)

Type: Reference (Bibliographic, Referral)
Subject: Biomedicine; Health Care & Social Services-Directories
Producer: U.S. National Institutes of Health (NIH), National Cancer Institute, International Cancer Research Data Bank
Online Service: Mead Data Central, Inc. (as a MEDIS database (see)); National Library of Medicine (NLM)
Conditions: Subscription to Mead Data Central required
Content: Contains information on cancer treatment methods and active treatment programs.
Cancer Information. Contains prognostic and treatment information for major cancer types. Provides capsule and detailed summaries for each type of cancer, including prognosis, staging and cellular classification systems, treatment options for each type or stage of disease, and ongoing investigational approaches under evaluation in clinical research trials. Also contains citations to the key medical literature on oncology.
Protocols. Contains information on over 1000 active treatment programs. Provides summaries of programs supported by the National Cancer Institute, as well as references to other nationwide programs. Includes study objectives and special study parameters, treatment regimen, patient entry criteria, and name and location of treating institution.
PDQ Directory. Contains references to about 10,000 physicians and about 2000 health-care organizations providing oncological disease care or treatment. Includes physician or organization name, address, and telephone, and professional affiliation (e.g., American Society of Clinical Oncology, Society of Surgical Oncology, American Association of Cancer Institutes, the Association of Community Cancer Centers).
Language: English
Coverage: U.S.
Time Span: Current information and programs
Updating: Monthly

PENINSULA TIMES-TRIBUNE

Type: Source (Full Text)
Subject: News
Producer: Peninsula Times-Tribune
Online Service: VU/TEXT Information Services, Inc. (to be available in 1987)
Conditions: Subscription to VU/TEXT required
Content: Contains news items and feature articles from *The Peninsula Times-Tribune* (California) newspaper.
Language: English
Coverage: U.S. (primarily Palo Alto and Redwood City, California area)
Updating: Daily

PEOPLE®

Type: Source (Full Text)
Subject: General Interest
Producer: Time Inc.
Online Service: Mead Data Central, Inc. (as part of NEXIS MAGAZINES *(see)*); VU/TEXT Information Services, Inc. (to be available in 1987)
Conditions: Subscription to Mead Data Central required; subscription to VU/TEXT required.
Content: Contains full text of *People*, a magazine covering noteworthy personalities in television, movies, the theater, literature, music, sports, and everyday life. Includes interviews and brief reviews of current films, books, musical recordings, and television shows.
Language: English
Coverage: Primarily U.S., with some international coverage
Time Span: Mead Data Central, December 1981 to date; VU/TEXT, 1985 to date.
Updating: Weekly

PEPSY

Type: Reference (Bibliographic)
Subject: Education & Educational Institutions; Psychology
Producer: Norwegian Centre for Informatics (in cooperation with Scandinavian educational and psychological libraries)
Online Service: Norwegian Centre for Informatics
Conditions: Subscription to Norwegian Center for Informatics required
Content: Contains about 10,000 citations, with some abstracts, to Nordic literature on education and psychology. Covers general education; didactics and teaching methods; social issues and processes; developmental and educational psychology; teacher, adult and vocational education; and educational systems in other countries. Sources include monographs, journal articles, and reports.
Language: Danish, English, Finnish, Norwegian, and Swedish
Coverage: Primarily Scandinavia, with some international coverage
Time Span: 1980 to date *(see NPSPEPSY for earlier information)*
Updating: Periodically, as new data become available

PESTDOC (Pest Control Literature Documentation)

Type: Reference (Bibliographic)
Subject: Agriculture
Producer: Derwent Publications Ltd.
Online Service: ORBIT Information Technologies Corporation
Conditions: Subscription to *PESTDOC ABSTRACTS JOURNAL* required
Content: Contains citations to the worldwide journal literature on pesticides, plant protection, and agricultural chemicals. Corresponds to the weekly publication, *PESTDOC ABSTRACTS JOURNAL*. Each record contains indepth keywording and fragmentation coding.

Language: English
Coverage: International
Time Span: 1968 to date
Updating: About 1000 records every 6 weeks

PESTDOC II

Type: Reference (Bibliographic)
Subject: Agriculture; Conferences & Meetings
Producer: Derwent Publications Ltd.
Online Service: ORBIT Information Technologies Corporation
Content: Contains about 17,000 citations, with abstracts, to conference papers on weed and pest control from the proceedings of relevant conferences held in North America. Sources are these conference proceedings: *Abstracts of the Meeting of the Weed Science Society of America; Pesticide Research Report; Research Progress Report; Western Society of Weed Science; Research Report, Canada Weed Committee, Eastern Section;* and *Research Report, Canada Weed Committee, Western Section.*
Language: English and French
Coverage: U.S. and Canada
Time Span: 1977 to date
Updating: Every 2 months

THE PESTICIDE DATABANK

Type: Source (Textual-Numeric)
Subject: Agriculture
Producer: British Crop Protection Council, in collaboration with C.A.B. International
Online Service: Pergamon InfoLine
Content: Contains data on over 5000 chemical compounds and products used in agricultural and horticultural pest control. Data for each product or compound include nomenclature, physical properties, Chemical Abstracts Service Registry Number, and Wiswesser Line Notation. Covers insecticides and acaricides, molluscicides, herbicides and fungicides, repellents, plant growth regulators, synergists, and crop safeners. Also contains names of pests and pathogens, host crops for particular compounds, and data from species tests. Corresponds to *The Pesticide Manual.*
Language: English
Coverage: International
Time Span: Current information
Updating: Quarterly

PESTICIDE RESEARCH INFORMATION SYSTEM

Type: Reference (Referral); Source (Textual-Numeric)
Subject: Agriculture; Research in Progress
Producer: Agriculture Canada, Research Branch
Online Service: Agriculture Canada, Research Branch
Content: Contains information on pest management products, organisms that are in experimental use or are registered in Canada, and beneficial insects for use in weed and pest control. Includes an inventory of pest management research projects, pesticide research data, maximum residue limits, and a glossary of pesticides, pests, and hosts. Sources of data include research scientists, chemical companies, and Health and Welfare Canada.
Language: English and French

Coverage: Canada
Time Span: 1981 to date
Updating: Periodically, as new data become available

PETERSON'S COLLEGE DATABASE

Type: Reference (Referral)
Subject: Education & Educational Institutions-Directories
Producer: Peterson's Guides, Inc.
Online Service: BRS (NATIONAL COLLEGE DATABANK); BRS After Dark (NATIONAL COLLEGE DATABANK); BRS/BRKTHRU (NATIONAL COLLEGE DATABANK); BRS/Colleague (NATIONAL COLLEGE DATABANK); CompuServe Information Service (PETERSON'S COLLEGE DATABASE); DIALOG Information Services, Inc. (PETERSON'S COLLEGE DATABASE); Dow Jones & Company, Inc. (PETERSON'S COLLEGE SELECTION SERVICE); TECH DATA (NATIONAL COLLEGE DATABANK)
Conditions: Annual minimum of $12 or monthly minimum of $3 to Dow Jones required
Content: Contains current information on approximately 3000 colleges and universities in the U.S. and Canada. Each record includes college name, size, and location; enrollment and admissions data; graduation requirements; athletics, including the availability of athletic scholarships; majors offered; special programs, such as college orientation and developmental courses for entering students; career services, including individual and group career counseling; costs; and availability of housing and financial aid. Corresponds in part to Peterson's *Annual Guide to Four-Year Colleges* and *Annual Guide to Two-Year Colleges,* which comprise the IPeterson's Annual Guides to Undergraduate Study series.
NOTE: On Dow Jones, the database includes additional textual information provided by college officials describing such topics as student housing, university facilities, the surrounding community, financial aid, foreign study, and the institution's history. On BRS, DIALOG, and CompuServe only the descriptive data collected by Peterson's are available.
Language: English
Coverage: U.S. and Canada
Time Span: Current information
Updating: Annually

PHARMAPROJECTS

Type: Reference (Bibliographic, Referral)
Subject: Pharmaceuticals & Pharmaceutical Industry
Producer: V & O Publications Ltd.
Online Service: DATA-STAR
Content: Contains descriptions of approximately 3500 pharmaceutical products, including new formulations and compounds, currently under development by more than 500 companies worldwide. For each product, includes generic name, trade name, and research code; chemical name and Chemical Abstracts Service (CAS) Registry Number; originating company and licensees; therapeutic activity descriptors; stages of development in any of 28 countries; and selected references to relevant literature. Covers pharmacological and clinical studies, registration progress, joint-development agreements, and licensing and marketing developments. Corresponds to *Pharmaprojects.*
Language: English
Coverage: International
Time Span: Current information
Updating: About 100 to 150 new compounds a month

PHARMLINE

Type: Reference (Bibliographic)

Subject: Biomedicine; Pharmaceuticals & Pharmaceutical Industry

Producer: National Health Services, Regional Drug Information Service

Online Service: DATA-STAR

Content: Contains approximately 35,000 citations, with abstracts (since 1983), to the worldwide journal literature on drugs and professional pharmacy practice. Covers adverse effects of drugs; bioavailability; clinical pharmacokinetics, including metabolism; drug interactions; drug modification of laboratory tests; information science, as applicable to drug information; new drugs and new uses of established drugs; new routes of administration and dosage schedules; pharmaceutics, pharmacology, and pharmacy practice; use of drugs in breastfeeding, pregnancy, and neonates; and liver and renal failure. Does not cover literature on animal studies.

Language: English

Coverage: International

Time Span: 1978 to date

Updating: Weekly

PHILADELPHIA DAILY NEWS

Type: Source (Full Text)

Subject: News

Producer: Philadelphia Newspapers, Inc.

Online Service: VU/TEXT Information Services, Inc.

Conditions: Subscription to VU/TEXT required

Content: Contains full text of news items and feature stories from the *Philadelphia Daily News* (Pennsylvania) newspaper. Day and date of item's publication, byline, headline, and section are also provided. Does not include weather, calendars, obituaries, and sports roundups.

Language: English

Coverage: U.S. (primarily Philadelphia, Pennsylvania area)

Time Span: 1980 to date

Updating: Daily, 48 hours after publication

PHILADELPHIA INQUIRER

Type: Source (Full Text)

Subject: News

Producer: Philadelphia Newspapers, Inc.

Online Service: VU/TEXT Information Services, Inc.

Conditions: Subscription to VU/TEXT required

Content: Contains the full text of news items and feature stories from the *Philadelphia Inquirer* (Pennsylvania) newspaper. Regional coverage emphasizes the insurance, banking, health care, legal services, shipping, and transportation industries. Day and date of item's publication, byline, and section are also provided. Does not include stock tables, weather, calendars, obituaries, and sports roundups.

Language: English

Coverage: Primarily U.S., with some international coverage

Time Span: 1981 to date

Updating: Daily

THE PHOENIX GAZETTE

Type: Source (Full Text)

Subject: News

Producer: Phoenix Newspapers, Inc.

Online Service: VU/TEXT Information Services, Inc.

Conditions: Subscription to VU/TEXT required

Content: Contains full text of news items and feature articles from *The Phoenix Gazette* (Arizona) newspaper. Regional coverage emphasizes the aerospace, high technology, and tourism industries.

Language: English

Coverage: U.S. (primarily southwestern states)

Time Span: April 1986 to date

Updating: Daily

PHYCOM® (Physician Communications Service)

Type: Reference (Referral); Source (Textual-Numeric)

Subject: Conferences & Meetings; Health Care; Pharmaceuticals & Pharmaceutical Industry

Producer: BRS/Colleague and others, including The Bureau of National Affairs, Inc. (NEWS BULLETINS), Medical Economics Company (PRODUCT INFORMATION), and various pharmaceutical companies

Online Service: BRS/Colleague (PHYCOM II)

Conditions: Subscription to BRS/Colleague required

Content: Consists of 4 files of pharmaceutical and medical information.

PDR ON-LINE. Contains full text of *Physicians' Desk Reference*, with prescribing information on over 1000 trade name pharmaceutical products. Includes manufacturer, generic description, clinical studies, abstracts of published papers, patient instruction information, pharmacology, dosage and administration, and contraindications. Source of data is product and labeling information supplied by manufacturers.

NEWS BULLETINS. Contains news stories relating to medicine, practice management, medicolegal events, and government developments affecting health care. Also contains a daily report of major stock market events. Prepared by The Bureau of National Affairs, Inc.

MESSAGES. Contains notices from pharmaceutical companies on such topics as changes in product availability, meeting announcements, and emergency messages.

REQUESTS. Contains pharmaceutical industry offers of literature and free samples, industry surveys, and information on registration for meetings and seminars.

Language: English

Coverage: U.S.

Time Span: Current information

Updating: Periodically, as new data become available

PHYTOMED

Type: Reference (Bibliographic)

Subject: Life Sciences

Producer: Biologische Bundesanstalt fuer Land- und Forstwirtschaft

Online Service: DIMDI

Content: Contains approximately 300,000 citations to the worldwide literature on phytomedicine, including phytopathology, plant protection, and protection of stored products. Covers bacteriology, biology, botany, ecological chemistry, entomology, mycology, nematology, plant physiology, toxicology, virology, and zoology. Corresponds to *Bibliography of Plant Protection*.

Language: English and German, with titles also in original languages

Coverage: International

Time Span: 1965 to date

Updating: About 3700 records a quarter

PHYTOTOX

Type: Reference (Bibliographic); Source (Textual-Numeric)

Subject: Toxicology

Producer: University of Oklahoma, Department of Botany and Microbiology, under a grant from the U.S. Environmental Protection Agency

Online Service: Chemical Information Systems, Inc., a subsidiary of Fein-Marquart Associates (CIS)

Conditions: Annual subscription fee of $300 to CIS required but fee is waived for educational institutions and non-profit public libraries worldwide

Content: Contains about 70,000 records providing data extracted from about 4000 published articles on the toxic effects of organic chemical substances on terrestrial vascular plants. Each record covers a single experiment with one chemical and one plant and includes a description of the chemical and the plant species, dosage level, method of application, and test results. A bibliographic reference is also provided.

Language: English

Coverage: U.S.

Time Span: Current information

Updating: Periodically, as new data become available

PNI℠ (Pharmaceutical News Index)

Type: Reference (Bibliographic)

Subject: Biomedicine; Biotechnology; Pharmaceuticals & Pharmaceutical Industry; Veterinary Sciences

Producer: Data Courier, an operating unit of UMI

Online Service: DIALOG Information Services, Inc.

Content: Contains citations to business, legislative, and product news items from major pharmaceutical and medical device newsletters: *FDC Reports* (Pink Sheet); *Drug Research Reports* (Blue Sheet); *Pharma Japan; Clinica World Medical Devices News; Medical Devices, Diagnostics and Instrumentation Reports* (Gray Sheet); *Quality Control Reports* (Gold Sheet); *Weekly Pharmacy Reports* (Green Sheet); *SCRIP World Pharmaceutical News*; *FDC Reports* (Rose Sheet); *Technology Reimbursement Reports* (Beige Sheet); *Animal Pharm World Animal Health News*; *Applied Genetics News*; *Biomedical Business International*; and *Health Devices*. Also covers *Washington Drug and Device Letter* and *PMA Newsletter* from December 1975 to November 1977. Topics covered include drugs and medical devices; sales and earnings reports; mergers and acquisitions; research developments; government regulations and legislation; and new product announcements.

Language: English

Coverage: U.S. and international

Time Span: *FDC Reports* (Pink), 1974 to date; *Drug Research Reports*, December 1975 to date; *Medical Devices, Diagnostics and Instrumentation Reports, Quality Control Reports*, and *Weekly Pharmacy Reports*, December 1977 to date; *SCRIP World Pharmaceutical News*, 1980 to date; *Pharma Japan* and *Clinica World Medical Devices News*, 1983 to date; *FDC Reports* (Rose), *Animal Pharm World Animal Health News*, *Biomedical Business International*, and *Health Devices*, December 1984 to date; *Technology Reimbursement Report*, early 1985 to date. *Washington Drug and Device Letter* and *PMA Newsletter*, December 1975 to November 1977.

Updating: About 2400 records a month

POLLUTION ABSTRACTS

Type: Reference (Bibliographic)

Subject: Environment

Producer: Cambridge Scientific Abstracts

Online Service: BRS; BRS/BRKTHRU; BRS/Colleague; DATA-STAR; DIALOG Information Services, Inc.; ESA-IRS; TECH DATA; University of Tsukuba

Content: Contains approximately 115,000 citations, with abstracts, to the worldwide technical and non-technical literature on pollution research, sources, and controls. Covers air, water, land, thermal, noise, and radiological pollution; pesticides; sewage and waste treatment; environmental action; and toxicology and health. Corresponds in coverage to *Pollution Abstracts*.

Language: English

Coverage: International

Time Span: Most services, 1970 to date; DATA-STAR, 1978 to date.

Updating: Most services, about 1500 records every 2 months; DATA-STAR, monthly.

POPLINE℠ (POPulation information onLINE)

Type: Reference (Bibliographic)

Subject: Biomedicine; Demographics & Population

Producer: Columbia University, Center for Population and Family Health, Library/Information Program; Johns Hopkins University, Population Information Program; Princeton University, Office of Population Research; University of North Carolina, Carolina Population Center

Online Service: National Library of Medicine (NLM)

Content: Contains citations, with abstracts, to the worldwide literature on family planning and population. Includes research in human fertility, contraceptive methods, community-based services, program evaluation, mortality, migration, censuses, vital statistics, and related health, law, and policy issues.

Language: English

Coverage: International

Time Span: 1970 to date, with earliest materials from 1831

Updating: About 1000 records a month

POPULATION BIBLIOGRAPHY

Type: Reference (Bibliographic)

Subject: Demographics & Population

Producer: University of North Carolina, Carolina Population Center

Online Service: DIALOG Information Services, Inc.

Content: Contains citations to the literature on population research and studies in the areas of abortion, demography, migration, family planning, fertility and, as well, in the general areas of population policy and law, population education, and population research methodology. Covers monographs, journals, technical reports, government documents, conference proceedings, dissertations, and many unpublished reports on population studies. Database focuses on the socioeconomic as opposed to the biomedical aspects of population, and on developing countries and the U.S. Corresponds to *CPC Microcatalog*.

Language: English, with some records in French and Spanish

Coverage: U.S. and developing countries

Time Span: 1966 to 1984

Updating: Not updated

PR NEWSWIRE

Type: Source (Full Text)
Subject: News
Producer: PR Newswire, National Press Communications Service
Online Service: BRS (as part of NEWSEARCH and TRADE AND INDUSTRY INDEX); BRS After Dark (as part of NEWSEARCH and TRADE AND INDUSTRY INDEX); BRS/BRKTHRU (as part of NEWSEARCH and TRADE AND INDUSTRY INDEX); Dialcom, Inc.; DIALOG Information Services, Inc. (as part of NEWSEARCH and TRADE AND INDUSTRY INDEX); Knowledge Index (as part of NEWSEARCH and TRADE AND INDUSTRY INDEX); Mead Data Central, Inc. (PRNEWS) (as part of NEXIS WIRE SERVICES *(see)*); NewsNet, Inc.; VU/TEXT Information Services, Inc.
Conditions: Subscription to Mead Data Central required; monthly subscription to NewsNet required; subscription to VU/TEXT required.
Content: Contains full text of news releases transmitted to the press by PR Newswire as issued by a variety of organizations, including corporations, public relations agencies, trade associations, labor unions, civic and cultural organizations, political parties, and government agencies. Covers primarily business and financial news, including information on mergers and acquisitions, tender offers, earnings, dividends, contracts, and management changes. Also covers sports, labor, medicine, science, and general interest news. News releases include name and telephone number of issuing organization.
Language: English
Coverage: Primarily U.S., with some international coverage
Time Span: Mead Data Central, January 21, 1980 to date; VU/TEXT, 1985 to date; other services, most current year.
Updating: Daily (Monday through Friday), within 2 days of publication

PREVENZIONE DEGLI INFORTUNI E SICUREZZA SUL LAVORO

Type: Reference (Bibliographic)
Subject: Occupational Safety & Health
Producer: Assolombarda
Online Service: SIRIO
Content: Contains about 1500 citations to laws, decrees, regulations, and technical documents on Italian industrial safety, industrial medicine, and accident prevention. Covers electricity, fire prevention, illumination, noise, machines, plant construction, and pollution.
Language: Italian
Coverage: Italy
Time Span: 1981 to date
Updating: Periodically, as new data become available

PRIMLINE

Type: Reference (Bibliographic)
Subject: Biomedicine; Health Care
Producer: Karolinska Institute, Department of Social Medicine
Online Service: MIC-KIBIC
Content: Contains approximately 5400 citations, with abstracts, to literature on Swedish research and development in primary health care, community medicine, and social medicine. Covers journal articles, monographs, pamphlets, and project records. Corresponds to *H-guiden*.

Language: English
Coverage: Primarily Sweden, with some international coverage
Time Span: 1982 to date
Updating: About 500 records a quarter

PRINCIPIOS ACTIVOS FARMACOLOGICOS COMERCIALIZADOS EN ESPANA

Type: Source (Textual-Numeric)
Subject: Pharmaceuticals & Pharmaceutical Industry
Producer: Consejo General de Colegios Oficiales de Farmaceuticos de Espana
Online Service: Consejo General de Colegios Oficiales de Farmaceuticos de Espana
Content: Contains information on about 2700 active ingredients in drugs available in Spain. Includes name, Chemical Abstracts Service Registry Number, type of substance (e.g., chemical compound, plant product, microorganism), clinical action and mechanism, indications and contraindications, precautions, interactions, side effects, posological data, pharmacokinetics, and notes on use during pregnancy and lactation. Sources include the pharameuticals register of the Ministerio de Sanidad y Consumo and the international scientific literature.
Language: Spanish
Coverage: Spain
Time Span: Current information
Updating: Periodically, as new data become available

PRODIL

Type: Reference (Referral)
Subject: Computers & Software
Producer: Centrale des Bibliotheques
Online Service: IST-Informatheque Inc.
Content: Contains references to about 400 producers and distributors of software described in LOGIBASE *(see)*. Includes company name, address, telephone number, telex, and contact person.
Language: French
Coverage: Canada (Quebec)
Time Span: 1984 to date
Updating: Quarterly

PsycALERT®

Type: Reference (Bibliographic)
Subject: Psychology
Producer: American Psychological Association
Online Service: BRS; BRS After Dark; BRS/BRKTHRU; BRS/Colleague; DIALOG Information Services, Inc.
Content: Contains citations, with preliminary indexing, to literature in psychology and the behavioral sciences, published in 1300 journal and serial publications worldwide. Complements PsycINFO *(see)* in coverage. When abstracting and final indexing are completed, records are transferred to PsycINFO.
Language: English
Coverage: International
Time Span: In-process records only
Updating: About 600 records a week

PsycFILE

Type: Reference (Bibliographic)

Subject: Psychology

Producer: American Psychological Association (APA)

Online Service: Executive Telecom System, Inc., Human Resource Information Network

Conditions: Annual subscription to Executive Telecom System required

Content: Contains about 19,000 citations, with abstracts, to journal literature and technical reports in psychology. Covers such topics of interest to human resource professionals as employee relations, job satisfaction, recruiting, occupational stress, communication, and organizational behavior. Source of information is PsycINFO *(see)*.

Language: English

Coverage: Primarily U.S., with some international coverage

Time Span: 1974 to date

Updating: About 200 records a month

PsycINFO®

Type: Reference (Bibliographic)

Subject: Psychology

Producer: American Psychological Association

Online Service: BRS; BRS After Dark; BRS/BRKTHRU; BRS/Colleague; DATA-STAR; DIALOG Information Services, Inc.; DIMDI; Knowledge Index; TECH DATA; University of Tsukuba

Content: Contains over 500,000 citations, with abstracts, to the worldwide literature (primarily journals) in psychology and the behavioral sciences. Includes both human and animal aspects in most of these fields: animal psychology; applied psychology; communication and language; cultural influences and social issues; developmental psychology; education; neurology and physiology; perception and motor performance; personality; physical and psychological disorders; psychometrics and statistics; treatment and prevention; and personnel and professional issues. Covers the psychology and behavior of groups and organizations in addition to that of individuals. From 1967 to 1979, corresponds to *Psychological Abstracts*. Beginning in 1980 the database contains more references than the printed publication.

Language: English

Coverage: International

Time Span: 1967 to date

Updating: About 3200 records a month

PSYNDEX

Type: Reference (Bibliographic)

Subject: Psychology

Producer: Trier University, Zentralstelle fuer Psychologische Information und Dokumentation (ZPID)

Online Service: DIMDI

Content: Contains citations, with abstracts, to literature on psychology and related behavioral and social science disciplines. Source materials include dissertations, books, reports, and articles from about 160 journals. Covers clinical psychology and psychotherapy, comparative psychology, cognitive processes, communication, developmental psychology, education and counseling, industrial-organizational psychology, learning, measurement and statistics, motivation, perception, personality, physiological psychology, social psychology, psychoanalysis, and philosophy of science. Corresponds to *Psychologischer Index*.

Language: Citations in German and English; abstracts in German, with English abstracts also available in about 50% of the records.

Coverage: German-speaking countries

Time Span: Most materials, 1977 to date; dissertations, 1968 to date.

Updating: Monthly

PTS NEW PRODUCT ANNOUNCEMENTS™

Type: Source (Full Text)

Subject: News

Producer: Predicasts, Inc.

Online Service: BRS (to be available in 1987); DATA-STAR; DIALOG Information Services, Inc.

Content: Contains full text of about 10,000 press releases from over 15,000 companies on new products and technologies. Covers announcements of new products and services, product modifications, and new technologies and processes from manufacturers, distributors, and service companies in nearly 30 industries (e.g., communications, medical and health services, textiles). Includes product description, specifications, and applications; information on trade names, prices, model numbers, availability, and licensing agreements; and the name, address, and telephone number of a company contact. Some records also include data on distribution channels, joint ventures, and market demographics. Information may be searched by product codes based on 2- to 7-digit Standard Industrial Classification (SIC) codes, company name or symbol, product trade name, product uses and applications, location of company, and special feature codes indicating discussions of price or performance specifications.

Language: English

Coverage: International

Time Span: 1985 to date

Updating: About 600 records a week

PUBLIC ACCESS MESSAGE SYSTEMS

Type: Reference (Referral)

Subject: Information Systems & Services-Directories

Producer: Robert M. Nebiker

Online Service: THE SOURCE

Conditions: Monthly minimum of $10 to THE SOURCE required, with $9 credited toward online usage charges

Content: Provides descriptions of about 400 publicly accessible electronic bulletin boards and message systems. Descriptions include name, location, hours of operation, type of system (e.g., games, messages, ring-back), communications protocol required, telephone number, and download or upload capabilities. Also indicates whether the entry is a new system or a new access number to an existing system and whether the message system has a religious or sexual orientation.

Coverage: Primarily U.S., with some international coverage

Time Span: Current information

Updating: Quarterly

PUBLIC AFFAIRS INFORMATION®

Type: Reference (Referral)

Subject: Legislative Tracking

Producer: Information for Public Affairs

Online Service: Information for Public Affairs

Conditions: Subscriptions range from $2000 to $35,000, depending on information to be accessed

Content: Contains status information on bills currently before state legislatures in the U.S. Includes PAI-prepared summaries of bills. Administrative regulations are summarized and compliance requirements are noted for federal, state, and territorial rules.

Language: English

Coverage: U.S.

Time Span: Current legislative session

Updating: Daily, while legislatures are in session

PULSE

Type: Source (Full Text)

Subject: News

Producer: New York Pulse, a New York Times Company

Online Service: Covidea

Conditions: Subscription to Covidea required

Content: Contains news, general interest information, and entertainment guides for the New York City area. Provides schedules and reviews of art exhibits, new and revived films, music, theater, dance performances, and restaurants; book reviews, best-seller lists, and reviews of books recommended by *The New York Times* during the past year; and worldwide travel information, including reviews of hotels and restaurants. Includes international and national news, sports, weather, and business stories on over 100 major companies in 30 different industries. Sources include *The New York Times* and major newswire services.

Language: English

Coverage: U.S. (primarily New York metropolitan area) , with some international coverage

Time Span: Varies by file, with earliest information from 1982

Updating: Continuously, throughout the day

QUALITY OF WORKLIFE

Type: Reference (Bibliographic)

Subject: Families & Family Life

Producer: Management Directions

Online Service: BRS (WORK/FAMILY LIFE DATABASE) ; Executive Telecom System, Inc., Human Resource Information Network

Conditions: Annual subscription to Executive Telecom System required

Content: Contains about 2500 citations, with abstracts, to U.S. literature on the relationships between work and family life, including how each is affected by the other and what families and companies are doing to address problems in these relationships. Topics covered include alternatives to traditional work arrangements, dual-career families, health, child care, retirement, industrial social work, working wives and mothers, relocation, and employer concerns and programs. Sources include journals, books, conference proceedings, research reports, newspapers, pamphlets, company publications, and bibliographies.

Language: English

Coverage: U.S.

Time Span: 1970 to date

Updating: About 200 records a month

QUEBEC-ACTUALITES

Type: Reference (Bibliographic)

Subject: News

Producer: Microfor-CEJ

Online Service: IST-Informatheque Inc.

Content: Contains about 62,000 citations, with abstracts, to articles from the newspapers *Le Devoir, La Presse*, and *Le Soleil*. Covers a broad range of subjects, including national and international events, and political, economic, social, and cultural issues. Corresponds to *Index de L'Actualite vue a Travers la Presse Ecrite*.

Language: French

Coverage: Canada

Time Span: 1982 to date

Updating: About 2000 records a month

QUIP

Type: Source (Full Text)

Subject: Information Systems & Services

Producer: ACI Computer Services

Online Service: ACI Computer Services

Conditions: Monthly minimum to ACI required; fees vary depending on service selected.

Content: Contain full text of *Information Retrieval Systems Newsletter*, a newsletter for users of ACI Computer Services online service. Includes announcements of new databases, system upgrades, and training schedules.

Language: English

Coverage: Primarily Australia

Time Span: August 1981 to date

Updating: Monthly

RADIOLOGY & IMAGING LETTER

Type: Reference (Referral) ; Source (Full Text)

Subject: Biomedicine; Biotechnology; Conferences & Meetings

Producer: Quest Publishing Company

Online Service: NewsNet, Inc.

Conditions: Monthly subscription to NewsNet required; differential charges for subscribers and non-subscribers to *Radiology & Imaging Letter*.

Content: Contains full text of the *Radiology & Imaging Letter*, a newsletter covering technological, clinical, and regulatory developments in the fields of medical imaging and radiation therapy. Includes new product announcements, reports of research on new technology and procedures, news of legal and regulatory activities (e.g., recalls, safety hazard notices) , business news on the medical imaging equipment and supplies industry, and interviews with industry and government figures. Also includes a calendar of conferences and continuing education courses, descriptions of new publications (e.g., *The Pocket Atlas of Cranial Magnetic Resonance Imaging*) , relevant information sources, and news of key industry personnel.

Language: English

Coverage: Primarily U.S.

Time Span: November 15, 1985 to date

Updating: Every 2 weeks

RARE DISEASE DATABASE

Type: Reference (Bibliographic, Referral) ; Source (Full Text)
Subject: Biomedicine; Health Care & Social Services-Directories; Research in Progress
Producer: Robert L. Walter Communications, in cooperation with the National Organization for Rare Diseases, Inc.
Online Service: CompuServe Information Service
Content: Contains information on approximately 200 rare diseases (e.g., Huntington's Disease, Tay-Sachs Disease, lupus). Includes general description, nomenclature, symptoms, etiology, related disorders, standard and experimental therapy, and, for some diseases, references to the medical literature. Also provides information on current research, including contact information for researchers engaged in studying rare diseases, as well as lists of agencies and organizations offering support to victims of rare diseases or serving as information clearinghouses. Data are accessible by approximately 15,000 keywords, including 1500 disease names and Current Medical Information and Terminology (CMIT) numbers. All information is reviewed by the National Organization for Rare Diseases.
Language: English
Coverage: Primarily U.S.
Time Span: October 1985 to date
Updating: Weekly

RCA HotlineSM

Type: Source (Numeric, Full Text)
Subject: General Interest; News
Producer: RCA Global Communications, Inc.
Online Service: RCA Global Communications, Inc.
Content: Consists of 6 files of general and special interest information and news.
Business & Finance. Contains international financial news reports, commentaries, and bulletins; London and New York spot and futures rates for major world currencies; gold prices; and key U.S. financial and money interest rates. Also includes London shipping and cargo information and prices.
International Markets. Contains stock and options prices for the New York, American, and NASDAQ Over-The-Counter stock exchanges and all major world stock exchanges, as well as market commentary for the U.S., London, and Tokyo exchanges.
Commodities, Futures, & Metals. Contains market activity updates in cocoa, coffee, copper, cotton, grains, livestock, metals, and sugar futures; London and New York gold and silver futures; U.S. Treasury bond and note futures; Government National Mortgage Association (GNMA) futures; and petroleum, foods, grains, textiles, metals, rubber, and tin spot prices.
World News, Sports, Science, & Weather. Contains world news headlines, bulletins, and features, including U.S. legislative and regulatory activity, U.S. and world sports scores, general science and technology stories, and weather conditions and forecasts for 60 world cities and 20 major U.S. cities.
General Interest. Contains weekly fiction and non-fiction best-seller list; U.S. and U.K. record charts; top films playing worldwide and box office grosses; movie reviews, profiles, and features; theater reviews; astrological and Chinese horoscopes; latest medical developments; trivia questions and answers; and "this day in history" feature.
Personal Messages. Contains graphics and greetings, to be printed on a user's terminal, for holidays and personal (e.g., birthday, anniversary, bon voyage) events.

Language: English and Spanish; graphics, user instructions, and file descriptions, variously, also in French, German, and Portuguese.
Coverage: International
Time Span: Current information
Updating: Varies by file; continuously for some and daily to weekly for others.

READERS' GUIDE TO PERIODICAL LITERATURESM

Type: Reference (Bibliographic)
Subject: General Interest
Producer: The H.W. Wilson Company
Online Service: WILSONLINE
Content: Contains more than 136,500 citations to articles of at least one column in length from more than 180 general interest and popular magazines. Includes feature articles, book reviews, selected editorials and letters to the editor, photographic essays, and such original works as short stories and poetry. Corresponds to *Readers' Guide to Periodical Literature*.
Language: English
Coverage: Primarily U.S., with some international coverage
Time Span: 1983 to date
Updating: Twice a week; about 5300 records a month.

REBK (Repertoire des banques de donnees en conversationnel)

Type: Reference (Referral)
Subject: Information Systems & Services-Directories
Producer: Association Nationale de la Recherche Technique (ANRT)
Online Service: G.CAM Serveur
Content: Contains references to over 800 databases available online in France. Each reference includes the database name, producer, subject matter, type of data, growth rate, corresponding printed publications, prices, conditions of access, and other services offered in connection with the database. Corresponds to *Repertoire des banques de donnees en conversationnel*.
Language: French
Coverage: International
Time Span: Current information
Updating: About 100 records twice a year

REGISTRY NOMENCLATURE AND STRUCTURE SERVICE

Type: Source (Textual-Numeric)
Subject: Chemistry-Structure & Nomenclature
Producer: Chemical Abstracts Service (CAS)
Online Service: DATA-STAR (CHEMICAL NOMENCLATURE) ; DIALOG Information Services, Inc. (CHEMNAME) ; ORBIT Information Technologies Corporation (CHEMDEX) ; STN International (REGISTRY FILE); Telesystemes-Questel (CANOM) (*see DARC for additional Registry data available through Telesystemes-Questel*)
Content: Contains data that are based on the CAS Registry Nomenclature and Structure Service, an authority file of names and structural data that have been registered by CAS. The coverage and size of the databases on each online service are somewhat different, but entries have in common the following data items: full nomenclature and synonyms; substructure search via nomenclature; preferred, alternate, replaced, and

replacing Registry Numbers, molecular formula; and ring system information.

CHEMDEX. Covers all substances cited in *Chemical Abstracts*, 1972 to date.

CHEMNAME. Covers substances that have been cited 2 or more times in *Chemical Abstracts*, 1967 to date. Additional search terms generated by DIALOG specifically for CHEMNAME are also included. *See also CHEMSEARCH, CHEMSIS, and CHEMZERO.*

CHEMICAL NOMENCLATURE. Covers all substances cited in *Chemical Abstracts*, 1967 to date.

CANOM. Contains Registry Number, preferred name, and molecular formula for substances appearing in CAS *(see CA SEARCH).*

EURECAS. *(see DARC)*

REGISTRY FILE. Covers all substances registered by CAS since 1965. Structure searching is conducted by selecting structure fragments from a menu, drawing on a graphics terminal, or typing commands on the keyboard. Users retrieve the structure diagram, molecular formula, CAS index name and Registry Number, and up to 50 synonyms. Retrieved Registry Numbers can then be transferred to the CA FILE *(see CA SEARCH)* for retrieving bibliographic information or to the CAOLD FILE *(see)* for retrieving CA reference numbers for documents cited in *Chemical Abstracts* from 1962-1966.

Time Span: DIALOG, STN International, and Telesystemes-Questel, 1965 to date; DATA-STAR, 1967 to date; ORBIT, 1972 to date.

Updating: Varies by online service, from quarterly to less frequently

REMARC® (REtrospective MARC)

Type: Reference (Bibliographic)
Subject: Library Holdings-Catalogs
Producer: Utlas International U.S. Inc.
Online Service: DIALOG Information Services, Inc.; Utlas International Canada Inc. (as part of UTLAS CATSS *(see)*) ; Utlas International U.S. Inc. (as part of UTLAS CATSS *(see)*)
Content: A companion file to LC MARC *(see)* that contains over 5.2 million bibliographic records on works cataloged by the Library of Congress (LC) prior to 1979 that are not included in LC MARC. Covers items in English prior to 1968; in French, prior to 1973; in German, Spanish, and Portuguese, prior to 1975; in Dutch, Scandinavian, Italian, and Rumanian, prior to 1976; in other Roman alphabet languages, prior to 1977; and in non-Roman alphabet languages, prior to 1979. All major bibliographic elements from LC catalog cards are included along with appropriate MARC tags, indicators, and subfield codes for each element.
Language: Primarily English
Coverage: International
Time Span: All LC cataloging prior to 1979 that is not in MARC
Updating: Irregularly

REPERE

Type: Reference (Bibliographic)
Subject: General Interest
Producer: Bibliotheque Nationale du Quebec (Canada), in conjunction with Centrale des Bibliotheques (Canada)
Online Service: IST-Informatheque Inc.
Content: Contains about 144,000 citations, with abstracts, to general interest articles from over 350 French-language magazines. Covers current affairs, leisure-time activities, arts, sports, recreation and travel, education, history, business, science and technology, politics, philosophy, religion, and other general topics. Corresponds to *Point de Repere*.

Language: French
Coverage: Canada (Quebec)
Time Span: 1972 to date
Updating: About 6800 records twice a year

RESAGRI

Type: Reference (Bibliographic)
Subject: Agriculture
Producer: Caisse National de Credit Agricole; Institut National de la Recherche Agronomique; Ministere de l'Agriculture; Union des Caisses Centrales de Mutualite Agricole
Online Service: Ministere de l'Agriculture
Conditions: Subscription fee of $130 required
Content: Contains 3 files of bibliographic information on various aspects of agriculture.

TECAGRI. Contains over 50,000 citations to literature on the technical aspects of agriculture.

RESADEC-ECO. Contains about 100,000 citations to the economic, social, and financial aspects of agriculture.

RESADEC-JUR. Contains about 60,000 citations to the legal aspects of agriculture.

Covers books, conference proceedings, reports, theses, research reports, and over 900 journals. Corresponds in part to *Economie et Techniques Agricoles, Droit Rural*. Some items are also included in AGRIS *(see)*.

Language: English and French
Coverage: Primarily France and Europe, with some international coverage
Time Span: RESADEC-ECO and RESADEC-JUR, 1974 to date; TECAGRI, 1978 to date.
Updating: RESADEC-ECO and RESADEC-JUR, every 2 weeks; TECAGRI, monthly.

RESOURCES IN VOCATIONAL EDUCATION

Type: Reference (Referral)
Subject: Education & Educational Institutions; Research in Progress
Producer: The National Center for Research in Vocational Education
Online Service: BRS; BRS After Dark; BRS/BRKTHRU; BRS/Colleague; TECH DATA
Content: Contains about 11,000 summary descriptions of ongoing and recently completed research and development projects in vocational education, covering project proposals, completed project descriptions, and resulting products. Includes exemplary and curriculum development projects that are federally funded and administered through state research coordinating units, and federally administered projects related to career and vocational education.
Language: English
Coverage: U.S.
Time Span: 1978 to date
Updating: About 250 records a quarter

RESTRICTION ENZYME DATABASE

Type: Reference (Bibliographic) ; Source (Textual-Numeric)
Subject: Biotechnology
Producer: Dr. Richard J. Roberts
Online Service: Bionet; IntelliGenetics, Inc., An IntelliCorp Company

Conditions: To access through Bionet, users must be qualified principal investigators employed by a non-profit organization

Content: Contains descriptions of more than 500 restriction enzymes. Includes microorganism name, enzyme (including isoschizomers and corresponding prototypes), recognition sequence, site of methylation, and site of cleavage. Also includes citations, with abstracts, to published and unpublished sources of data. Corresponds to *Nucleic Acids Research*, Volume 13 Supplement, "Restriction and modification enzymes and their recognition sequences."

Language: English
Coverage: International
Time Span: Current information
Updating: Periodically, as new data become available

REUTER NEWS REPORTS

Type: Source (Full Text)
Subject: News
Producer: Reuters U.S. Inc.
Online Service: NewsNet, Inc.
Conditions: Monthly subscription to NewsNet required
Content: Contains full text of items from the Reuter News Reports newswire service. Covers international news, U.S. general news, financial news, and standing features and commentaries. Includes brief excerpts of the full text for selected international news items.
NOTE: News items are accessible only through a selective dissemination service, NewsFlash, and are retained 2 weeks for each user.
Language: English
Coverage: International
Time Span: Most current 2 weeks
Updating: Continuously, throughout the day

RICHMOND NEWS LEADER

Type: Source (Full Text)
Subject: News
Producer: Richmond Newspapers, Inc.
Online Service: VU/TEXT Information Services, Inc.
Conditions: Subscription to VU/TEXT required
Content: Contains full text of news items and feature articles from the *Richmond News Leader* (Virginia) newspaper. Regional coverage emphasizes news of the agriculture, banking, and tobacco industries and of state government activities.
Language: English
Coverage: U.S. (primarily Richmond, Virginia area)
Time Span: June 1985 to date
Updating: Daily

RICHMOND TIMES-DISPATCH

Type: Source (Full Text)
Subject: News
Producer: Richmond Newspapers, Inc.
Online Service: VU/TEXT Information Services, Inc.
Conditions: Subscription to VU/TEXT required
Content: Contains full text of news items and feature articles from the *Richmond Times-Dispatch* (Virginia) newspaper. Regional coverage emphasizes news of state government activities.

Language: English
Coverage: U.S. (primarily Richmond, Virginia area)
Time Span: June 1985 to date
Updating: Daily

RINGDOC (Pharmaceutical Literature Documentation)

Type: Reference (Bibliographic)
Subject: Pharmaceuticals & Pharmaceutical Industry
Producer: Derwent Publications Ltd.
Online Service: DIALOG Information Services, Inc.; ORBIT Information Technologies Corporation
Conditions: Subscription to *RINGDOC ABSTRACTS JOURNAL* required
Content: Contains citations, with abstracts, to the worldwide journal literature on pharmaceuticals. Covers topics ranging from chemistry through pharmacology to medicine. Corresponds to the weekly publication, *RINGDOC ABSTRACTS JOURNAL*. Each record contains indepth keywording and fragmentation coding.
Language: English
Coverage: International
Time Span: 1964 to date
Updating: About 4500 records a month

RLIN

Type: Reference (Bibliographic)
Subject: Library Holdings-Catalogs
Producer: Library of Congress (LC); National Library of Medicine (NLM); U.S. Government Printing Office (GPO); member and participant libraries of The Research Libraries Group (RLG), Inc.
Online Service: RLIN
Content: A database system that provides technical support to member libraries for shared cataloging, acquisitions, and reference. The database comprises nearly 19 million cataloging records from LC MARC tapes, CONSER, GPO tapes, NLM tapes, and original cataloging conforming to RLG standards for member libraries. All 6 MARC formats-books, serials, films, maps, music (sound recordings and musical scores), and archives and manuscripts-are covered. Both member libraries and subscribing libraries have searching access to the database and may use the shared-cataloging capabilities, e.g., to change a record for their own use or generate catalog cards. Access points include personal name, corporate name, title, subject heading, LC card number, local call number, ISBN, and ISSN. Boolean operators and truncation of words, phrases, and numbers can be used to search across fields. RLIN may also be used by member libraries for sending interlibrary loan requests.
Language: Primarily English
Coverage: International
Time Span: 1968 to date
Updating: LC records, weekly; other records, continuously, throughout the day.

RTECS (Registry of Toxic Effects of Chemical Substances)

Type: Source (Textual-Numeric)
Subject: Toxicology
Producer: U.S. Department of Health and Human Services, Public Health Service, National Institute for Occupational Safety and Health, Registry of Toxic Effects of Chemical Substances (NIOSH)

Online Service: Australian Medline Network; Chemical Information Systems, Inc., a subsidiary of Fein-Marquart Associates (CIS); DIMDI; Information Consultants, Inc. (ICI) (as part of The Integrated Chemical Information System); MIC-KIBIC; National Library of Medicine (NLM)

Conditions: Annual subscription fee of $300 to CIS required but fee is waived for educational institutions and non-profit public libraries worldwide; differential charges for subscribers and non-subscribers to ICI.

Content: Contains over 135,000 unevaluated toxicological measurements pertaining to approximately 80,000 chemicals. Each entry contains the Chemical Abstracts Service (CAS) name and Registry Number, synonyms, molecular formula, and one or more measures of toxicity, including acute and chronic *in vivo* data, *in vitro* mutagenesis data, and skin and eye irritation data. Searchable fields include animal species, dosage methods, toxicity measures (e.g., LD50), special toxic effects (e.g., carcinogenic), and range of toxicity values (CIS only). The NLM and CIS versions of this file both contain searchable CAS and NIOSH/RTECS numbers, chemical names and synonyms, name fragments, Wiswesser Line Notation, threshold limit values, International Agency for Research on Cancer (IARC) carcinogenic determinations, recommended and existing standards and regulations, National Toxicology Program bioassay status, EPA Toxic Substances Control Act (TSCA) status, and EPA GENE-TOX data. Corresponds to the printed and microfiche RTECS publication available from the U.S. Government Printing Office.

Language: English
Updating: Quarterly

THE SACRAMENTO BEE

Type: Source (Full Text)
Subject: News
Producer: Advanced Search Concepts
Online Service: VU/TEXT Information Services, Inc.
Conditions: Subscription to VU/TEXT required
Content: Contains full text of news items, feature articles, stories, and editorials from *The Sacramento Bee* (California) newspaper. Covers local, state, and national news, including government, law, business and industry, economics, transportation, education, sports, leisure, and the arts. Does not include illustrations or classified ads.
Language: English
Coverage: U.S. (primarily California)
Time Span: March 1984 to date
Updating: Daily

SAFETY SCIENCE ABSTRACTS

Type: Reference (Bibliographic)
Subject: Safety
Producer: Cambridge Scientific Abstracts
Online Service: Pergamon InfoLine
Content: Contains approximately 34,500 citations to the worldwide literature on safety science and hazard control, with an emphasis on the identification, evaluation, and elimination or control of hazards. Covers industrial and occupational safety, transportation safety, aviation and aerospace safety, environmental and ecological safety, and medical safety. Includes such topics as environmental pollution and waste disposal, radiation, pesticides, natural disasters, toxicology, genetics, epidemics, drugs, injuries, diseases, and criminal acts (e.g., arson). Also covers issues related to liablity. Sources include books, periodicals, government reports, conference proceedings, patents, and dissertations. Corresponds to *Safety Science Abstracts*.

Language: English
Coverage: International
Time Span: 1981 to date
Updating: Quarterly

SAN JOSE MERCURY-NEWS

Type: Source (Full Text)
Subject: News
Producer: San Jose Mercury/News
Online Service: VU/TEXT Information Services, Inc.
Conditions: Subscription to VU/TEXT required
Content: Contains full text of news items and feature articles from the *San Jose Mercury-News* (California) newspaper. Regional coverage emphasizes commercial real estate, high technology industries, medicine, and science.
Language: English
Coverage: U.S. (primarily San Jose, California area)
Time Span: June 1985 to date
Updating: Daily

SANSS (Substructure and Nomenclature Searching System)

Type: Source (Textual-Numeric)
Subject: Chemistry-Structure & Nomenclature
Producer: Chemical Information Systems, Inc. (CIS), a subsidiary of Fein-Marquart Associates for CIS and Information Consultants, Inc. (ICI) for ICI, from data provided by Chemical Abstracts Service, U.S. Environmental Protection Agency, and U.S. National Institutes of Health

Online Service: Chemical Information Systems, Inc., a subsidiary of Fein-Marquart Associates (CIS); Information Consultants, Inc. (ICI) (as part of The Integrated Chemical Information System)

Conditions: Annual subscription fee of $300 to CIS required but fee is waived for educational institutions and non-profit public libraries worldwide; differential charges for subscribers and non-subscribers to ICI.

Content: Contains chemical nomenclature and substructure data for over 348,000 substances represented in the Toxic Substances Control Act (TSCA) Inventory *(see TSCA INITIAL INVENTORY)*, the databases available through CIS and ICI, and 101 other files produced by the U.S. Environmental Protection Agency, National Bureau of Standards, National Cancer Institute, and other sources. Each entry contains the Chemical Abstracts Service name and Registry Number and a connection table, i.e., a 2-dimensional representation of the non-hydrogen atoms in the molecule, their neighbors, and bonds. Searching is done by "drawing" a molecule, through a series of commands to the system, to generate a connection table for a compound that is to be matched against the connection tables contained in the database. Users can also search by molecular weight, molecular formula, compound name, name fragments, English- and non-English-language synonyms, or standard fragment codes. A list of pointers to other sources of information on the compounds is included with the information retrieved in each search.

Language: English
Updating: Periodically, as new data become available

SCARABEE

Type: Reference (Bibliographic)

Subject: Environment

Producer: Agence Nationale pour la Recuperation et l'Elimination des Dechets

Online Service: Agence Nationale pour la Recuperation et l'Elimination des Dechets

Content: Contains about 6500 citations, with abstracts, to the worldwide literature on waste management. Covers legislation, measuring and monitoring techniques, statistics, and the recovery, recycling, and treatment of agricultural, household, and industrial wastes. Sources include books, periodicals, technical reports, and government publications.

Language: English, French, German, and Spanish

Coverage: Primarily Europe, with some international coverage

Time Span: 1975 to date

Updating: About 50 items a week

SCHOOL PRACTICES INFORMATION FILE

Type: Reference (Referral)

Subject: Education & Educational Institutions

Producer: BRS

Online Service: BRS; BRS After Dark; BRS/BRKTHRU; BRS/Colleague; TECH DATA

Content: Contains about 24,000 descriptions of educational resource programs, practices, materials, and products from public organizations and commercial publishers. Covers nationally- and state-validated or exemplary programs, special education programs and materials, school business practices, administrator and teacher inservice education programs, curriculum materials in all subject areas and grade levels, audiovisual aids including films and videotapes, testing materials, and microcomputer educational software for all major brands of microcomputers. Each description contains availability, ordering, and cost information.

Language: English

Coverage: U.S.

Time Span: 1980 to date

Updating: Monthly

SCIENCE EDUCATION FORUM

Type: Reference (Referral); Source (Full Text, Software)

Subject: Education & Educational Institutions

Producer: Rick Needham

Online Service: CompuServe Information Service

Content: Contains information related to science education of interest to users in schools and in the home. Includes newsletters, summaries of current science news, ideas for student science experiments, hardware and software reviews, and utility and science tutorial software, including some software in Spanish and French, that can be downloaded. Also provides references to job openings for science teachers at the high school and college levels, as well as information for graduate students about available fellowships and research assistantships.

Language: English

Coverage: Primarily U.S., with some international coverage

Time Span: Current information

Updating: Daily

SCISEARCH®

Type: Reference (Bibliographic)

Subject: Agriculture; Biomedicine; Environment; Life Sciences

Producer: Institute for Scientific Information (ISI)

Online Service: DATA-STAR; DIALOG Information Services, Inc.; DIMDI

Conditions: Differential charges for subscribers and non-subscribers to *Science Citation Index*

Content: Contains citations to worldwide literature across a wide range of scientific and technological disciplines. Covers approximately 4500 journals. Topics covered include life sciences, physical sciences, chemistry, earth sciences, agriculture, environmental sciences, clinical medicine, engineering, technology, and applied sciences. Corresponds to coverage in *Science Citation Index*. Also includes additional journal coverage drawn from ISI's *Current Contents* series of publications.

Language: English

Coverage: International

Time Span: DATA-STAR and DIALOG, 1974 to date; DIMDI, 1974 to 1978 *(see ISI/BIOMED and ISI/MULTISCI for 1979 to date)*.

Updating: DATA-STAR, about 14,000 records a week; DIALOG, about 26,500 records every 2 weeks; DIMDI, not updated *(see ISI/BIOMED and ISI/MULTISCI for current information (1979 to date))*.

SCRIPPS HOWARD NEWS SERVICE

Type: Source (Full Text)

Subject: News

Producer: Scripps Howard News Service

Online Service: THE SOURCE

Conditions: Monthly minimum of $10 to THE SOURCE required, with $9 credited toward online usage charges

Content: Contains full text of about 50 news and sports stories, editorials, and reviews of books, movies, and the theater. Sources include newspapers owned by Scripps Howard (e.g., *The Detroit News, The Providence Journal and Horizon* (Rhode Island), *Rocky Mountain News* (Denver, Colorado), *Pittsburgh Press*), other newspapers (e.g., *Fort Worth Star-Telegram* (Texas), *The San Francisco Examiner*), news services distributed by Scripps Howard (e.g., The London Observer News Service, The London Express Service), and stories written by reporters at Scripps Howard's Washington bureau.

Language: English

Coverage: Primarily U.S., with some international coverage (about 7 or 8 stories a day)

Time Span: Current day

Updating: About 50 stories a day, Monday through Saturday

SDF (Standard Drug File)

Type: Source (Textual-Numeric)

Subject: Pharmaceuticals & Pharmaceutical Industry

Producer: Derwent Publications Ltd.

Online Service: ORBIT Information Technologies Corporation

Conditions: Available only to RINGDOC *(see)* subscribers

Content: Is a companion dictionary to RINGDOC *(see)* and covers approximately 7500 known drugs and other commonly occurring compounds. Includes full name, Derwent Standard Registry Name, activities, chemical substructure, and chemical ring codes.

Language: English
Coverage: International
Time Span: Current information
Updating: Periodically, as new data become available

SEATTLE POST–INTELLIGENCER

Type: Source (Full Text)
Subject: News
Producer: Hearst Corporation
Online Service: VU/TEXT Information Services, Inc.
Conditions: Subscription to VU/TEXT required
Content: Contains full text of news items, feature stories, and editorials from the *Seattle Post-Intelligencer* newspaper. Regional coverage emphasizes high technology, aviation, and timber industries.
Language: English
Coverage: U.S. (primarily Seattle, Washington area)
Time Span: June 1986 to date
Updating: Daily

THE SEATTLE SHUTTLE®

Type: Reference (Referral); Source (Full Text)
Subject: News
Producer: The Shuttle Corp. and others, including the Associated Press
Online Service: The Shuttle Corp.
Conditions: Annual subscription of $24.95 required for THE SHUTTLE INFORMATION SERVICE; access to THE SHUTTLE EXPRESS is free.
Content: Contains news and information of interest in the Seattle (Washington) area.
THE SHUTTLE EXPRESS. Includes news and sports from the Associated Press, weather information from the National Oceanic and Atmospheric Administration, and financial and stock quote data. Also contains columns from professional writers, entertainment and restaurant information, as well as descriptions of local businesses, including products and services offered and, in some cases, current prices and other relevant information. An electronic mail service is also available.
THE SHUTTLE INFORMATION SERVICE. A membership service providing enhanced access to THE SHUTTLE EXPRESS.
Language: English
Coverage: U.S. (primarily Seattle, Washington area)
Time Span: Current information
Updating: Periodically, as new data become available

SEGURIDAD E HIGIENE EN EL TRABAJO

Type: Reference (Bibliographic)
Subject: Occupational Safety & Health
Producer: Instituto Nacional de Seguridad e Higiene en el Trabajo
Online Service: Instituto Nacional de Seguridad e Higiene en el Trabajo
Content: Contains approximately 40,000 citations to the worldwide journal literature on industrial health and safety. Covers industrial hygiene and medicine, industrial toxicology, legislation, psycho-social factors, risk prevention, and safety training.
Language: Spanish

Coverage: International
Time Span: 1972 to date
Updating: Monthly

SERIX (Swedish Environmental Research Index)

Type: Reference (Bibliographic, Referral)
Subject: Environment; Research in Progress
Producer: The Swedish National Environmental Protection Board
Online Service: ARAMIS (a cooperative service of the Swedish Center for Working Life, Swedish National Board of Occupational Safety and Health, and The Swedish National Environmental Protection Board)
Content: Contains approximately 17,500 citations, most with abstracts, to research reports, including descriptions of research projects, on environmental issues in Sweden. Topics covered include air, water, and soil pollution; toxic wastes; natural resources and wildlife; environmental monitoring and technology; environmental hygiene; epidemiology; ergonomics; and occupational medicine and hygiene. Each record includes project or report title, project leader or report author, sponsoring organization, research organization, abstract (when available), and subject and geographical area codes. Corresponds to *Swedish Environmental Research*.
Language: Swedish, with some titles and abstracts (about 30%) also in English
Coverage: Sweden
Time Span: 1975 to date
Updating: About 50 records 40 times a year

SERLINE™ (SERials onLINE)

Type: Reference (Bibliographic)
Subject: Biomedicine; Library Holdings-Catalogs
Producer: National Library of Medicine
Online Service: Australian Medline Network; National Library of Medicine (NLM)
Content: Contains citations to approximately 65,000 serial titles, including all serials and numbered congresses that are on order, in process, or currently received at NLM. Many records contain locator information for approximately 150 major biomedical libraries in the Regional Medical Library Network that have the publications. Corresponds to the microfiche publication, *Health Sciences Serials*.
Language: English
Coverage: International
Updating: About 300 records a month

SIGLE (System for Information on Grey Literature in Europe)

Type: Reference (Bibliographic)
Subject: Science & Technology
Producer: European Association for Grey Literature Exploitation (EAGLE)
Online Service: BLAISE-LINE; FIZ Karlsruhe
Conditions: Annual subscription of 49 pounds (UK) for U.K. users or 56 pounds (UK) for other users to BLAISE Online Services required
Content: Contains citations to the grey literature (e.g., reports, conference papers, and other non-conventional literature issued informally and not available through normal channels) published in European Economic Community member

countries. Covers these fields: aeronautics; agriculture; behavioral and social sciences; biology and medicine; chemistry; earth science; electronics and electrical engineering; energy; materials; mathematics; mechanical, industrial, civil, and marine engineering; methods and equipment; military science; missile technology; navigation, communications, detection, and counter measures; physics; propulsion and fuels; and space technology.

Language: English, with titles also in original languages

Coverage: European Economic Community (Belgium, Denmark, Federal Republic of Germany, France, Greece, Ireland, Italy, Luxembourg, The Netherlands, Portugal, Spain, and U.K.)

Time Span: 1981 to date

Updating: BLAISE-LINE, about 3000 records a month; FIZ, about 4000 records every 2 months.

SILICON MOUNTAIN REPORT

Type: Source (Full Text)

Subject: Science & Technology

Producer: Silicon Mountain Associates

Online Service: NewsNet, Inc.

Conditions: Monthly subscription to NewsNet required; differential charges for subscribers and non-subscribers to *Silicon Mountain Report*.

Content: Contains full text of *Silicon Mountain Report*, a newsletter covering companies in high-technology industries located in Colorado, especially in the region between Colorado Springs and Fort Collins. Covers such industries as biotechnology, communications, data processing, electronics, medical instrumentation, robotics, optics, and software. Includes news of corporate expansion or acquisitions, product announcements, contract awards, personnel changes, and financial and economic developments. Also includes profiles of selected companies.

Language: English

Coverage: U.S. (Colorado)

Time Span: March 1984 to date

Updating: Monthly

SITADEX

Type: Reference (Referral)

Subject: Patents

Producer: Registro de la Propiedad Industrial

Online Service: Registro de la Propiedad Industrial

Content: Contains information on the current status of approximately 400,000 applications for patents, registrations, and trademarks in Spain.

Language: Spanish

Coverage: Spain

Time Span: 1964 to date

Updating: Twice a month

SLUDGE NEWSLETTER

Type: Source (Full Text)

Subject: Environment

Producer: Business Publishers, Inc.

Online Service: NewsNet, Inc.

Conditions: Monthly subscription to NewsNet required; differential charges for subscribers and non-subscribers to *Sludge Newsletter*.

Content: Contains full text of *Sludge Newsletter*, a newsletter on sludge management, treatment, disposal, generation, and use. Covers legislative and regulatory developments in the U.S. Congress and the U.S. Environmental Protection Agency; sludge management industry news; new product introductions; and announcements of personnel changes, meetings, and publications.

Language: English

Coverage: U.S.

Time Span: 1982 to date

Updating: Every 2 weeks

SOCIAL PLANNING, POLICY & DEVELOPMENT ABSTRACTS (SOPODA)

Type: Reference (Bibliographic)

Subject: Social Services; Sociology

Producer: Sociological Abstracts, Inc.

Online Service: BRS; DIALOG Information Services, Inc.

Content: Contains about 9500 citations, with abstracts, to articles from over 1200 journals and serials covering the social sciences, including social welfare, planning and policy, and development, as applied to specific settings and situations. Covers such topics as welfare services, helping techniques (e.g., case work, community organization), social security programs (e.g., unemployment insurance, company pension plans), problems in industrialized and developing countries, policy administration, activism and action research, voluntarism, demographic change, and urban and rural community development.

NOTE: On DIALOG, SOPODA is part of SOCIOLOGICAL ABSTRACTS *(see)*.

Language: English

Coverage: International

Time Span: 1979 to date

Updating: Twice a year; about 2500 records a year.

SOCIAL SCIENCES INDEX^{SM}

Type: Reference (Bibliographic)

Subject: Social Sciences & Humanities

Producer: The H.W. Wilson Company

Online Service: WILSONLINE

Content: Contains over 35,000 citations to articles and book reviews in over 300 English-language periodicals in the social sciences. Covers anthropology, economics, environmental sciences, geography, law and criminology, planning and public administration, political science, psychology, social aspects of medicine, sociology, international relations and related subjects. Also includes coverage of current events.

Language: English

Coverage: International

Time Span: February 1984 to date

Updating: Twice a week

SOCIAL SCISEARCH®

Type: Reference (Bibliographic)

Subject: Social Sciences & Humanities

Producer: Institute for Scientific Information (ISI)

Online Service: BRS; BRS After Dark; BRS/BRKTHRU; BRS/Colleague; DIALOG Information Services, Inc.; DIMDI; TECH DATA

Conditions: Differential charges for subscribers and non-subscribers to *Social Sciences Citation Index*

Content: Contains over 1.5 million citations to significant articles from the 1400 most important social sciences journals worldwide and social sciences articles from 3300 journals in the natural, physical, and biomedical sciences. Covers anthropology, archaeology, area studies, business and finance, communications, community health, criminology, economics, demographics, education, ethnic group studies, geography, history, information and library science, international relations, law, linguistics, management, marketing, philosophy, political science, psychology, psychiatry, sociology, statistics, and urban planning and development. Corresponds to *Social Sciences Citation Index*.

Language: English

Coverage: International

Time Span: Most services, 1972 to date; DIMDI, 1973 to date.

Updating: About 10,000 records a month

SOCIAL SECURITY

Type: Source (Full Text)

Subject: Social Services

Producer: U.S. Department of Health and Human Services, Social Security Administration, Office of Information

Online Service: CompuServe Information Service

Content: Contains information for the general public on U.S. Social Security benefits and services. Covers such topics as check eligibility, how to build coverage, and how and when to contact the Social Security office. Sources include various Social Security public information publications. Corresponds in part to *Your Social Security*.

Language: English

Coverage: U.S.

Time Span: Current information

Updating: Periodically, as new data become available

SOCIAL WORK ABSTRACTS

Type: Reference (Bibliographic)

Subject: Social Services

Producer: National Association of Social Workers, Inc.

Online Service: BRS; BRS After Dark; BRS/BRKTHRU; BRS/Colleague

Content: Contains about 13,000 citations, with abstracts, to journal articles, doctoral dissertations, and other materials on social work and related fields. Covers such topics as alcoholism and drug abuse, crime and delinquency, schools, family and child welfare, employment and economic security, aging, health and medical care, mental health, and housing and urban development. Also covers social policy, social work service methodology, as well as issues from such related disciplines as psychology, psychiatry, economics, and sociology. Includes journal articles, doctoral dissertations, and other source materials.

Language: English

Coverage: International

Time Span: July 1977 to date

Updating: About 500 records a quarter

SOCIOLOGICAL ABSTRACTS

Type: Reference (Bibliographic)

Subject: Sociology

Producer: Sociological Abstracts, Inc.

Online Service: BRS; BRS After Dark; BRS/BRKTHRU; BRS/Colleague; DATA-STAR; DIALOG Information Services, Inc.; TECH DATA

Content: Contains over 170,000 citations, with abstracts (1973 to date), to articles from over 1400 journals and serial publications in the field of sociology and related disciplines in the social and behavioral sciences. Provides coverage of original research, reviews, discussions, monographic publications, theory, and conference reports in these areas: methodology and research; history and theory of sociology; social psychology and group interaction; culture and social structure; management and complex organization; social change and economic development; mass phenomena and political interactions; social differentiation; rural and urban sociology; sociology of the arts, religion and science; health and knowledge; demography and human biology; the family and social welfare; community development; policy; planning; forecasting and speculation; radical sociology; Marxist sociology; studies in violence, poverty and feminism; and environmental interaction.

Language: English

Coverage: International

Time Span: 1963 to date

Updating: Most services, 5 times a year; DIALOG, 3 times a year.

SOFT

Type: Reference (Referral)

Subject: Computers & Software

Producer: Online, Inc.

Online Service: BRS; BRS After Dark; BRS/BRKTHRU; BRS/Colleague; TECH DATA

Content: Contains descriptions of over 5000 software packages available for microcomputers. Includes software name, version, date released, and cost; producer name, address, telephone number, and contact; a brief product description (e.g. word processing); application information, including a detailed description of the product's capabilities; central processing unit, operating system, disk size, and other hardware requirements; other software used with the package; documentation available; where the product may be purchased; citations to reviews, if any, with an indication of whether the review was favorable; and producer comments. Sources of information include supplier literature and reviews. Games and other types of entertainment software are not covered.

Language: English

Coverage: International

Time Span: Current information

Updating: Monthly

SOFTWARE LOCATOR

Type: Reference (Referral)

Subject: Computers & Software

Producer: John Fairfax & Sons

Online Service: ACI Computer Services

Conditions: Monthly minimum to ACI required; fees vary depending on service selected.

Content: Contains approximately 1000 descriptions of computer software available in Australia. Corresponds to information published in *Todays Computers* and *The Australian Software Guide*.

Language: English
Coverage: Australia
Time Span: May 1984 to date
Updating: Monthly

SOFTYME EXPRESS

Type: Source (Software)
Subject: Computers & Software
Producer: Softyme
Online Service: Tymshare, Inc.
Conditions: Access limited to retail software dealerships; initiation fee of $1500 and monthly fee of $500 to Softyme required.
Content: Contains more than 200 programs for personal computers that can be downloaded for purchase at participating retail software dealerships. Programs selected by the retail customer are downloaded onto disks by the dealer for immediate purchase. Partial documentation is included when a program is downloaded; full printed documentation is mailed after sale. Also includes a list of frequently asked questions and answers about specific software items and a bulletin board for dealers to report program problems.
Updating: Daily

SOLIS (Social Sciences Literature Information System)

Type: Reference (Bibliographic)
Subject: Social Sciences & Humanities; Sociology
Producer: Informationszentrum Sozialwissenschaften
Online Service: FIZ Karlsruhe
Content: Contains over 58,000 citations, with abstracts, to social science literature. Covers sociology, social research methods, social psychology, social history, social problems, demography, and social science contributions in such areas as work, education, women, families, youth, communication, recreation, law, culture, religion, economics, technology assessment, politics, medicine, and the environment. Each record includes data on methodology and, where applicable, on the period covered and the availability of relevant published quantitative data. Sources include monographs, grey literature (e.g., reports, conference proceedings), and journals.
Language: German, with some abstracts also in English
Coverage: Austria, Federal Republic of Germany, German Democratic Republic, and Switzerland
Time Span: 1945 to date, with abstracts from 1976 to date
Updating: About 3000 records a quarter

SOLO (Supply On-Line Option)

Type: Source (Textual-Numeric)
Subject: Health Care
Producer: IMS America, Ltd.
Online Service: IMS America, Ltd.
Conditions: Subscription to *Hospital Supply Index* and annual online subscription required
Content: Contains information on 100,000 hospital supply products. Product descriptions include catalog number, price guidelines, pack description, material, sterility, and disposability. Purchase data include dollar and unit volume, market share, and growth, aggregated by product class, manufacturer, and corporation. Users can form other aggregations. Product descriptions are based on industry promotional literature and purchase data are gathered from invoices to selected hospitals.

Language: English
Coverage: U.S.
Time Span: Current 6 years
Updating: Monthly

SOMED

Type: Reference (Bibliographic)
Subject: Health Care; Social Sciences & Humanities
Producer: Institut fuer Dokumentation und Information ueber Sozialmedizin und Offentliches Gesundheitswesen (IDIS)
Online Service: DIMDI
Content: Contains about 160,000 citations, with abstracts (in about 60% of the records), to the worldwide literature on social medicine. Covers epidemiology, evaluation and quality assurance in public health, health politics, organization of health care, industrial hygiene, industrial toxicology, vital statistics, medical rehabilitation (through 1985 only), preventive medicine, school health, social pediatrics, social psychology, drug abuse and misuse, alcoholism, smoking, and environmental toxicology. Sources include journals, books, German dissertations, technical reports, and the grey literature.
Language: Primarily English, French, and German, with all keywords in German
Coverage: International, with emphasis on German and other European literature
Time Span: 1978 to date
Updating: About 1800 records a month

SpecialNet®

Type: Reference (Referral); Source (Full Text)
Subject: Education & Educational Institutions
Producer: National Systems Management, Inc.
Online Service: SpecialNet
Conditions: Annual subscription of $200 to National Systems Management required
Content: Contains news and information on trends and developments in educational services and programs. Covers legislation (e.g., congressional committee notices), Department of Education policies, litigation (e.g., court cases, hearing decisions), funding (e.g., federal grants and contracts), and technology (e.g., cable television, computer software). Includes descriptions of promising practices, current research studies, curriculum materials, and conferences, as well as the full text of *Education Daily (see EDUCATION DAILY ONLINE)* and a directory of private schools. A number of state, regional, and group-specific electronic bulletin boards and conferencing facilities (e.g., for employment opportunities, rural special education programs, programs involving parents) produced by a number of educational institutions are also available.
Language: English
Coverage: Primarily U.S., with some coverage of Canada
Time Span: Current information
Updating: Daily

SPF (Standard Pesticide File)

Type: Reference (Referral)
Subject: Agriculture
Producer: Derwent Publications Ltd.
Online Service: ORBIT Information Technologies Corporation
Conditions: Available only to PESTDOC *(see)* subscribers

Content: Contains references to about 3900 known pesticides and other common compounds. Includes full name, standard registry name, phamacological classification or standard activities, chemical substructure terms, chemical ring codes, and other codes.

Language: English

Coverage: International

Time Span: Current information

Updating: Periodically, as new data become available

SPORT

Type: Reference (Bibliographic)

Subject: Sports Medicine

Producer: Sport Information Resource Centre

Online Service: BRS; BRS After Dark; BRS/BRKTHRU; BRS/Colleague; CISTI, Canadian Online Enquiry Service (CAN/OLE) (SPORTS AND FITNESS DATABASE); DIMDI; ORBIT Information Technologies Corporation; TECH DATA

Conditions: CISTI accessible only in Canada

Content: Contains over 170,000 citations, with some abstracts, to the worldwide scientific and practical literature in the areas of sports, recreation, sports medicine, and physical education. Covers practice, training and equipment, sports facilities (including management and architecture), and international sport history. Sources in English and French are covered completely, but for those in other languages, only the more scientific items are referenced. Corresponds to *Sport Bibliography* and *SportSearch*.

Language: English

Coverage: International

Time Span: Monographs, 1949 to date; serials, 1975 to date.

Updating: Most services, quarterly; BRS services and CISTI, monthly.

SSIE CURRENT RESEARCH

Type: Reference (Referral)

Subject: Research in Progress

Producer: National Technical Information Service

Online Service: DIALOG Information Services, Inc.

Content: Contains descriptions of and references to research in progress and recently completed research sponsored primarily by federal government agencies. Also includes some research sponsored by state and local governments, major foundations, individuals, and universities and colleges. Covers basic and applied research in all areas of the life, physical, social, behavioral, and engineering sciences.

Language: English

Coverage: U.S.

Time Span: 1978 to February 1982 *(see FEDERAL RESEARCH IN PROGRESS for current information)*

Updating: Not updated

STARTEXT®

Type: Reference (Referral); Source (Textual-Numeric, Full Text)

Subject: Flight Schedules; Computers & Software; Encyclopedias; General Interest; News

Producer: STARTEXT, A Division of the Fort Worth Star-Telegram

Online Service: STARTEXT, A Division of the Fort Worth Star-Telegram

Conditions: Monthly subscription of $9.95 to STARTEXT required

Content: Provides a variety of files of information and electronic services, with an emphasis on items of interest in the Fort Worth, Texas area.

ACADEMIC AMERICAN ENCYCLOPEDIA. *(see)*

General Information. Contains international and national news stories from the Associated Press and Knight-Ridder newswire services; news items of general interest (e.g., health and medical news, religious news); local news items from the *Fort Worth Star-Telegram*; current weather and forecasts for Texas and various U.S. cities; and sports news. Also includes feature items on a variety of consumer topics (e.g., gardening, stamp collecting, motorcycle maintenance), references to sources of travel data, discussion columns for adolescents, and reviews of books and records.

Business Information. Contains closing prices for stocks traded on the American, New York, and NASDAQ Over-The-Counter markets, as well as prices for mutual funds, bonds, U.S. Treasury issues, gold, silver, and other commodities. Also includes foreign exchange rates, money rates, Moore Diversified mortgage rates, wildcat well reports, money supply reports, and real estate news.

Entertainment Guide. Contains information on concerts, nightclub performances, plays, art and museum exhibits, and films currently scheduled in the Dallas-Fort Worth area. Also provides synopses of over 6000 movies available on network or cable television and reviews of current films.

Reference Services. Contains Dallas-Fort Worth International Airport flight schedules for American and Delta Airlines; Fort Worth police information on stolen checks and credit cards, crime statistics, and top accident locations; school calendars for the Dallas, Fort Worth, and Richardson school districts; and telephone numbers for local self-help organizations. Also contains court reports from the Texas Court of Criminal Appeals, the Texas Supreme Court, and the U.S. Supreme Court.

Computer Information. Contains news and product information on Apple, Atari, Commodore, IBM, Tandy, and Texas Instruments computers; user group directories; reviews of local bulletin board systems; and other computer-related information.

Language: English

Coverage: U.S. (primarily Fort Worth, Texas area)

Time Span: Current information

Updating: Stock prices, 4 times daily; other data, varies by file.

STATE REGULATION REPORT: TOXICS

Type: Source (Full Text)

Subject: Environment; Legislative Tracking

Producer: Business Publishers, Inc.

Online Service: NewsNet, Inc.

Conditions: Monthly subscription to NewsNet required; differential charges for subscribers and non-subscribers to *State Regulation Report: Toxic Substances & Hazardous Waste*.

Content: Contains full text of *State Regulation Report: Toxic Substances & Hazardous Waste*, a newsletter on hazardous wastes and toxic substances in the environment, marketplace, and workplace. Covers state legislative, regulatory, and judicial developments and programs.

Language: English

Coverage: U.S.

Time Span: 1985 to date

Updating: Every 2 weeks

STREAMLINE: WATER INFORMATION DATABASE

Type: Reference (Bibliographic, Referral)

Subject: Aquatic Sciences; Environment; Research in Progress

Producer: Department of Resources and Energy (Australia), Water Branch

Online Service: ACI Computer Services

Conditions: Monthly minimum to ACI required; fees vary depending on service selected.

Content: Contains citations to Australian literature and research projects on all aspects of water, waste water, and the aquatic environment. Covers water quality and supply, water and the land environment, wastes, research and development, and water planning, design, and engineering. Corresponds in part to *Streamline Update* and *Water Research in Australia: Current Projects*.

Language: English

Coverage: Australia

Time Span: 1982 to date

Updating: Every 2 months; about 3000 citations and 1050 research projects a year.

SUPERINDEX

Type: Reference (Bibliographic)

Subject: Biomedicine; Science & Technology

Producer: Supersearch, Inc.

Online Service: BRS; BRS/BRKTHRU; BRS/Colleague; TECH DATA

Content: Contains back-of-the-book indexes from approximately 3000 English-language professional-level scientific, technical, engineering, and medical reference books. Covers reference works produced by over 33 major publishers, including the American Chemical Society; Annual Reviews, Inc.; Computer Science Press; CRC Press; Elsevier Science Publishers; McGraw-Hill Book Company; Prentice-Hall; Springer-Verlag; Van Nostrand; and John Wiley & Sons. Covers such reference works as *The Merck Index* and *Physicians Desk Reference*. Records include the title, author, subject index entry, page location, publisher, and the International Standard Book Number (ISBN) for the referenced publication. Types of information referenced include state-of-the-art data, standards, formulae, tables, properties, and descriptions of methods, applications, and procedures.

Language: English

Coverage: International

Time Span: Current reference works

SUPPLIER DATABASE

Type: Reference (Referral)

Subject: Information Systems & Services

Producer: DIMDI

Online Service: DIMDI

Content: Contains information on organizations that provide document delivery services for databases available through DIMDI. For each organization, includes name and address, document holdings, databases supported, and document ordering information, including available formats (e.g., photocopy, microfilm, microfiche), prices, terms of delivery, and any applicable restrictions.

Language: English

Coverage: International

Time Span: Current information

Updating: Periodically, as new data become available

SURGEON GENERAL'S INFORMATION SERVICE

Type: Reference (Bibliographic, Referral); Source (Full Text)

Subject: Biomedicine

Producer: American Medical Association (AMA), in conjunction with the U.S. Public Health Service, Office of the Surgeon General

Online Service: AMA/NET

Conditions: Subscription fee of $50 to AMA/NET required

Content: Contains news and information on public health issues from the Office of the Surgeon General, as well as references to literature on public health topics.

Excerpts from *Public Health Reports*. Contains synopses of articles from the current issue of *Public Health Reports*.

Surgeon General's Advisories. Contains official health notices from the Surgeon General's Office alerting physicians to critical health care conditions (e.g., shortages in supplies of vaccines).

Bulletins from the Surgeon General. Provides news of current activities and research.

Disease Prevention Information. Contains information provided by the Office of Disease Prevention and Health Promotion (ODPHP). Includes citations to ODPHP publications and abstracts of disease prevention research reports. "Healthfinders" provides names and addresses of clearinghouses for specific health care problems.

Language: English

Coverage: Primarily U.S. and Canada

Time Span: Current information

Updating: Periodically, as new data become available

SWEMED

Type: Reference (Bibliographic)

Subject: Biomedicine

Producer: MIC-KIBIC

Online Service: MIC-KIBIC

Content: Contains approximately 5000 citations to Swedish biomedical literature not referenced in MEDLINE *(see)*. Covers Swedish biomedical journals and reports and medical dissertations from Swedish universities.

Language: English, with titles in original Scandinavian languages

Coverage: Sweden

Time Span: 1982 to date

Updating: About 80 items every 2 weeks

TANDY NEWSLETTER

Type: Source (Full Text)

Subject: Computers & Software

Producer: Tandy Corp.

Online Service: CompuServe Information Service

Content: Contains information on Radio Shack computer products and selected other items. Includes product descriptions and information about new products, product delivery and availability, and software updates.

Language: English

Coverage: U.S.

Time Span: Current information

Updating: Weekly

TECHNO-SEARCH

Type: Reference (Bibliographic)

Subject: Science & Technology; Technology Transfer

Producer: Heiwa Information Center Co., Ltd.; Informatic Research Inc.

Online Service: Heiwa Information Center Co., Ltd.

Content: Contains about 215,000 citations, abstracts, and edited news stories from 5 major Japanese industrial and technical newspapers, including *Nikkan Kogyo Shimbun, Nippon Kogyo Shimbun, Kagaku Kogyo Nippo, Denpa Shimbun*, and *Joho Sangyo Shimbun*. Emphasis is on the development and exchange of technology in the chemical, electronics, energy, computer, and food technology industries.

Language: Japanese

Coverage: Primarily Japan, with some international news

Time Span: September 1982 to date, with some data from 1981

Updating: About 1200 records a week

TELEGEN®

Type: Reference (Bibliographic)

Subject: Biotechnology

Producer: EIC/Intelligence Inc.

Online Service: DIALOG Information Services, Inc. (TELEGEN) (as part of SUPERTECH *(see)*); DIMDI (TELE-GENLINE); ESA-IRS (TELEGENLINE)

Content: Contains citations, with abstracts, to the worldwide literature on all aspects of biotechnology and genetic engineering. Covers business and economics; social impacts and constraints; patents and legal issues; policy and regulatory issues; general and historical aspects; international discussions and general policy; industrial microbiology; applications to chemistry, energy and mining, the environment, food processing and production, crops, livestock, pharmacy, and medicine; and general research and research by specific type of gene (i.e., human, animal, plant, yeast and fungus, bacterial, or viral). Sources of data include over 7000 journals, conference papers, government reports, newspapers, and research reports. Corresponds to the *Telegen Reporter*.

Language: English

Coverage: International

Time Span: 1973 to date

Updating: Monthly; about 3600 records a year.

Teleresource

Type: Reference (Referral); Source (Software)

Subject: Computers & Software

Producer: Infotran Teleresource

Online Service: THE SOURCE

Conditions: Monthly minimum of $10 to THE SOURCE required, with $9 credited toward online usage charges

Content: Contains about 70 descriptions of software packages for personal computers that can be purchased online and downloaded. Descriptions include type of computer (e.g., Apple, IBM, Radio Shack, Texas Instruments), software language, price of program, time necessary to download program, and description of program. Program categories include games and entertainment, business and finance, education, and mathematics and science.

Time Span: Current information

Updating: Every 2 months

TERMDOK®

Type: Reference (Bibliographic, Referral)

Subject: Science & Technology; Terminology & Translations

Producer: Swedish Center for Technical Terminology

Online Service: Swedish Center for Technical Terminology (TNC)

Content: Contains translations and definitions of over 27,000 scientific and technical terms standardized by TNC or the Swedish Standards Institute. Each record contains the term in up to 10 languages (e.g., Danish, Swedish, Norwegian, Finnish, English, French, German, and Spanish) with definitions, notes and explanations about term usage, and cross-references to broader and narrower terms in Swedish.

Language: Swedish, with index terms in Danish, English, Finnish, French, German, Norwegian, and Spanish

Updating: About 500 terms a month

TERMINALS Guide

Type: Reference (Referral)

Subject: Computers & Software

Producer: Commission of the European Communities (CEC)

Online Service: ECHO Service

Content: Contains descriptions of over 350 terminals, including microcomputers, primarily those that function in asynchronous mode and are teletype compatible. Information on each terminal includes make and model; address of supplier and service offices in Europe; lease, purchase, and maintenance prices; date of first production; compatibility with Euronet; PTT approval (where applicable, e.g., Belgium, Federal Republic of Germany, United Kingdom); print and/or display characteristics; functions (e.g., cursor control, insert/delete modes, scroll mode, tab stops); ancillary devices (e.g., cassette tape, diskette drive); and communications elements (e.g., mode, interfaces, procedures, codes, parity, speeds, and connections). Corresponds to *EURONET-Diane Terminal User Guide*, published by Diebold Deutschland GmbH. Diebold obtains information from promotional literature and through contacts with manufacturers and suppliers.

Language: English

Coverage: European Economic Community (Belgium, Denmark, Federal Republic of Germany, France, Greece, Ireland, Italy, Luxembourg, The Netherlands, and U.K.)

Time Span: Current information

Updating: Periodically, as new data become available

TEXNET

Type: Reference (Referral); Source (Software)

Subject: Computers & Software

Producer: Don Bynum

Online Service: THE SOURCE

Conditions: Monthly minimum of $10 to THE SOURCE required, with $9 credited toward online usage charges

Content: Contains information of interest to users of Texas Instruments (TI) equipment, especially users of the TI 99/4. Includes software that users can download, product news and information, addresses of TI service centers, and a directory to TI users' groups.

Language: English

Time Span: Current information

Updating: Periodically, as new data become available

TIME®

Type: Source (Full Text)

Subject: General Interest; News

Producer: Time Inc.

Online Service: Mead Data Central, Inc. (as part of NEXIS MAGAZINES *(see)*); VU/TEXT Information Services, Inc.

Conditions: Subscription to Mead Data Central required; subscription to VU/TEXT required.

Content: Contains full text of *Time*, a magazine covering current national and international events, trends in economics and business, politics, sports, science and technology, medicine, religion, law, education, lifestyle patterns, and reviews of books, films, and plays.

Language: English

Coverage: International

Time Span: Mead Data Central, 1981 to date; VU/TEXT, 1985 to date.

Updating: Weekly

TITLE-SEARCH

Type: Reference (Bibliographic)

Subject: Science & Technology

Producer: Heiwa Information Center Co., Ltd.; Science & Engineering Information Center Co., Ltd.

Online Service: Heiwa Information Center Co., Ltd.

Content: Contains about 230,000 citations to Japanese scientific and technical literature. Covers government and university technical publications and articles from about 1000 journals. Includes electrical, energy, architectural, general, mechanical, and traffic engineering; chemistry and chemical engineering; environmental and sanitation engineering; nucleonics; electronics and telecommunications; computer science; metals and metal mining; and physical and life sciences. Corresponds in part to *Quick Titles of R&D in Japan*, with additional information available online.

Language: Japanese

Coverage: Japan

Time Span: September 1982 to date

Updating: About 6000 records a month

TOXIC MATERIALS NEWS

Type: Source (Full Text)

Subject: Legislative Tracking; Occupational Safety & Health

Producer: Business Publishers, Inc.

Online Service: NewsNet, Inc.

Conditions: Monthly subscription to NewsNet required; differential charges for subscribers and non-subscribers to *Toxic Materials News*.

Content: Contains full text of *Toxic Materials News*, a newsletter on the toxic substances control program of the U.S. Environmental Protection Agency. Covers the progress of regulations, from rough draft to final rulemaking, in such areas as pesticide and hazardous waste programs, toxic air and water pollutants, workplace and household product carcinogens, and transportation of hazardous materials.

Language: English

Coverage: U.S.

Time Span: 1982 to date

Updating: Weekly

TOXIC MATERIALS TRANSPORT

Type: Source (Full Text)

Subject: Environment; Legislative Tracking

Producer: Business Publishers, Inc.

Online Service: NewsNet, Inc.

Conditions: Monthly subscription to NewsNet required; differential charges for subscribers and non-subscribers to *Toxic Materials Transport*.

Content: Contains full text of *Toxic Materials Transport*, a newsletter on the legal aspects of transporting toxic, flammable, corrosive, radioactive, and other hazardous substances. Covers investigations, litigations, legislation, and regulations concerning carriers, packagers, and shippers. Also covers routing requirements, technological developments, and compliance efforts and costs.

Language: English

Coverage: U.S.

Time Span: 1985 to date

Updating: Every 2 weeks

TOXICO

Type: Reference (Bibliographic)

Subject: Toxicology

Producer: Centre de Toxicologie du Quebec

Online Service: IST-Informatheque Inc.

Content: Contains approximately 14,000 citations to the worldwide literature on toxicology. Covers clinical toxicology, including acute or chronic poisoning from drugs, medicines, and chemicals; toxic risks in the workplace; and environmental toxicology. Sources include about 2500 periodicals.

Language: French, with titles in original languages

Coverage: International

Time Span: 1974 to date

Updating: About 250 articles a month

TOXICS LAW REPORTER

Type: Source (Full Text)

Subject: Legislative Tracking; Occupational Safety & Health

Producer: The Bureau of National Affairs, Inc. (BNA)

Online Service: Executive Telecom System, Inc., Human Resource Information Network

Conditions: Annual subscription to Executive Telecom System required

Content: Contains full text of *Toxics Law Reporter*, covering major developments in federal and state legislation, litigation, and insurance issues related to hazardous substances. Covers personal injury and property damage liability, the Comprehensive Environmental Response, Compensation, and Liability Act (Superfund), the Resource Conservation and Recovery Act (RCRA), and tort law reform.

Language: English

Coverage: U.S.

Time Span: July 1986 to date

Updating: Weekly

TOXLINE®

Type: Reference (Bibliographic)

Subject: Agriculture; Biomedicine; Toxicology

Producer: National Library of Medicine, Toxicology Information Program

Online Service: DIMDI; The Japan Information Center of Science and Technology (JICST); National Library of Medicine (NLM)

Content: Contains citations, with abstracts, to the worldwide literature in all areas of toxicology, including chemicals and pharmaceuticals, pesticides, environmental pollutants, and mutagens and teratology. Comprises 13 discrete files:

Abstracts on Health Effects of Environmental Pollutants (HEEP). Contains records from the BIOSIS PREVIEWS database *(see)*, and corresponds to the *HEEP* publication. Covers effects of environmental chemicals or substances, other than medicinals, on human health. Includes abstracts and Chemical Abstracts Service (CAS) registry numbers. (1970 to date)

Aneuploidy. *(see)*

Chemical-Biological Activities (CBAC). Contains records from *Chemical Abstracts (see CA SEARCH)* that cover interactions of chemical substances with biological systems in vivo and in vitro. All records contain CAS registry numbers. (1965 to date)

Environmental Mutagen Information Center File (EMIC). *(see ENVIRONMENTAL MUTAGENS)*

Environmental Teratology Information Center File (ETIC). *(see ENVIRONMENTAL TERATOLOGY)*

Hayes File on Pesticides. Contains citations to published articles on health aspects of pesticides. Is essentially a backfile for *Pesticides Abstracts*. Does not include abstracts. (1940-1968)

Hazardous Materials Technical Center Bulletin (HMTC). Contains citations to published literature on the management of hazardous materials, including disposal, storage, and transportation. Corresponds in part to the quarterly *HMTC Abstract Bulletin*.

International Labour Office. *(see CISDOC)*

International Pharmaceutical Abstracts (IPA). *(see)*

Pesticides Abstracts. Covers published reports on the epidemiological effects of pesticides on humans, from more than 1000 journals published in the U.S. and other countries. All records contain Chemical Abstracts Service Registry Numbers. (1967 to December 1981)

Toxic Materials Information Center File (TMIC). Contains citations and abstracts on toxic materials prepared by the TMIC, Oak Ridge National Laboratory. (1940 to 1973)

Toxicity Bibliography. Is a subset of the MEDLINE database *(see)*. Covers adverse effects, toxicity, poisoning, or environmental effects caused by drugs and chemicals, as well as disease conditions induced by chemical substances or radiation. Records contain Chemical Abstracts Service Registry Numbers, when applicable. (1965 to date)

Toxicology/Epidemiology Research Projects (RPROJ). Contains descriptions of research projects supported by research grants and contracts programs of the Public Health Service, or conducted intramurally by the U.S. National Institutes of Health (NIH) and the National Institute of Mental Health in the areas of toxicology and epidemiology. Information is obtained from the NIH, Division of Research Grants, CRISP system (Computer Retrieval of Information on Scientific Projects). (1983 to date)

Toxicology Document and Data Depository (TD3). Contains citations to the report literature dealing with toxicology and related subjects. Information is obtained from the NTIS database *(see)*. (1979 to date)

Language: English
Coverage: International
Time Span: Varies by file *(see Content)*
Updating: About 12,000 records a month

TRANSIN
Type: Reference (Referral)
Subject: Technology Transfer
Producer: Transinove International
Online Service: Telesystemes-Questel
Content: Contains approximately 3500 descriptions of offers and requests for transferable technologies, including new products, processes, and techniques. Each item is described by the country of patent or country in which a license is available or sought; title; name, position, and address of patent holder or item announcer; abstract describing the technology and its advantages; country of origin; international patent classification codes that identify industrial and scientific areas of interest; developmental stage of the technology offered or sought; and technical skills required or developed. Information is obtained from such sources as research centers, public laboratories, private industry, and independent inventors. Corresponds to *La Lettre de Transinove*.
Language: Primarily English, with some records also in French, German, Italian, and Spanish
Coverage: International
Time Span: 1982 to date
Updating: About 60 records every 2 weeks

TROPAG (ATA)
Type: Reference (Bibliographic)
Subject: Agriculture
Producer: Royal Tropical Institute
Online Service: ORBIT Information Technologies Corporation
Content: Contains citations, with abstracts, to the worldwide literature on the practical aspects of tropical and subtropical agriculture. Topics covered include crop production and protection; crop processing and storage; fertilizers and soil as they relate to plant nutrition; and agricultural techniques. Also covers such areas as the social and cultural aspects of agricultural development, research and development in farming systems, and environmental aspects. References are drawn from journals, books, research reports, intergovernmental and governmental publications, symposia papers and proceedings, and extension bulletins. Corresponds to *Abstracts on Tropical Agriculture*.
Language: English
Coverage: International
Time Span: 1975 to date
Updating: About 1000 records a quarter

TSCA INITIAL INVENTORY
Type: Source (Textual-Numeric)
Subject: Toxicology
Producer: U.S. Environmental Protection Agency (EPA), Office of Pesticides and Toxic Substances
Online Service: DIALOG Information Services, Inc. (TSCA INITIAL INVENTORY); ORBIT Information Technologies Corporation (TSCA PLUS)
Content: Contains information on the approximately 60,000 chemical substances in commerce in the U.S. covered in the Toxic Substances Control Act (TSCA) Initial Inventory published June 1, 1979. Each record, providing information on one substance, includes the Chemical Abstracts Service (CAS) Registry Number, preferred name, molecular formula, and synonyms. Synonyms in the records are only those received in the inventory reports; additional synonyms provided in the corresponding printed version are not included. Confidential substances and definitions of complex substances are also excluded.
NOTE: Through ORBIT, TSCA Plant and Production *(see TSCAPP)* data are also available.

Language: English
Coverage: U.S.
Time Span: Inventory current as of May 1, 1983
Updating: Irregularly

TSCAPP (TSCA Plant and Production)

Type: Reference (Referral); Source (Textual-Numeric)
Subject: Toxicology
Producer: U.S. Environmental Protection Agency (EPA), Office of Pesticides and Toxic Substances
Online Service: Chemical Information Systems, Inc., a subsidiary of Fein-Marquart Associates (CIS); Information Consultants, Inc. (ICI) (as part of The Integrated Chemical Information System); ORBIT Information Technologies Corporation (as part of the TSCA INITIAL INVENTORY database *(see)*)
Conditions: Annual subscription fee of $300 to CIS required but fee is waived for educational institutions and non-profit public libraries worldwide; differential charges for subscribers and non-subscribers to ICI.
Content: Contains about 127,000 references to non-confidential plant and production information for approximately 55,000 unique chemical substances on the Toxic Substances Control Act (TSCA) Inventory *(see TSCA INITIAL INVENTORY)*, published June 1, 1979, plus the 1981 supplement. Data on each substance include manufacturer's name and address, chemical name, Chemical Abstracts Service Registry Number, volume produced at each site, manufacturing and import information, and the manufacturer's identification number.
Language: English
Coverage: U.S.
Updating: Periodically, as new data become available

TSCATS (Toxic Substances Control Act Test Submissions)

Type: Reference (Bibliographic); Source (Textual-Numeric)
Subject: Environment; Toxicology
Producer: U.S. Environmental Protection Agency (EPA), Office of Pesticides and Toxic Substances
Online Service: Chemical Information Systems, Inc., a subsidiary of Fein-Marquart Associates (CIS)
Conditions: Annual subscription fee of $300 to CIS required but fee is waived for educational institutions and non-profit public libraries worldwide
Content: Contains over 5000 references to chemical substances mentioned in about 1600 unpublished health and safety reports submitted by chemical manufacturers, users, and importers to the EPA under the provisions of the Toxic Substances Control Act (TSCA). Approximately 1200 different chemical substances are referenced. Each record contains chemical tracking information (e.g., TSCA section code, Chemical Abstracts Service Registry Number) on one substance, with descriptors covering health effects, environmental effects, environmental fate, study design (e.g., study type, subject organism/test system, route of exposure, test substance), and microfiche location. Users can place orders online with CIS for microfiche copies of studies.
Language: English
Coverage: U.S.
Time Span: November 1982 to date
Updating: Quarterly

TT-NYHETSBANKEN

Type: Source (Full Text)
Subject: News
Producer: Tidningarnas Telegrambyra (TT)
Online Service: DataArkiv AB
Content: Contains the full text (in Swedish) of the TT news wire. Covers international news and Swedish national, regional, and local news, weather, and sports.
Language: Swedish
Coverage: International
Time Span: July 1980 to date
Updating: About 300 records a day

U.S. GOVERNMENT PUBLICATIONS

Type: Source (Full Text)
Subject: Publishers & Distributors-Catalogs
Producer: U.S. Government Printing Office
Online Service: CompuServe Information Service
Content: Contains full text of selected U.S. government publications in the areas of food preparation and storage, fitness and health, personal finances, energy conservation, and consumer information.
Language: English
Coverage: U.S.
Time Span: Current information
Updating: Periodically, as new data become available

UKMARC

Type: Reference (Bibliographic)
Subject: Publishers & Distributors-Catalogs
Producer: The British Library
Online Service: BLAISE-LINE
Conditions: Annual subscription of 49 pounds (UK) for U.K. users or 56 pounds (UK) for other users to BLAISE Online Services required
Content: Contains bibliographic information on all books and first issues of serials published in Great Britain since 1950 and deposited with the Copyright Receipt Office of the British Library. Covers all types of publications and includes some Cataloging in Publication data. Corresponds to *British National Bibliography*.
Language: English
Coverage: U.K.
Time Span: 1950 to date
Updating: About 700 records a week

ULRICH'S INTERNATIONAL PERIODICALS DIRECTORY

Type: Reference (Bibliographic)
Subject: Publishers & Distributors-Catalogs
Producer: R.R. Bowker Company
Online Service: BRS; BRS/BRKTHRU; BRS/Colleague; DIALOG Information Services, Inc.; ESA-IRS; TECH DATA
Content: Contains citations to approximately 128,000 serial publications, including international magazines, newsletters, and general interest publications published regularly as well as annuals, continuations, conference proceedings, and other serial publications that are published at least once every 3 years. Also includes approximately 16,000 discontinued publications from 1974 to date. Corresponds to *Ulrich's International Periodicals Directory, Irregular Serials and Annuals,*

Ulrich's Quarterly, and *Sources of Serials*. Subject classification scheme utilizes Dewey Decimal numbers, abstracting and indexing services, and approximately 500 Bowker subject headings.
Language: English
Coverage: International
Time Span: Current information, with some earlier material
Updating: About 5000 records every 6 weeks

UMI ARTICLE CLEARINGHOUSE
Type: Reference (Bibliographic)
Subject: Publishers & Distributors-Catalogs
Producer: University Microfilms International (UMI)
Online Service: BRS; BRS/BRKTHRU; Dialcom, Inc.; OCLC Online Computer Library Center, Inc.; Utlas International Canada Inc.
Content: Contains citations to approximately 9000 periodicals and serials from which articles can be ordered from UMI. Publications cover such topics as chemistry, computer science, earth sciences, engineering, life sciences, mathematics, medicine, physics, arts, business and management, communications, current events, economics, education, general interest, history, and nursing. For each publication, includes title, available years, International Standard Book Number (ISBN) or International Standard Serial Number (ISSN), CODEN, UMI order number, imprint, and other bibliographic information. Users can order articles online. Corresponds to *UMI Article Clearinghouse Catalog*.
Language: English, with titles in original languages
Coverage: International
Time Span: Primarily 1978 to date, with selected coverage of earlier materials
Updating: Monthly

UMWELTFORSCHUNGSDATENBANK (UFOR)
Type: Reference (Bibliographic)
Subject: Environment; Research in Progress
Producer: Umweltbundesamt
Online Service: DATA-STAR
Content: Contains about 20,000 citations, with abstracts, to planned, ongoing, and completed environment-related research projects in Austria and the Federal Republic of Germany. Covers ecology; environmental aspects of the agriculture, fishing, forestry, food, and energy industries; government policy; environmental education; air, water, soil, and noise pollution; pollutants, including chemicals, fumes, and waste; environment and the economy; landscape protection; and rural and urban development. Provides name and academic qualifications of project leader, name and address of institution where research is being done, information on total cost of project, location of research subject (e.g., Rhine valley), sponsoring institution name, contract or grant number (Foerderungskennzeichen (FKZ)), Umweltbundesamt's Ufokat (Umweltforschungskatalog) reference number, names of cooperating institutions, and publications related to the project. Sources include Federal Republic of Germany governmental departments and the Austrian Ministry for Health Care in Vienna.
Language: German, with some titles and abstracts also in English
Coverage: Austria and Federal Republic of Germany
Time Span: 1974 to date
Updating: About 1000 records twice a year

UMWELTLITERATURDATENBANK (ULIT)
Type: Reference (Bibliographic)
Subject: Environment
Producer: Umweltbundesamt
Online Service: DATA-STAR
Content: Contains about 60,000 citations, with abstracts, to primarily German-language literature on environmental topics relating to the Federal Republic of Germany. Covers ecology; environmental aspects of the agriculture, fishing, forestry, food, and energy industries; government policy; environmental education; air, water, soil, and noise pollution; pollutants, including chemicals, fumes, and waste; environment and the economy; landscape protection; and rural and urban development. Sources include Bundesforschungsanstalt fuer Naturschutz und Landschaftsoekologie, Informationsdienst Technischer Umweltschutz, Institut fuer Paedagogik der Naturwissenschaften, Landesanstalt fuer Immissionsschutz des Landes Nordrhein-Westfalen, as well as monographs, journals, and literature on research and development projects sponsored by the German Ministry of Internal Affairs and the Umweltbundesamt (Federal Environmental Agency, Federal Republic of Germany).
Language: German, with some titles and abstracts also in English
Coverage: Federal Republic of Germany
Time Span: 1976 to date
Updating: About 1000 records a month

UNION (Union List of Scientific Serials in Canadian Libraries)
Type: Reference (Bibliographic)
Subject: Library Holdings-Catalogs
Producer: CISTI
Online Service: CISTI, Canadian Online Enquiry Service (CAN/OLE)
Conditions: CISTI accessible only in Canada
Content: Contains citations to approximately 76,000 scientific, technical, and medical serials held by more than 295 Canadian libraries. Information on each serial includes title, place of publication, issuing/sponsoring body, notes, and standard interlibrary loan code for each library that owns the serial. Corresponds to *Union List of Scientific Serials in Canadian Libraries. (See also DOBIS)*
Language: English
Coverage: International
Updating: Every 2 weeks

UNION CATALOGUE OF BIOMEDICAL SERIALS
Type: Reference (Bibliographic)
Subject: Library Holdings-Catalogs
Producer: Secretariat RPM/VMZ
Online Service: DATA-STAR
Content: Contains over 13,000 references for biomedical journals held in about 300 Swiss libraries. Also covers forthcoming and discontinued titles. Titles are cataloged in accordance with International Standard Bibliographic Description (Serials) (ISBD(S)). Information is also provided on each holding library, including name, address, and availability of journal photocopies.
Language: English
Coverage: Primarily Switzerland, with some international coverage

Time Span: 1985 to date
Updating: Quarterly

UNITED STATES LAW WEEK

Type: Source (Full Text)
Subject: Legislative Tracking
Producer: The Bureau of National Affairs, Inc. (BNA)
Online Service: Mead Data Central, Inc. (as part of LEXIS GENERAL FEDERAL LIBRARY); West Publishing Company (to be available in 1987)
Conditions: Subscription to Mead Data Central required; subscription to West Publishing Company required.
Content: Contains full text of Sections 1, 2, and 3 of *United States Law Week*, providing an overview of precedent-setting cases in all areas of law and from all jurisdictions. Includes detailed reports of key legislation and regulatory actions and U.S. Supreme Court proceedings from docketing through denial or formal review. Covers criminal law, labor law, civil rights, taxation, court reform, environmental law, energy law, consumer protection, economic controls, trade regulation, and procedural amendments. Excludes Supreme Court opinions available in the printed version.
Language: English
Coverage: U.S.
Time Span: 1982 to date
Updating: Weekly

UPI DataBase

Type: Source (Full Text)
Subject: News
Producer: Comtex Scientific Corporation, as the licensee for United Press International
Online Service: Dialcom, Inc. (UPI); DIALOG Information Services, Inc. (UPI NEWS); Mead Data Central, Inc. (UPI) (as part of NEXIS WIRE SERVICES *(see)*); NewsNet, Inc. (UPI); THE SOURCE (UPI); Western Union Telegraph Company (UPI NEWS) (as an FYI NEWS SERVICE database *(see)*)
Conditions: Subscription to Mead Data Central required; monthly subscription to NewsNet required; monthly minimum of $10 to THE SOURCE required, with $9 credited toward online usage charges.
Content: Contains full text of items from the United Press International (UPI) newswire service. Covers international news; U.S. general, regional, and state news; columns, standing features, and commentaries; and financial news. Also includes the stock market service, business text wire, and all-sports wire.
NOTE: On NewsNet, news items are accessible only through NewsFlash, a selective dissemination service, and are retained 2 weeks for each user.
Language: English
Coverage: International
Time Span: DIALOG, April 1983 to date; NewsNet, most current 2 weeks; THE SOURCE, current 7 days.
Updating: Most services, continuously, throughout the day; DIALOG, daily, with records added 48 hours after they appear on the newswire.

USA TODAY BROADCAST

Type: Source (Full Text)
Subject: News
Producer: Gannett New Media Services

Online Service: THE SOURCE
Conditions: Monthly fee of $75 includes 3 hours of connect time
Content: Contains topical news features and summary reports gathered and written for radio broadcast by *USA Today* reporters. Covers lifestyles, health, personal finance, travel, entertainment, sports, and weather.
Language: English
Coverage: Primarily U.S.
Time Span: Current information
Updating: Daily

USA TODAY UPDATE™

Type: Source (Full Text)
Subject: News
Producer: Gannett New Media Services
Online Service: Dialcom, Inc.; General Electric Information Services Company (GEISCO); GTE Telemail; Quantum Computer Services, Inc.
Conditions: Subscription to individual DECISIONLINES reports required on most services; fees for access vary by service.
Content: Contains 3 files of news reports, HOTLINES, DECISIONLINES, and SPECIAL REPORTS, excerpted from *USA Today* newspaper and 200 other sources, including major U.S. newspapers (e.g., *The Boston Globe*, *The New York Times*, *The Philadelphia Inquirer*), news services, newsletters, and trade magazines. HOTLINES contains hourly reports on general, business, and financial news and the weather. DECISIONLINES contains summaries of the current day's news in selected industry areas (e.g., banking, energy, insurance, real estate) and features on trends and issues affecting U.S. business. SPECIAL REPORTS contains in-depth reports on stories of topical interest.
NOTE: Specific subject coverage within each file varies among the online services.
Language: English
Coverage: Primarily U.S., with some international news
Time Span: Current information
Updating: HOTLINES, hourly; DECISIONLINES, daily; SPECIAL REPORTS, periodically, as new reports become available.

USCLASS

Type: Reference (Bibliographic)
Subject: Patents
Producer: Derwent Inc.
Online Service: ORBIT Information Technologies Corporation
Content: Contains current classification information for over 4.7 million patents issued by the U.S. Patent and Trademark Office since 1790. Covers all U.S. Classifications, Cross-Reference Classifications, and Unofficial Classifications. Searching can be performed by classification or by patent number.
Language: English
Coverage: U.S.
Time Span: 1790 to date
Updating: Twice a year

USDA ONLINE

Type: Reference (Bibliographic, Referral) ; Source (Full Text)

Subject: Agriculture; Conferences & Meetings; Food Sciences & Nutrition; Government-U.S. Federal; Veterinary Sciences

Producer: U.S. Department of Agriculture (USDA) , Office of Governmental and Public Affairs (OGPA)

Online Service: Dialcom, Inc. (as a FEDNEWS database)

Content: Contains information on a variety of topics prepared by the USDA and its agencies. Includes national and state agricultural statistics, from *Crop and Livestock Reports*; reports on world agricultural trade, from the Foreign Agricultural Service; the *Outlook and Situation Summary*, from the Economic Research Service; commodity analyses, from the Cooperative Extension Services; synopses of USDA-sponsored research and a file of frequently requested facts on U.S. agriculture and USDA-sponsored programs (e.g., the number of children fed through school lunch programs, the number of people fed by production from the average U.S. farm) . Also includes a daily summary of agricultural news from major news publications (e.g., *The New York Times, Time Magazine*) and wire services.

Provides a calendar of meetings, conferences, and exhibitions sponsored by the USDA, agricultural agencies, and related organizations (e.g., the American Farm Bureau, land-grant universities with agricultural extension services) . Includes the name of the event, sponsoring organization, date, location, and speakers. Also provides a directory of food and nutrition experts (e.g., dieticians, nutritionists) within USDA, land-grant universities, or state extension services; a bibliography of U.S. government publications on food and nutrition; and press releases and publications on nutrition. Information from USDA and the Food and Drug Administration on veterinary sciences (e.g., citations to agency publications, press releases, reports) is also available.

Language: English

Coverage: U.S.

Time Span: Press releases, current month; news summary, current week; calendar of events, to 1988; other information, varies by file.

Updating: Varies by file

USPATENTS

Type: Reference (Bibliographic)

Subject: Patents

Producer: Derwent Inc.

Online Service: ORBIT Information Technologies Corporation

Content: Contains citations, with abstracts, to U.S. patents, reissues, continuations, divisionals, defense documents, and designs issued since 1970. Includes information listed on the front page of the patent and the text of all claims, which describe aspects of the patent in legal terms. Searchable elements of information include patent and application number; filing date; publication date; terms from the title, abstract, and full text of the claim; inventor and assignee name and location; earlier foreign priority filings; prior application information, including application number, patent number (when granted) , status, and dates; examiner and attorney names; all cited references, including those of U.S. patents, non-U.S. patents, and other literature; and all U.S. and international patent classifications.

NOTE: Patents issued in the most recent 18 to 24 months are listed in USPATENTS ALERT (USPA) .

Language: English

Coverage: U.S.

Time Span: 1970 to date

Updating: Weekly

UTLAS CATSS (CATalog Support Service)

Type: Reference (Bibliographic)

Subject: Library Holdings-Catalogs

Producer: Utlas International Canada Inc. and client libraries

Online Service: Utlas International Canada Inc.; Utlas International U.S. Inc.

Content: Contains over 32 million cataloging records from the National Library of Canada, Bibliotheque Nationale du Quebec, U.S. Library of Congress, U.S. National Library of Medicine, The British Library, Universite Laval, CONSER, and other source agencies. Also includes REMARC *(see)* records and original cataloging records and order records from client libraries. Covers books, serials, audiovisual materials, music, maps, and manuscripts. The system provides technical support to libraries in shared cataloging (including authority control) , interlibrary loan services, acquisitions, reference, and online catalogs.

Language: Primarily English and French, with representation of over 70 other languages

Coverage: International

Time Span: 1968 to date, with some earlier materials

Updating: Continuously, throughout the day

VANYTT

Type: Reference (Bibliographic)

Subject: Environment; Library Holdings-Catalogs

Producer: K-Konsult

Online Service: K-Konsult

Content: Contains approximately 38,000 citations, with abstracts, to literature on the environment and environmental technology from the holdings of the k-Konsult library. Topics covered include conservation; air, noise, and water pollution; pollution control; water supply and treatment; sewage systems and treatment; industrial waste and waste water; sludge handling and treatment; solid waste treatment and recovery; and the occupational environment. Sources covered include monographs, technical reports, and over 300 technical journals.

Language: Primarily English, German, Norwegian, and Swedish

Coverage: International

Time Span: 1970 to date

Updating: About 300 records 8 times a year

VectorBank®

Type: Source (Textual-Numeric)

Subject: Biotechnology; Life Sciences

Producer: IntelliGenetics, Inc., An IntelliCorp Company

Online Service: Bionet; IntelliGenetics, Inc., An IntelliCorp Company

Conditions: To access through Bionet, users must be qualified principal investigators employed by a non-profit organization

Content: Contains 135 maps of the 27 most frequently used cloning vectors. Sources include GenBank *(see)*, EMBL NUCLEOTIDE SEQUENCE DATA LIBRARY *(see)* and NBRF-PIR PROTEIN SEQUENCE DATABASE *(see)*.

Language: English
Coverage: International
Time Span: 1967 to date
Updating: Twice a year

VENDOR INFORMATION FILE®
Type: Reference (Referral)
Subject: Products & Vendors
Producer: Information Handling Services (IHS)
Online Service: BRS; BRS/BRKTHRU; BRS/Colleague; TECH DATA
Content: Contains references to over 32,000 manufacturers and vendors of industrial products, including components, equipment, and machinery related to architectural engineering, transportation and materials handling, medicine and health care, construction, electrical and electronic engineering, and marine and metric design. Provides manufacturer or vendor name, address, addresses of sales offices, brand and trade names, tables of content from vendor catalog, and a reference to the cartridge and frame location in IHS's VSMF (Visual Search Microfilm System) for the complete catalog page.
Language: English
Coverage: U.S., with selected coverage of non-U.S. vendors that have major corporate sales offices located in the U.S.
Time Span: Current information
Updating: About 250 records a month

VERTICAL FILE INDEX℠
Type: Reference (Bibliographic)
Subject: General Interest; Publishers & Distributors-Catalogs
Producer: The H.W. Wilson Company
Online Service: WILSONLINE (to be available in 1987)
Content: Contains citations to English-language non-book materials of general interest, including charts and posters, booklets, pamphlets, museum catalogs, exhibition bulletins, and government and university publications. Covers agriculture, art, business, careers, current events, energy conservation, food and nutrition, geography, history, hobbies, home repair, law, medicine and health, personal finance, and travel. Complete ordering information is provided for each item. Corresponds to *Vertical File Index*.
Language: English
Coverage: International
Time Span: Fall 1985 to date
Updating: Twice a week

VETDOC (Veterinary Literature Documentation)
Type: Reference (Bibliographic)
Subject: Veterinary Sciences
Producer: Derwent Publications Ltd.
Online Service: ORBIT Information Technologies Corporation
Conditions: Subscription to *VETDOC ABSTRACTS JOURNAL* required
Content: Contains citations, with abstracts, to the worldwide journal literature on veterinary drugs, vaccines, growth promotants, toxicology, and hormonal control of breeding. Subject areas covered include analysis, biochemistry, chemistry, endocrinology, microbiology, pathology, pharmacology, zoology, and management. Corresponds to the biweekly *VETDOC ABSTRACTS JOURNAL*. Each record contains indepth keywording and fragmentation codes.

Language: English
Coverage: International
Time Span: 1968 to date
Updating: About 400 records a month

VETERINARY COMPUTERIZED INFORMATION SYSTEM (VCIS)
Type: Reference (Referral); Source (Full Text)
Subject: Products & Vendors; Veterinary Sciences
Producer: The Veterinary Information Company, Inc.
Online Service: The Veterinary Information Company, Inc. (as a database on Dialcom, Inc.)
Conditions: Initiation fee of $495 to The Veterinary Information Company, Inc. required; access limited to individuals in the animal health field.
Content: Contains a variety of information services for animal health professionals.

Veterinary Stock*Finder. Contains information on about 15,000 products of use in animal health care and research, available from over 800 different vendors. Covers drugs, medical devices, diagnostic aids, dressings, vitamins, and other products. Information on each product includes name, unit price, and vendor name, address, and telephone number. Sources are manufacturers' and distributors' catalogs. Users may order products online.

Also provides a variety of electronic services, including forums on animal health and veterinary medicine, announcements from the Society of Veterinary Hospital Pharmacists, listings of computer hardware or software for rent or sale, listings of employment and business opportunities, electronic mail, and software programs for statistical manipulation of research data.

NOTE: Users may also access OAG-EE *(see)*, TRAVEL SCAN *(see)*, FDA ELECTRONIC BULLETIN BOARD *(see)*, and USDA ONLINE *(see)* available through Dialcom, Inc., as well as databases available through DIALOG Information Services, Inc.
Language: English
Coverage: Primarily U.S., with international coverage of products to be added
Time Span: Current information
Updating: Monthly

VITIS (Viticulture and Enology Abstracts)
Type: Reference (Bibliographic)
Subject: Agriculture
Producer: Bundesforschunganstalt fuer Rebenzuechtung; International Food Information Service (IFIS)
Online Service: DIALOG Information Services, Inc. (as part of FSTA *(see)*); DIMDI
Content: Contains approximately 25,000 citations to the worldwide literature on the science and technology of wine production. Covers viticulture, enology, microbiology, biochemistry, plant pathology, soils, trade, and economics. Provides references to journals, books, pamphlets, standards and specifications, legislation, patents, and reports. Corresponds to *Vitis*.
Language: English
Coverage: International
Time Span: 1969 to date
Updating: About 400 records a quarter

VOCATIONAL EDUCATION CURRICULUM MATERIALS

Type: Reference (Bibliographic, Referral)
Subject: Education & Educational Institutions
Producer: The National Center for Research in Vocational Education
Online Service: BRS; BRS After Dark; BRS/BRKTHRU; BRS/Colleague; TECH DATA
Content: Contains over 5000 citations, with abstracts, to print and non-print instructional materials in vocational and technical education. Covers guides, textbooks, workbooks, catalogs, films, and computer courseware. Each reference provides the title, year of publication, sponsoring agency, name of developer, intended users, educational level, subject descriptors, name and address of organization from which the item is available, and cost. Information is collected by 6 regional centers of the National Network for Curriculum Coordination in Vocational and Technical Education. Subject descriptors are assigned from *A Classification of Instructional Programs*, a thesaurus of the National Center for Education Statistics.
Language: English
Coverage: U.S.
Time Span: 1980 to date, with some coverage of earlier materials
Updating: About 250 records a quarter

WAIT INDEX TO NEWSPAPERS

Type: Reference (Bibliographic)
Subject: News
Producer: Western Australian Institute of Technology, T.L. Robertson Library
Online Service: ACI Computer Services
Conditions: Monthly minimum to ACI required; fees vary depending on service selected.
Content: Contains citations, with abstracts, to items in *The National Times* newspaper. Covers all major articles and book and film reviews. Also includes selected items from *The Business Review* for the period when it was a supplement to *The National Times* (September 1980-March 1981).
Language: English
Coverage: Australia
Time Span: 1980 to date
Updating: Every 2 months

WASTE MANAGEMENT AND RESOURCE RECOVERY

Type: Reference (Bibliographic)
Subject: Environment
Producer: International Research & Evaluation
Online Service: International Research & Evaluation
Content: Contains citations, with abstracts, to the worldwide literature covering solid, liquid, hazardous, and nuclear waste management; water quality; toxic substances; land reclamation; and resources recovery. Emphasis in these areas is on air pollution, agricultural engineering, civil engineering, food science, geology, and nuclear science. Sources include government reports, journal articles, monographs, proceedings, news items, patents, and other databases.
Language: English
Coverage: International
Time Span: March 1971 to date, with some materials from 1934
Updating: Every 2 weeks; about 67,250 records a year.

WATER RESOURCES ABSTRACTS

Type: Reference (Bibliographic)
Subject: Aquatic Sciences; Environment
Producer: U.S. Department of the Interior, Geological Survey
Online Service: DIALOG Information Services, Inc.
Content: Contains about 180,000 citations, with abstracts, to scientific and technical literature on the water-resource-related aspects of the physical, social, and life sciences. Also covers related engineering and legal aspects of the characteristics, conservation, control, use, and management of water resources. Topics covered include the nature of water and water cycles; water supply augmentation and conservation; water quantity management and control; water quality management and protection; water resources planning; and engineering works. Corresponds to *Selected Water Resources Abstracts*.
Language: English
Coverage: International
Time Span: 1968 to date
Updating: About 500 records a month

WATERLIT

Type: Reference (Bibliographic)
Subject: Aquatic Sciences
Producer: South African Water Information Centre
Online Service: Pergamon InfoLine
Content: Contains over 105,000 citations to the worldwide literature on water and related subjects. Covers hydrology and limnology, ecology, wastewater and pollution, recycling, desalinization, engineering and construction, and planning and management. Sources include journals, conference proceedings, government reports, and patents.
Language: English
Coverage: International
Time Span: 1976 to date
Updating: About 1300 records a month

WATERNET™

Type: Reference (Bibliographic)
Subject: Aquatic Sciences; Environment
Producer: American Water Works Association (AWWA)
Online Service: DIALOG Information Services, Inc.
Content: Contains over 18,000 citations, with abstracts, to literature on water quality, water utility management, analytical procedures for water quality testing, energy-related economics, water system materials, water and wastewater treatment and reuse, industrial and potable uses of water, and environmental issues related to water. Includes these specific topics: the drinking water industry, water pollution, health effects, toxicology, water rates, water conservation, energy costs, and the history of water supply. Items are selected from books, conference proceedings, journals, newsletters, standards, handbooks, water quality standard test methods, and all AWWA and AWWA Research Foundation (AWWARF) publications, e.g., *Annual Conference Proceedings, Water Quality Technology Conference Proceedings, Distribution System Symposium Proceedings, Conference Seminars*, and *AWWARF Quality Research Newsletter* from 1973 to date. Also covers selected non-AWWA items. Corresponds in part to the index of the *Journal AWWA*.
Language: English
Coverage: Primarily North America, with some coverage of Europe, Australia, and South Africa

Time Span: 1971 to date
Updating: About 750 records every 2 months

WETLAND VALUES BIBLIOGRAPHIC DATABASE

Type: Reference (Bibliographic)
Subject: Aquatic Sciences; Environment
Producer: U.S. Army Corps of Engineers, Waterways Experiment Station; U.S. Department of the Interior, Fish and Wildlife Service, Division of Biological Services
Online Service: EG & G Idaho, through a contract with U.S. Department of Energy, Idaho National Engineering Laboratory
Conditions: Available to U.S. federal, state, and local government agencies, universities, and firms under contract to the U.S. federal government
Content: Contains approximately 5000 citations, with abstracts, to literature on functions and values of wetlands in the U.S. Covers food chain, habitat, human use, hydrologic and water quality values, as well as wetland value assessment techniques, economic models, and related bibliographies. In addition to standard bibliographic information, each record contains subject, hydrologic unit, ecoregion, landform, land surface form, location, U.S. Army Corps of Engineers Districts, and wetland type. Sources include scientific journals, government publications, and theses.
Language: English
Coverage: U.S.
Time Span: Varies, with most data from 1950 to date
Updating: Monthly

WICHITA EAGLE-BEACON

Type: Source (Full Text)
Subject: News
Producer: Wichita Eagle and Beacon Publishing Co., Inc.
Online Service: VU/TEXT Information Services, Inc.
Conditions: Subscription to VU/TEXT required
Content: Contains full text of news items, columns, feature articles, and editorials from the *Wichita Eagle-Beacon* (Kansas) newspaper.
Language: English
Coverage: U.S. (primarily Wichita, Kansas area)
Time Span: October 1984 to date
Updating: Daily

WILDSCAPE

Type: Reference (Bibliographic)
Subject: Environment
Producer: Nature Conservancy Council
Online Service: Datasolve Limited
Conditions: Monthly subscription to Datasolve required
Content: Contains citations, with abstracts, to British books, reports, periodicals, and unpublished papers on ecology. Covers nature conservation, wildlife management, farming and wildlife, and landscape planning. Sources also include commissioned research papers and unpublished reports from the Nature Conservancy Council.
Language: English
Coverage: International
Time Span: 1983 to date
Updating: Periodically, as new data become available

WILEY CATALOG/ONLINE

Type: Reference (Bibliographic, Referral)
Subject: Publishers & Distributors-Catalogs
Producer: John Wiley & Sons, Inc.
Online Service: DIALOG Information Services, Inc.
Content: Contains citations to products published, sold, or distributed by John Wiley & Sons, Inc., as well as to selected products from other Wiley divisions and subsidiaries. Covers about 10,000 available and 20,000 forthcoming and out-of-print books, journals, other types of publications, software, and databases. Each record contains table of content (for publications), order information, and details on market rights, book-trade discounts, and special pricing. References to former Wiley products now handled by others are also included. Covers a wide range of subjects, including business, medicine, computer science, mathematics, architecture, chemistry, engineering, and life sciences. Users can order available items online. Corresponds to Wiley's *General Catalog*.
Language: English
Coverage: U.S.
Time Span: 1908 to date, with data on out-of-print materials retained indefinitely
Updating: About 200 records every 2 months

WLN (Western Library Network)

Type: Reference (Bibliographic)
Subject: Library Holdings-Catalogs
Producer: Member libraries of the Western Library Network and Library of Congress (LC)
Online Service: Western Library Network (WLN)
Conditions: Available only to subscribing libraries in the Pacific Northwest and Southwest United States and British Columbia and Alberta, Canada.
Content: A database system that provides reference, technical support (including authority control) and interlibrary loan services to libraries, through an integrated, shared cataloging and acquisition system. The basic Bibliographic File comprises approximately 3.5 million cataloging records from the Library of Congress MARC tapes, Government Printing Office Tapes, and original cataloging of member libraries. This collection of records covers books, serials, audiovisual media, music scores, and sound recordings. Users may draw upon existing cataloging records or create original records for items that have not previously been cataloged. Access points to the Bibliographic File include author, keywords in title, and corporate/conference headings, subject, series, LC card number, ISBN, and ISSN. Output may be requested for online display and offline, for catalog cards, bibliographies, or COM fiche or film catalog production. Records may also be produced on magnetic tape. The Bibliographic File is linked with the Acquisitions File for easy retrieval of bibliographic data that will be used in acquisitions. It is also linked with the Authority File which contains name, subject, and series headings. The linked Acquisitions System allows users to send purchase orders for library materials online from WLN to 14 U.S. book and serial vendors; also provides full online fund accounting.
Language: Primarily English
Coverage: International
Updating: About 9000 records a week

WORLD ENVIRONMENT REPORT®

Type: Source (Full Text)

Subject: Environment

Producer: Business Publishers, Inc.

Online Service: NewsNet, Inc.

Conditions: Monthly subscription to NewsNet required; differential charges for subscribers and non-subscribers to *World Environment Report*.

Content: Contains full text of *World Environment Report*, a newsletter covering environmental issues and trends worldwide. Topics include new methods of controlling air and water pollution; new methods for controlling toxic substances; waste management; land use planning; and natural resources development.

Language: English

Coverage: International

Time Span: 1982 to date

Updating: Every 2 weeks

WORLD REPORTER℠

Type: Source (Full Text)

Subject: News

Producer: Datasolve Limited and others

Online Service: Datasolve Limited; Info Globe; VU/TEXT Information Services, Inc.

Conditions: Initiation fee of $125 to Info Globe includes user manual and one-half hour of online connect time; subscription to VU/TEXT required.

Content: Contains full text of about 475,000 news items, articles, and broadcast transcripts from press, radio, and news agencies. Newspapers include the *Financial Times* (London and Frankfurt) since February 28, 1985; *The Economist* since December 26, 1981; *The Guardian* (Manchester) since May 1, 1984; *The Washington Post (see THE ELECTRONIC WASHINGTON POST LIBRARY)* since 1984; and the British tabloid *Today* since March 1986. Also includes *Keesing's Contemporary Archives* since 1983 and *New Scientist* since August 29, 1985. News agencies include The Associated Press (Europe wire) since September 9, 1983; Agence France-Presse since February 1985; TASS since November 17th, 1985; and Asahi News Service since August 2, 1982. Sources of radio transcripts include the BBC "Summary of World Broadcasts and Monitoring Reports" and the BBC "External Services News" since 1982.

Language: English

Coverage: International

Time Span: Varies by source *(see Content)*

Updating: BBC, *Financial Times*, *The Guardian*, *Today*, and news services, daily; *The Washington Post*, twice a week; *The Economist* and *New Scientist*, weekly; *Keesing's*, monthly.

WORLD TRANSINDEX

Type: Reference (Bibliographic)

Subject: Science & Technology

Producer: Centre National de la Recherche Scientifique, Centre de Documentation Scientifique et Technique (CNRS/CDST); International Translations Centre

Online Service: ESA-IRS

Content: Contains about 150,000 citations to translations of scientific and technical literature. Covers translations from all languages into Western languages. All fields of science and technology are covered. Corresponds to *World Transindex*.

Language: English

Coverage: International

Time Span: 1977 to date

Updating: About 25,000 records a year

WPI (World Patents Index)

Type: Reference (Bibliographic)

Subject: Patents

Producer: Derwent Publications Ltd.

Online Service: DIALOG Information Services, Inc.; ORBIT Information Technologies Corporation; SDC of Japan, Ltd.; Telesystemes-Questel

Conditions: Differential charges for subscribers and non-subscribers to Derwent printed publications

Content: Contains citations, with abstracts, to chemical, electrical, and mechanical patents issued by 29 major patent-issuing authorities. Data elements include title; patent assignee and inventor name; patent numbers; ICIREPAT country; priority and publication dates; and various classification and subject codes. Corresponds to coverage in the abstracts publications, *Chemical Patents Index* (CPI), *World Patents Abstracts* (WPA), and *Electrical Patents Index* (EPI).

NOTE: WPIL (WORLD PATENTS INDEX-LATEST) contains all basic and corresponding equivalent patent records, 1981 to date. Beginning in 1982, Japanese electrical patents are included.

Coverage: International

Time Span: Varies by subject area, with earliest data from 1963

Updating: About 6800 new patents and 6200 equivalent filings a week

ZOOLOGICAL RECORD ONLINE®

Type: Reference (Bibliographic)

Subject: Life Sciences

Producer: BioSciences Information Service, in cooperation with The Zoological Society of London

Online Service: BRS; BRS After Dark; BRS/BRKTHRU; BRS/Colleague; DIALOG Information Services, Inc.

Content: Contains more than 300,000 citations to the worldwide literature on zoology, with systematic and taxonomic information for 25 animal groups, including Mammalia, Aves, Reptilia, Amphibia, Pisces, Protochordata, Hemiptera, Insecta, Crustacea, and Protozoa. Subject areas covered include taxonomy, physiology, morphology, parasitology, biochemistry, biophysics, evolution, ecology, genetics, behavior, biometrics, communication, disease, habitat, histology, immunology, life cycle and development, locomotion, nomenclature, techniques, and zoogeography. Includes items from over 6000 sources, including journals, books, monographs, newsletters, and conference proceedings. Up to 6 levels of names from a systematic classification are assigned for each biological organism that is the subject of a record. Corresponds to *Zoological Record*.

Language: English

Coverage: International

Time Span: 1978 to date

Updating: Monthly

3rd Base, Division of STEL Enterprises
P.O. Box 6354
Lafayette, IN 47903
   317/742-5369

ABA
   (see American Bar Association)

ACI Computer Services
AUSINET
310 Ferntree Gully Road
Clayton, VIC 3168
Australia
   61 (3) 544-8433
   Telex 33852 ACICS AA

Agence Nationale pour la Recuperation
et l'Elimination des Dechets
  (ANRED)
Centre National de Documentation sur
  les Dechets
2 Square Lafayette
B.P. 406
49004 Angers Cedex
France
   33 (41) 87 29 24
   Telex 721325 F

Agenzia ANSA
94, via della Dataria
00187 Rome
Italy
   39 (6) 677 41
   Telex 612220 I

AGNET
University of Nebraska
Lincoln, NE 68583
   402/472-1892
   Telex 484340 UNL COMM LCN

Agriculture Canada, Research Branch
K.W. Neatby Building, Room 1133
Ottawa, Ontario K1A 0C6
Canada
   613/995-9073
   Telex 0533283

AgriData Network
AgriData Resources, Inc.
330 East Kilbourne Avenue
Milwaukee, WI 53202
   414/278-7676
   800/558-9044
   800/242-6001 (in WI)
   TWX 910-262-3360

AMA/NET
535 North Dearborn Street
Chicago, IL 60610
   312/645-5000

American Bar Association (ABA)
750 North Lake Shore Drive
Chicago, IL 60611
   312/988-5158
   800/621-6159

ANRED
   *(see Agence Nationale pour la
   Recuperation et l'Elimination des
   Dechets)*

Applied Videotex Systems
490 Trapelo Road
Belmont, MA 02178
   617/484-6814

ARAMIS
Swedish Center for Working Life
Box 5606
114 86 Stockholm
Sweden
   46 (8) 22 99 80

ARAMIS
Swedish National Board of Occupa-
  tional Safety and Health
Library/CIS Service
171 84 Solna
Sweden
   46 (8) 730 90 00
   Telex 15816 ARBSKY S

ARAMIS
The Swedish National Environmental
  Protection Board
Library and Documentation Section
Box 1302
171 24 Solna
Sweden
   46 (8) 799 10 00

Asian Institute of Technology
P.O. Box 2754
Bangkok 10501
Thailand
   66 (2) 5920100-13
   Telex 84276 TH

Australian Medline Network
National Library of Australia
Parkes Place
Canberra ACT 2600
Australia
   61 (62) 62-1523
   Telex 62100 NATLIBAUST AA

Battelle, Centre de Recherches
7 route de Drize
1277 Carouge/Geneva
Switzerland
   41 (22) 27 02 70
   Telex 423472 BATEL CH

BELINDIS
Belgian Ministry of Economic Affairs
Rue J.A. de Mot 30
1040 Brussels
Belgium
   32 (2) 233 67 37
   Telex 23509 ENERGI B

Bertelsmann InformationsService GmbH
Rosenkavalierplatz 4
8000 Munich 81
Federal Republic of Germany
   49 (89) 9 26 90 70
   Telex 17898331 D

Beth Israel Hospital
   (see PaperChase)

Bibliographic Retrieval Services
   (see BRS)

Bionet
c/o IntelliGenetics
124 University Avenue
Palo Alto, CA 94301
   415/382-4870

BLAISE-LINE
The British Library
Marketing and Support Group
Bibliographic Services
2 Sheraton Street
London W1V 4BH
England
   44 (1) 636-1544 x258 or x290
   Telex 21462 BLREF G

BLAISE-LINK
The British Library
Marketing Office
Bibliographic Services
2 Sheraton Street
London W1V 4BH
England
   44 (1) 636-1544 x245 or x253
   Telex 21462 BLREF G

Bolt, Beranek & Newman, Inc.
Computer Systems Division
10 Moulton Street
Cambridge, MA 02238
   617/497-2742
   Telex 921470
   TWX 710-320-7700

The British Library
   (see BLAISE-LINK)

The British Library
   (see BLAISE-LINE)

BRS
BRS Information Technologies
1200 Route 7
Latham, NY 12110
   518/783-1161
   800/345-4277
   TWX 710-444-4965

ADDRESSES OF ONLINE SERVICES AND GATEWAYS

BRS After Dark
1200 Route 7
Latham, NY 12110
  518/783-1161
  800/345-4277
  TWX 710-444-4965

BRS/BRKTHRU
1200 Route 7
Latham, NY 12110
  518/783-1161
  800/345-4277
  TWX 710-444-4965

BRS/Colleague
555 East Lancaster Avenue, 4th Floor
St. Davids, PA 19087
  212/765-4840
  800/833-4707
  800/553-5566 (in NY)

BT Dialcom
(see Dialcom, Inc.)

Business Connection
(see DIALOG Information Services, Inc.)

CAB International
Farnham House
Farnham Royal
Slough SL2 3BN
England
  44 (2814) 2281
  Telex 847964 COMAGG G

CAN/OLE CAN/SDI
(see CISTI, Canadian Online Enquiry Service)

CAN/SND
(see CISTI, Canadian Scientific Numeric Database Service)

Capitol Information Management
A division of Electronic Data Systems
11060 White Rock Road
Rancho Cordova, CA 95670
  916/636-4400

CEDIB
(see Universidad de Valencia, Facultad de Medicina, Centro de Documentacion e Informatica Biomedica)

Central Institute for Scientific and Technical Information
52 A.G. Nasser
Sofia 1040
Bulgaria
  359 / 88-08-41
  Telex 22404 ZINTI BG

Central Medical Library
Haartmaninkatu 4
00290 Helsinki
Finland
  358 (90) 418544
  Telex 121498 LKK SF

Centre de Documentation de l'Armement
26 boulevard Victor
75996 Paris Armees
France
  33 (1) 45 52 45 04
  Telex 202778 CEDOCAR F

Centre National de la Recherche Scientifique
Centre de Documentation Sciences Humaines
54 boulevard Raspail
75260 Paris Cedex 06
France
  33 (1) 45 44 38 49 x357
  Telex 203104 MSH F

Centro Nacional de informacion y Documentacion en Salud
A.P. 19-471
Delegacion Benito Juarez
03910 Mexico, D.F.
Mexico
  52 (5) 534 48 20

Chemical Abstracts Service
(see STN International)

Chemical Information Systems, Inc.
A subsidiary of Fein-Marquart Associates
7215 York Road
Baltimore, MD 21212
  301/321-8440
  800/247-8737

Chunichi Shimbun Company
1-chome, Sannomaru
Naka-ku, Nagoya 460
Japan
  81 (52) 201-8811

CILEA
Via R. Sanzio 4
20090 Segrate
Milan
Italy
  39 (2) 213 25 41
  Telex 310330 CILEAM I

CISTI
Canadian Online Enquiry Service (CAN/OLE)
National Research Council Canada
Ottawa, Ontario K1A 0S2
Canada
  613/993-1210
  Telex 0533115 CA

CISTI
Canadian Scientific Numeric Database Service (CAN/SND)
National Research Council Canada
Ottawa, Ontario K1A 0S2
Canada
  613/993-3294
  Telex 0533115 CA

Compusearch Corporation
Federal Systems Division
7631 Leesburg Pike
Falls Church, VA 22043
  703/893-7200

CompuServe Information Service
5000 Arlington Centre Blvd.
Columbus, OH 43220
  614/457-8600
  800/848-8990
  TWX 810-482-1709 CPS A COL

Congressional Quarterly Inc., Washington Alert Service
1414 22nd Street, N.W.
Washington, DC 20037
  202/887-6353

Consejo General de Colegios Oficiales de Farmaceuticos de Espana
Calle Villanueva 11
28001 Madrid
Spain
  34 (1) 431 25 60

Consejo Superior de Investigaciones Cientificas
Instituto de Informacion y Documentacion en Ciencia y Tecnologia (ICYT)
Calle Joaquin Costa 22
28002 Madrid
Spain
  34 (1) 261 48 08

Council of Scientific Research
Scientific Documentation Center
Jadiriyah
P.O.B. 2241
Baghdad
Iraq
  964 (1) 776-0023
  Telex 2187

Covidea
300 Jericho Quadrangle, 3rd Floor
Jericho, NY 11753
  212/310-5900

Data Resources, Inc.
Data Products Division Headquarters
1750 K Street NW, 9th Floor
Washington, DC 20006
  202/663-7720
  Telex 440480 DRI WASHDC

DATA-STAR
D-S Marketing Ltd.
Plaza Suite
114, Jermyn Street
London SW1Y 6HJ
England
  44 (1) 930-5503

DataArkiv AB
P.O. Box 12079
102 22 Stockholm
Sweden
  46 (8) 54 02 00
  Telex 8105030 S

Datacentralen
DC Host Centre
Retortvej 6-8
2500 Valby
Copenhagen
Denmark
    45 (1) 46 81 22
    Telex 27122 DC DK

DATANETWORK
A division of Applied Business
  Systems, Inc.
400 Embassy Square
Louisville, KY 40299
    502/491-1050
    800/626-2358

Datasolve Limited
99 Staines Road West
Sunbury-on-Thames
Middlesex TW16 7AH
England
    44 (932) 785566
    Telex 8811720 DSOLVE G

Delphi
  (see General Videotex Corporation/
    DELPHI)

Deutsches Institut fuer Normung e.V.
  (DIN)
Deutsches Informationszentrum fuer
  technische Regeln (DITR)
Burggrafenstrasse 6
Postfach 11 07
1000 Berlin 30
Federal Republic of Germany
    49 (30) 26 01 - 6 00
    Telex 185269 DITR D

Dialcom, Inc.
1109 Spring Street, Suite 410
Silver Spring, MD 20910
    301/588-1572
    800/435-7342
    TWX 710-825-9601

DIALOG Business Connection
  (see DIALOG Information Services,
    Inc.)

DIALOG Information Services, Inc.
3460 Hillview Avenue
Palo Alto, CA 94304
    415/858-3785
    800/334-2564
    800/387-2689 (in Canada)
    Telex 334499 DIALOG
    TWX 910-339-9221

DIMDI
Weisshausstrasse 27
P.O. Box 420580
5000 Cologne 4I
Federal Republic of Germany
    49 (221) 47 24 - 1
    Telex 8881364 DIM D

DIN
  (see Deutsches Institut fuer
    Normung e.V., Deutsches Informa-
    tionszentrum fuer technische
    Regeln)

Direct-Net
31220 La Baya Drive, Suite 110
Westlake Village, CA 91362
    805/495-0901
    800/223-0822
    800/824-5526 (in CA)

DITR
  (see Deutsches Institut fuer
    Normung e.V., Deutsches Informa-
    tionszentrum fuer technische
    Regeln)

Dow Jones & Company, Inc.
P.O. Box 300
Princeton, NJ 08543
    609/452-2000
    800/257-5114

Dr. Dvorkovitz & Associates
P.O. Box 1748
Ormond Beach, FL 32074
    904/677-7033

EasyNet
134 North Narberth Avenue
Narberth, PA 19072
    215/296-1793
    800/841-9553

ECHO Service
177 route d'Esch
1471 Luxembourg
Luxembourg
    352 / 48 80 41
    Telex 2181 EUROL LU

EDICLINE
Economic Documentation and Informa-
  tion Centre Ltd.
84 Temple Chambers
Temple Avenue
London EC4Y 0HP
England
    44 (273) 813238
    Telex 295833 EMS G

EG & G Idaho
Idaho National Engineering Laboratory
P.O. Box 1625
Idaho Falls, ID 83415
    208/526-0757

The Electric Pages
P.O. Box 2550
Austin, TX 78768
    512/472-6432

ENTEL, S.A.
Paseo de la Castellana 141
28046 Madrid
Spain
    34 (1) 450 90 96

ESA-IRS
C.P. 64 Via Galileo Galilei
00044 Frascati
Italy
    39 (6) 940 11
    Telex 610637 ESRIN I

European Patent Office
Erhardtstrasse 27
8000 Munich 2
Federal Republic of Germany
    49 (89) 23 99 - 0
    Telex 523656 EPMU D

EXCHANGE Service
  (see Mead Data Central, Inc.)

Executive Telecom System, Inc.
Human Resource Information Network
9585 Valparaiso Court
Indianapolis, IN 46268
    317/872-2045
    800/421-8884

Exis Limited
38 Tavistock Street
London WC2E 7PB
England
    44 (1) 240-0837

The Faxon Company, Inc.
15 Southwest Park
Westwood, MA 02090
    617/329-3350
    800/225-6055
    Telex 6817238

Finsbury Data Services Ltd.
68-74 Carter Lane
London EC4V 5EA
England
    44 (1) 248-9828
    Telex 892520 FINDAT G

FIZ Karlsruhe
c/o Fachinformationszentrum Energie,
  Physik, Mathematik GmbH
7514 Eggenstein-Leopoldshafen 2
Federal Republic of Germany
    49 (7247) 82 46 00
    800/247-3825 (in U.S.)
    Telex 17724710 FIZE D

FIZ Technik
Ostbahnhofstrasse 13
Postfach 60 05 47
6000 Frankfurt am Main 1
Federal Republic of Germany
    49 (69) 43 08 - 2 25
    Telex 4189459 FIZT D

FUNDACION OFA
Para el Avance de las Ciencias
  Biomedicas
Carrera 11-A, No. 93A-62
Bogata, DE
Colombia

ADDRESSES OF ONLINE SERVICES AND GATEWAYS

G.CAM Serveur
Tour Maine-Montparnasse
33 avenue du Maine
75755 Paris Cedex 15
France
    33 (1) 45 38 70 72
    Telex 203933 GCAMSER F

General Electric Information Services
  Company
401 North Washington Street
Rockville, MD 20850
    301/294-5405
    Telex 898431

General Videotex Corporation/DELPHI
3 Blackstone Street
Cambridge, MA 02139
    617/491-3393
    800/544-4005

GENIOS Wirtschaftsdatenbanken
German Economic Network
Kasernenstrasse 67
4000 Duesseldorf 1
Federal Republic of Germany
    49 (211) 8 38 81 83
    Telex 17211308 HBL VERL D

GID-SfT
Sektion fuer Technik
Herriotstrasse 5
Postfach 710370
6000 Frankfurt am Main 71
Federal Republic of Germany
    49 (69) 6 68 71
    Telex 414351 GIDFM D

Global Villages, Incorporated
One Kendall Square
Cambridge, MA 02139
    617/494-0189
    800/225-0750

GTE Telemail
12490 Sunrise Valley Drive
Reston, VA 22096
    800/368-4215

Heiwa Information Center Co., Ltd.
9-2, Nishi-Shinjuku-3
Shinjuku-ku
Tokyo 160
Japan
    81 (3) 374-8673

Human Resource Selection Network,
  Inc.
3 Cabot Place
Stoughton, MA 02072
    617/341-1968

Hydrocomp, Inc.
201 San Antonio Circle
Mountain View, CA 94040
    415/948-3919
    Telex 348357

I.P. Sharp Associates
Suite 1900, Exchange Tower
2 First Canadian Place
Toronto, Ontario M5X 1E3
Canada
    416/364-5361
    800/387-1588
    Telex 0622259

ICYT
    (see Consejo Superior de Investi-
    gaciones Cientificas, Instituto de
    Informacion y Documentacion en
    Ciencia y Tecnologia)

Idaps Information Services Pty. Ltd.
30 Bowden Street
Postal Bag 30
Alexandria 2015
Australia
    61 (2) 699-9955
    Telex 72394 AA

IGME
    (see Instituto Geologico y Minero de
    Espana)

IMS America, Ltd.
Butler Pike & Maple Avenue
Ambler, PA 19002
    215/283-8500
    800/523-5333
    Telex 685-1007

Info Globe
The Globe and Mail
444 Front Street West
Toronto, Ontario M5V 2S9
Canada
    416/585-5250
    Telex 06219629

Information Consultants, Inc.
1133 15th Street, NW, Suite 300
Washington, DC 20005
    202/822-5200

Information for Public Affairs
1900 14th Street
Sacramento, CA 95814
    916/444-0840

INKA Karlsruhe
    (see FIZ Karlsruhe)

INSERM
Centre du Documentation
Hospital de Bicetre
78 rue du General le Clerc
94270 Le Kremlin Bicetre
Paris
France
    33 (1) 46 71 86 87

Institute for Medical Literature
South African Medical Research
  Council
P.O. Box 70
Tygerberg 7505
South Africa

Instituto Geologico y Minero de Espana
  (IGME)
Calle Rios Rosas 23
28003 Madrid
Spain
    34 (1) 441 65 00

Instituto Nacional de Seguridad e
  Higiene en el Trabajo
Centro Nacional de Informacion y
  Documentacion
Calle Dulcet s/n
08034 Barcelona
Spain
    34 (3) 204 45 00

IntelliGenetics, Inc.
An IntelliCorp Company
1975 El Camino Real West
Mountain View, CA 94040
    415/965-5575
    Telex 171596 AAACOM SUVL

International Atomic Energy Agency
Vienna International Centre
P.O. Box 100
1400 Vienna
Austria
    43 (222) 2360 2882
    Telex 12645 A

International Computing Centre
1211 Geneva 10
Switzerland
    41 (22) 98 58 50 x287
    Telex 289696 CH

International Patent Documentation
  Center
INPADOC, Sales Department
Mollwaldplatz 4
1040 Vienna
Austria
    43 (222) 65 87 84
    Telex 136337 A

International Research & Evaluation
21098 IRE Control Center
Eagan, MN 55121
    612/888-9635
    Telex 29-1008

IQuest
5000 Arlington Centre Blvd.
Columbus, OH 43220
    614/457-8600
    800/848-8990
    TWX 810-482-1709 CPS A COL

IRS
    (see ESA-IRS)

IST-Informatheque Inc.
1611 boulevard Cremazie East
Montreal, Quebec H2M 2P2
Canada
    514/383-1611
    800/361-1611 (in Canada)

ADDRESSES OF ONLINE SERVICES AND GATEWAYS

Istituto Superiore di Sanita
Viale Regina elena 299
00161 Rome
Italy

Japan Computer Technology Co. Ltd.
4-3, Kanda-Surugadai
Chiyoda-ku
Tokyo 101
Japan
    81 (3) 233-1111

The Japan Information Center of
  Science and Technology (JICST)
2-5-2 Nagatacho
Chiyoda-ku, Tokyo 100
Japan
    81 (3) 581-6411
    Telex 02223604 JICST J

JICST
    (see The Japan Information Center
    of Science and Technology)

JOIS
    (see The Japan Information Center
    of Science and Technology)

K-Konsult
Documentation and Library
117 80 Stockholm
Sweden
    46 (8) 744 00 00
    Telex 17150 TEAMCON S

Knowledge Index
DIALOG Information Services, Inc.
3460 Hillview Avenue
Palo Alto, CA 94304
    415/858-3796
    800/227-5510
    Telex 334499 DIALOG
    TWX 910-339-9221

Kuwait University
Libraries Department Director
P.O. Box 17140
Kuwait

Leatherhead Food Research Associa-
  tion (LFRA)
Randalls Road
Leatherhead
Surrey KT22 7RY
England
    44 (372) 376761
    Telex 929846 FOODRA G

LEGI-SLATE, Inc.
111 Massachusetts Avenue, NW
Washington, DC 20001
    202/898-2300

Legi-Tech Corporation
The Senator Hotel
1121 L Street, Suite 207
Sacramento, CA 95814
    916/447-1886

LEXIS Service
    (see Mead Data Central, Inc.)

LFRA
    (see Leatherhead Food Research
    Association)

Library of Congress Information System
  (LOCIS)
General Reading Rooms Division
Washington, DC 20540
    202/287-6560

Lockheed Information Services, Inc.
    (see DIALOG Information Services,
    Inc.)

Longman Cartermill Limited
Technology Centre
Saint Andrews
Fife KY16 9EA
Scotland
    44 (334) 77660

Mead Data Central, Inc.
P.O. Box 933
Dayton, OH 45401
    513/865-6800
    800/227-4908

Medical Literature Review Inc.
Building # 1, Suite 6A
Flowerfield Industrial Park
St. James, NY 11780
    516/862-6160

MIC-KIBIC
Medical Information Center
P.O. Box 60201
104 01 Stockholm
Sweden
    46 (8) 23 22 70
    Telex 171 79 KIBIC S

Ministere de l'Agriculture
RESAGRI
78 rue de Varenne
75700 Paris
France
    33 (1) 45 55 95 50 x2310 or
    x2799

Ministerio de Cultura
Secretaria General Tecnica
Plaza del Rey 1
28004 Madrid
Spain
    34 (1) 429 24 44
    Telex 27286 CULTURA E

Ministerio de Educacion y Ciencia
Centro de Proceso de Datos
Calle Vitruvio 4
28006 Madrid
Spain
    34 (1) 262 96 11

Ministerio de Industria y Energia
Paseo de la Castellana 160
28046 Madrid
Spain
    34 (1) 458 80 10 x1211

NASA/RECON
    (see National Aeronautics and
    Space Administration, RECON)

National Aeronautics and Space
  Administration, RECON
Scientific and Technical Information
  Branch (NTT-2)
Washington, DC 20546
    202/453-2906

National Data Corporation
Health Care Data Services Division
One National Data Plaza
Corporate Square
Atlanta, GA 30329
    404/329-8500 x430
    800/554-3000
    Telex 542785

National Library of Canada
Library Systems Centre
395 Wellington Street
Ottawa, Ontario K1A ON4
Canada
    613/994-6949

National Library of Medicine
MEDLARS Management Section
8600 Rockville Pike
Bethesda, MD 20209
    301/496-6193

National Pesticide Information Retrieval
  System
Purdue University
Entomology Hall
West Lafayette, IN 47907
    317/494-6614

National Planning Data Corporation
P.O. Box 610
20 Terrace Hill
Ithaca, NY 14850
    607/273-8208

National Water Well Association
500 West Wilson Bridge Road
Worthington, OH 43085
    614/846-9355

NewsNet, Inc.
945 Haverford Road
Bryn Mawr, PA 19010
    215/527-8030
    800/345-1301

NEXIS Service
    (see Mead Data Central, Inc.)

ADDRESSES OF ONLINE SERVICES AND GATEWAYS

NIKKEI
(see NKS)

Nippon Telegraph and Telephone
  Corporation
1-6-6 Uchisaiwai-Cho
Chiyoda-ku
Tokyo
Japan
  81 (3) 509-5111
  Telex 2225300 J

NKS (Nihon Keizai Shimbun)
Databank Bureau
1-9-5 Otemachi
Chiyoda-ku, Tokyo 100
Japan
  81 (3) 270-0251
  Telex 22308 NIKKEI J

Norwegian Centre for Informatics
P.O. Box 350 Blindern
0314 Oslo 3
Norway
  47 (2) 45 20 10
  Telex 72042 NSI N

NSI, Inc.
333 East River Drive
East Hartford, CT 06108
  203/528-9021
  800/624-5916
  800/624-5958 (in CT)
  Telex 6711649 NAICO UW

Oak Ridge National Laboratory
P.O. Box X
Oak Ridge, TN 37831
  615/576-1743

Occupational Health Services, Inc.
400 Plaza Drive
P.O. Box 1505
Secaucus, NJ 07094
  201/865-7500
  800/223-8978
  Telex 4754124

OCLC Gateway
6565 Frantz Road
Dublin, OH 43017
  614/764-6000
  TWX 810-339-2026

OCLC LINK
6565 Frantz Road
Dublin, OH 43017
  614/764-6000
  TWX 810-339-2026

OCLC Online Computer Library Center,
  Inc.
6565 Frantz Road
Dublin, OH 43017
  614/764-6000
  TWX 810-339-2026

Official Airline Guides, Inc.
2000 Clearwater Drive
Oak Brook, IL 60521
  312/654-6000
  800/323-3537
  Telex QHOAGXD

ORBIT Information Technologies
  Corporation
8000 Westpark Drive, Suite 400
McLean, VA 22102
  703/442-0900
  800/336-7575
  Telex 901811

PaperChase
Beth Israel Hospital
330 Brookline Avenue
Boston, MA 02215
  617/735-2253
  800/722-2075

Pergamon InfoLine
12 Vandy Street
London EC2A 2DE
England
  44 (1) 377-4650
  Telex 8814614 PERINF G

PIR
  *(see Protein Identification Resource,
  National Biomedical Research
  Foundation)*

Planning Research Corporation
1500 Planning Research Drive
McLean, VA 22102
  703/556-1000

PRC
  (see Planning Research Corporation)

Protein Identification Resource (PIR)
National Biomedical Research Foundation (NBRF)
Georgetown University Medical Center
3900 Reservoir Road, NW
Washington, DC 20007
  202/625-2121

QL Systems Limited
112 Kent Street
Suite 205, Tower B
Ottawa, Ontario K1P 5P2
Canada
  613/238-3499

Quantum Computer Services, Inc.
8620 Westwood Center Drive
Vienna, VA 22180
  703/448-8700
  800/392-8200

RCA Global Communications, Inc.
RCA Hotline
60 Broad Street
New York, NY 10004
  201/885-4310
  800/526-3969
  Telex 219901 RCAC UR

Reference Service
  (see Mead Data Central, Inc.)

Registro de la Propiedad Industrial
Calle Panama 1
28036 Madrid
Spain
  34 (1) 458 22 00 x260

RLIN
The Research Libraries Group, Inc.
Jordan Quadrangle
Stanford, CA 94305
  415/328-0920

RPI
  *(see Registro de la Propiedad Indus-
  trial)*

Scicon Limited
49 Berners Street
London W1P 4AQ
England
  44 (1) 580-5599
  Telex 24293 SCICON G

SDC Information Services
  *(see ORBIT Information Technolo-
  gies Corporation)*

SDC of Japan, Ltd.
Nishi-Shinjuku Showa Building
13-12 Nishi-Shinjuku
1-Chome
Shinjuku-ku
Tokyo 160
Japan
  81 (3) 349-8521

SEMI
248 avenue Roger Salengro
13015 Marseille
France
  33 (91) 84 48 00

Serveur Universitaire National de
  l'Information Scientifique et Technique (SUNIST)
Chemin Saint-Hubert
L'Isle d'Abeau
B.P. 112
38303 Bourgoin-Jallieu Cedex
France
  33 (74) 27 28 10

The Shuttle Corp.
2569 152nd Avenue, NE
Redmond, WA 98052
  206/882-3447

SIPE Optimation S.p.A.
Via Silvio D'Amico 40
Rome
Italy
  39 (6) 54 76
  Telex 613362 I

Online Databases in the Medical and Life Sciences

SIRIO
Via Orazio 2
Milan
Italy
  39 (2) 8 82 31

THE SOURCE
Source Telecomputing Corporation
1616 Anderson Road
McLean, VA 22102
  703/734-7500
  800/336-3366
  800/572-2070 (in VA)

SpecialNet
National Association of State Directors
  of Special Education
2021 K Street, NW, Suite 315
Washington, DC 20006
  202/296-1800

STARTEXT, A Division of the Fort
  Worth Star-Telegram
P.O. Box 1870
Fort Worth, TX 76101
  817/390-7892

STN International
c/o Fachinformationszentrum Energie,
  Physik, Mathematik GmbH
7514 Eggenstein-Leopoldshafen 2
Federal Republic of Germany
c/o Chemical Abstracts Service
2540 Olentangy River Road
P.O. Box 3012
Columbus, OH 43210
  49 (7247) 82 45 66
  614/421-3600
  800/848-6533
  800/848-6538
  Telex 7826487 FIZE D
  Telex 6842086 CHMAB
  TWX 810-482-1608

STSC, Inc.
2115 East Jefferson Street
Rockville, MD 20852
  301/984-5000
  TWX 710-828-9790 STSC ROVE

Swedish Center for Technical Terminology
Box 2303
103 17 Stockholm
Sweden
  46 (8) 24 92 90

The Swedish Institute for the Handicapped
Box 303
161 26 Bromma
Sweden
  46 (8) 87 91 40
  Telex 11926 HANDVIK S

Syracuse Research Corporation
Merrill Lane
Syracuse, NY 13210
  315/425-5100

TECH DATA
Information Handling Services
Department 438
15 Inverness Way East
P.O. Box 1154
Englewood, CO 80150
  303/790-0600
  800/241-7824
  TWX 910-935-0715

The Teledata Network
24 Camberwell Road
East Hawthorne, VIC 3123
Australia
  61 (3) 813-1133
  Telex 135042 AA

Telesystemes-Questel
83-85 boulevard Vincent Auriol
75013 Paris
France
  33 (1) 45 82 64 64
  Telex 204594 TELQUES F

Timeplace, Inc.
460 Totten Pond Road
Waltham, MA 02154
  617/890-4636
  800/544-4023

TNO Institute for Mathematics, Data
  Processing, and Statistics
P.O. Box 297
2501 BD The Hague
The Netherlands
  31 (70) 82 41 61
  Telex 31707 WSTNO NL

Tymshare, Inc.
20705 Valley Green Drive
Cupertino, CA 95014
  408/446-6000
  800/538-9350

U.S. Dept. of Energy
Idaho National Engineering Laboratory
550 2nd Street
Idaho Falls, ID 83401

Uninet Japan Ltd.
c/o Kokusai-Denshin-Denwa Co.
  (KDD)
Marunouchi Mitsu Building 1F
2-2-2, Marunouchi
Chiyoda-ku
Tokyo 100
Japan
  Telex 24700 KDDSALES J

Universidad de Valencia
Facultad de Medicina
Centro de Documentacion e Informa-
  tica Biomedica (CEDIB)
Avenida Blasco Ibanez 17
46010 Valencia
Spain
  34 (6) 369 24 66

Universitetsbiblioteket i Oslo
Drammensveien 42
0255 Oslo 2
Norway
  47 (2) 55 36 30

University of California, Los Angeles
University Research Library 11717A
Orion User Services Office
Los Angeles, CA 90024
  213/825-7557

University of Tsukuba
Science Information Processing Center
1-1-1 Tennodai
Sakuramura Niiharigun
Ibaraki-Ken 305
Japan
  81 (298) 53-2451
  Telex 3652580 UNTUKU J

University of Wisconsin
Department of Psychiatry
Lithium Information Center
600 Highland Avenue
Madison, WI 53792
  608/263-6171

Utlas International Canada Inc.
80 Bloor Street West
Toronto, Ontario M5S 2V1
Canada
  416/923-0890
  Telex 06524479

Utlas International U.S. Inc.
1611 North Kent Street
Suite 910
Arlington, VA 22209
  703/525-5940
  800/368-3008
  Telex 64340

VCIS
  (see The Veterinary Information
  Company, Inc.)

The Veterinary Information Company,
  Inc.
Suite 108-110
Langmuir Laboratory
Brown Road
Cornell Industry Research Park
Ithaca, NY 14850
  607/257-4303

VU/TEXT Information Services, Inc.
1211 Chestnut Street
Philadelphia, PA 19107
  215/665-3300
  800/258-8080

West Publishing Company
50 West Kellogg Blvd.
P.O. Box 43526
St. Paul, MN 55164
  612/228-2433
  800/328-0109
  800/328-9833

ADDRESSES OF ONLINE SERVICES AND GATEWAYS

Western Library Network
AJ-11
Olympia, WA 98504
  206/459-6518

Western Union InfoMaster
1 Lake Street
Upper Saddle River, NJ 07458
  201/825-5000
  800/527-5184
  Telex 642491

Western Union Telegraph Company
1 Lake Street
Upper Saddle River, NJ 07458
  201/825-5000
  800/527-5184
  Telex 642491

WILSONLINE
The H.W. Wilson Company
950 University Avenue
Bronx, NY 10452

  212/588-8400
  800/367-6770
  800/462-6060 (in NY)

Young Peoples' Logo Association
1208 Hillsdale Drive
Richardson, TX 75081
  214/783-7548

SUBJECT INDEX

SUBJECT INDEX

SUBJECT INDEX

SUBJECT INDEX

SUBJECT INDEX

ONLINE SERVICE/GATEWAY INDEX

ONLINE SERVICE/GATEWAY INDEX

ONLINE SERVICE/GATEWAY INDEX

ONLINE SERVICE/GATEWAY INDEX

ONLINE SERVICE/GATEWAY INDEX

Online Databases in the Medical and Life Sciences

ONLINE SERVICE/GATEWAY INDEX

ONLINE SERVICE/GATEWAY INDEX

MASTER INDEX

MASTER INDEX

Food Science and Technology
Abstracts (see FSTA)
FOODS ADLIBRA 55
FORENSIC SERVICES DIREC-
TORY 55
FORT LAUDERDALE NEWS 56
FoU 56
FoU-indeks (see FoU)
FOUNDATION DIRECTORY (see
FOUNDATIONS)
FOUNDATION GRANTS INDEX (see
FOUNDATIONS)
FOUNDATIONS 56
FRANCIS: EMPLOI ET FORMA-
TION 56
FRANCIS: RESHUS 56
FRANCIS: SCIENCES DE
L'EDUCATION 56
FRANCIS: SOCIOLOGIE 57
FRESNO BEE 57
FRIP (see FEDERAL RESEARCH IN
PROGRESS)
FROSTI 57
FRSS 57
Fruits Agro-Industrie Regions Chaudes
(see FAIREC)
FSTA 57
FUNDACION OFA . . . . G
FYI NEWS SERVICE 58
G.CAM Serveur . . . . O
GAMBIT 2 58
GARY POST-TRIBUNE 58
GASTROINTESTINAL ABSORPTION
DATABASE 58
GCR (see GENEVA CONSULTANTS
REGISTRY)
**GEISCO (see General Electric
Information Services Company)**
GenBank 58
The GenBank Software Clearing-
house 59
**General Electric Information
Services Company** . . . . O
General Electric Network for Informa-
tion Exchange (see GEnie)
GENERAL SCIENCE INDEX 59
**General Videotex Corporation/
DELPHI** . . . . O,G
Genetic Sequence Databank (see
GenBank)
GENETIC TOXICITY 59
GENETOX (see GENETIC TOXICITY)
GENEVA CONSULTANTS
REGISTRY 59
GEnie 59
**GENIOS Wirtschaftsdaten-
banken** . . . . O,G
Geriatrics and Gerontology (see
COLLEAGUE MAIL SERVICES)
**German Economic Network Informa-
tion Online Service (see GENIOS
Wirtschaftsdatenbanken)**
**German Institute for Medical Infor-
mation and Documentation (see
DIMDI)**
German Patent Database (see
PATDPA)
GIABS (see GASTROINTESTINAL
ABSORPTION DATABASE)
GID-SfT . . . . O
THE GILROY DISPATCH 59
Global Villages, Incorporated . . . O
**The Globe and Mail (see Info
Globe)**

GLOBE AND MAIL ONLINE 60
GOVERNMENT PUBLICATION INFOR-
MATION SERVICE (see GPO PUBLI-
CATIONS REFERENCE FILE)
GOVT (see INDEX TO U.S. GOVERN-
MENT PERIODICALS)
GPO MONTHLY CATALOG 60
GPO PUBLICATIONS REFERENCE
FILE 60
GPOM (see GPO MONTHLY
CATALOG)
GRADLINE 60
GRANTS 60
GRUPOS TERAPEUTICOS 61
GTE Telemail . . . . O
GUIDE TO MICROFORMS IN
PRINT 61
H.W. WILSON JOURNAL AUTHORITY
FILE 61
Hackers Q & A (see COLLEAGUE
MAIL SERVICES)
Handbuch fuer Internationale Zusam-
menarbeit (see INSTITUTIONEN-
VERZEICHNIS FUER INTERNATIONALE
ZUSAMMENARBEIT)
HANDICAPPED USERS DATA-
BASE 61
HARF (see INDUSTRY DATA
SOURCES)
HARFAX INDUSTRY DATA SOURCES
(see INDUSTRY DATA SOURCES)
HAVC (see HEALTH AUDIOVISUAL
ONLINE CATALOG)
HAZARD (see HAZARDLINE)
HAZARDLINE 61
Hazardous Cargo Contacts (see EXIS)
HAZARDOUS SUBSTANCES DATA
BANK 62
HAZARDOUS WASTE NEWS 62
HAZE (see DRUGINFO and ALCOHOL
USE/ABUSE)
HDOK 62
HEALTH AUDIOVISUAL ONLINE
CATALOG 62
HEALTH CARE AND ADMINISTRA-
TION (see HEALTH PLANNING AND
ADMINISTRATION)
Health Care Literature Information
Network (see HECLINET)
HEALTH EDUCATION (see COMBINED
HEALTH INFORMATION DATABASE)
HEALTH FORUM (see HEALTHCOM
MEDICAL INFORMATION SERVICE)
HEALTH PLANNING AND ADMINIS-
TRATION 62
HEALTHCARE EVALUATION
SYSTEM 63
HEALTHCOM MEDICAL INFORMA-
TION SERVICE 63
HEALTHLINE (see BNA EXECUTIVE
DAY)
HEALTHNET 63
HECLINET 63
HEILBRON 63
**Heiwa Information Center Co.,
Ltd.** . . . . O
HERA (see HERACLES)
HERACLES 64
HES (see HEALTHCARE EVALUATION
SYSTEM)
HIGH BLOOD PRESSURE (see
COMBINED HEALTH INFORMATION
DATABASE)

HIGH TECH EUROPE 64
HIGH TECH GERMANY (see HIGH
TECH INTERNATIONAL)
HIGH TECH INTERNATIONAL 64
HISTLINE 64
HLTH (see HEALTH PLANNING AND
ADMINISTRATION)
**Honeywell DATANETWORK (see
DATANETWORK, a division of
Applied Business Systems, Inc.)**
HOSPITAL DATABASE 64
HOUSTON POST 64
HSDB (see HAZARDOUS SUBSTANCES
DATA BANK)
HSELiNE 64
Human Genetics (see COLLEAGUE
MAIL SERVICES)
**Human Resource Selection Network,
Inc.** . . . . O
HUMAN SEXUALITY 65
Hydrocomp, Inc. . . . . O
HZDB (see HAZARDLINE)
I.P. Sharp Associates . . . . O,G
IAA (see NASA)
**IAEA (see International Atomic
Energy Agency)**
IALINE 65
IBM PC SIG 65
ICAR 65
ICIE DATABASE 65
ICR (see INTERNATIONAL CONSUMER
REPORTS)
**ICYT (see Consejo Superior de
Investigaciones Cientificas, Insti-
tuto de Informacion y Documenta-
cion en Ciencia y Tecnologia)**
ICYT (see INDICE ESPANOL DE
CIENCIA Y TECNOLOGIA)
**Idaps Information Services Pty.
Ltd.** . . . . O
IEC 65
IFIPAT (see CLAIMS/U.S. PATENTS)
IFIREF (see CLAIMS/CLASS)
IFIS (see INDUSTRY FILE INDEX
SYSTEM)
IFIUDB (see CLAIMS/UNITERM)
**IGME (see Instituto Geologico y
Minero de Espana)**
IHPD (see INTERNATIONAL HEALTH
PHYSICS DATA BASE)
IHS VENDOR INFORMATION DATA-
BASE (see VENDOR INFORMATION
FILE)
IME (see INDICE MEDICO ESPANOL)
Immunology (see COLLEAGUE MAIL
SERVICES)
IMO (see EXIS)
IMS America, Ltd. . . . . O
IMSPACT 66
IMTS (see INTERNATIONAL MEDICAL
TRIBUNE SYNDICATE)
INABS (see THE INFORMATION BANK
ABSTRACTS)
INDASO (see INDUSTRY DATA
SOURCES)
INDEX CHEMICUS ONLINE 66
INDEX MEDICUS ESPANOL (see
INDICE MEDICO ESPANOL)
INDEX TO READER'S DIGEST 66
Index to Scientific & Technical
Proceedings & Books (see
ISI/ISTP&B)
INDEX TO U.S. GOVERNMENT PERI-
ODICALS 66

MASTER INDEX

MASTER INDEX